Current Topics in Microbiology 157 and Immunology

Retroviruses

Strategies of Replication

Edited by
R. Swanstrom and P. K. Vogt

With 40 Figures

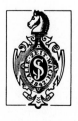

Springer-Verlag
Berlin Heidelberg New York
London Paris Tokyo Hong Kong

RONALD SWANSTROM, Ph.D.

Associate Professor of Biochemistry,
Dept. of Biochemistry,
Lineberger Cancer Research Ctr.,
CB#7295, 246 Lineberger Bldg.,
University of North Carolina at Chapel Hill,
Chapel Hill, NC 27599, USA

PETER K. VOGT, M.D.

Dept. of Microbiology,
University of Southern California,
School of Medicine,
2011 Zone Avenue HMR 401,
Los Angeles, CA 90033, USA

QR 1
E6
vol, 157

Cover illustration:
Graphic representation of the crystal structure of the HIV-1 protease bound to a substrate-based inhibitor. Provided by Dr. Alex Wlodawer, NCI, Frederick Cancer Research Facility, Frederick, MD.

ISBN 3-540-51895-9 Springer-Verlag Berlin Heidelberg New York
ISBN 0-387-51895-9 Springer-Verlag New York Berlin Heidelberg

© Springer-Verlag Berlin Heidelberg 1990
Library of Congress Catalog Card Number 15-12910
Printed in Germany

The use of registered names, trademarks, etc. in this publication does not imply, even in the absence of a specific statement, that such names are exempt from the relevant protective laws and regulations and therefore free for general use.

Product Liability: The publisher can give no guarantee for information about drug dosage and application thereof contained in this book. In every individual case the respective user must check its accuracy by consulting other pharmaceutical literature.

Typesetting: Thomson Press (India) Ltd., New Delhi. Offsetprinting: Saladruck, Berlin
Bookbinding: B. Helm Berlin
2123/3020-543210 – Printed on acid-free paper

Preface

Among the first diseases for which a viral etiology was established were tumors, lymphomas, and sarcomas in chickens, shown by Ellermann and Bang (1908) and Rous (1910) to be transmissible with cell-free filtrates. The broad significance of these discoveries was not fully recognized at first, mainly because chickens were perceived as too distantly related to humans to provide useful and relevant models for human disease. Change came slowly. In 1936 Bittner found that a viral agent is involved in the causation of mammary cancer in mice, and in 1957 Gross discovered the first murine leukemia virus. In the years following numerous tumor-inducing viruses, infecting all classes of vertebrates, were isolated.

The decisive impulse for the development of the RNA tumor virus field sprang from advances in cell culture. In 1958 Temin and Rubin, following initial observations of Manaker and Groupé, worked out the conditions for virus-induced tumorigenic transformation in cell culture and made this transformation the basis for a quantitative assay of viral infectivity and oncogenicity. The genetic and cell biological studies that grew out of Rubin's and Temin's groundwork quickly brought into focus two puzzling problems: a requirement for DNA synthesis early in the lifecycle of the RNA tumor viruses, and the existence of genetic information in the virus that is needed for oncogenesis but not for virus reproduction. Temin, Mizutani and Baltimore in 1969 clarified the role of DNA in the replication of RNA tumor viruses with the discovery of reverse transcription, catalyzed by an RNA-dependent DNA polymerase that is coded for by the viral genome and carried in RNA tumor virus particles. Reverse transcription marked the advent of an understanding of RNA tumor virus replication at the molecular level. RNA tumor viruses became known henceforth as retroviruses.

Genetic and biochemical studies defined the oncogenic information in retroviruses and showed that it was confined to a single gene, termed an oncogene, which was responsible for the induction and maintenance of the oncogenic cellular phenotype.

This work culminated in the demonstration by Stehelin, Bishop, Varmus, and Vogt that the *src* oncogene was a cellular and not a retroviral gene, a finding that was soon extended to all oncogenes of retroviruses. With this emancipation from virology the science of oncogenes grew into a separate, flourishing field concerned not only with cancer but also with the molecular components of normal growth control, cell differentiation, and cellular signal transduction.

In recent years retroviruses have assumed increasingly important roles in human disease. Human T lymphotropic virus (HTLV), found by Gallo and coworkers (1980), is the etiologic agent of adult T cell leukemia. Human immunodeficiency virus (HIV), isolated independently by Montagnier and Gallo in 1983 and 1984, has started a pandemic of acquired immunodeficiency disease which at the end of this century issues a major challenge to public health and antiviral therapy. HTLV and HIV have lent new urgency to the study of retrovirus replication.

In 1982 a landmark compendium on retroviruses and retroviral oncogenes was published by a collective of eminent authors (*RNA Tumor Viruses*, R. Weiss, N. Teich, H. Varmus, and J. Coffin (eds), Cold Spring Harbor Laboratory, New York). It was updated in 1985. These volumes are justifiably referred to as the "bible" of retrovirologists. But much progress in our knowledge of retrovirus replication has been made in the last five years. In the present volume of *Current Topics in Microbiology and Immunology* we will review the important aspects of these new developments. Unlike the "retroviral bible" this volume is not comprehensive but selective, concentrating on areas in which striking new advances have been made. These include key features of the viral growth cycle common to all retroviruses. The presentations of this volume assume familiarity with the growth cycle of retroviruses. Readers needing basic background are directed to the appropriate sections of the "bible."

The first chapter in this collection is by Russell Doolittle and colleagues and takes advantage of the abundant sequence data now available to formulate new insights into the origin and evolution of retroviruses. This is followed by Pat Brown's review of provirus integration. The development of an *in vitro* integration reaction that closely duplicates the steps occurring in the cell has been the key factor in this field. Integrated retroviral DNA represents a genetic element that is seen by the host cell as an RNA polymerase II transcription unit. The sequences in the viral LTR that interact with viral and host transcription factors are reviewed by John Majors. Retroviruses use several types of posttranscriptional modification in the control of viral gene expression. One type that has been illuminated recently is translational suppression resulting from a requirement for ribosomal frameshifting. Tyler Jacks discusses this phenomenon as it occurs in a variety of settings. Retroviral progeny RNA is specifically packaged into viral particles. This initial step of viral maturation is controlled by recognition sequences present in progeny RNA. An understanding of RNA packaging bears on our ability to develop retroviral vectors for cloned genes and is an important aspect in the acquisition and transduction of oncogenes by retroviruses. These issues are dealt with in the chapter by Maxine Linial and Dusty Miller. A late step in the viral lifecycle is the processing of precursor proteins coded for by the *gag* and *pol* sequences of the viral genome. This processing is mediated by a virus-coded protease. Much progress has been made in recent years in our understanding of retroviral proteinases and their origins and mechanisms of action. These results are reviewed in the chapter by Stephen Oroszlan and Ronald Luftig. The molecular biology of the viral envelope protein that bridges the virus lifecycle from one cell to another is reviewed in the final chapter by Eric Hunter and Ron Swanstrom.

As editors we have not imposed a uniform style and format on the chapters of this book. Such uniformity, although aesthetically appealing, would inevitably have delayed production and thereby lessened the value of this communication. We are grateful to the authors who are all actively working in the forefront of their fields for having accepted our invitation to contribute to this volume. May they find reward for their labors in a job well done.

This volume of *Current Topic in Microbiology and Immunology* is meant for all scientists who work with retroviruses directly or indirectly. We hope this collection of authoritative reviews will be especially useful to those who have joined the retrovirus community coming from other disciplines and attracted by the challenge of AIDS. We also hope that this book will fulfil a dual function: to inform about recent progress and to stimulate and inspire new advances.

Chapel Hill and Los Angeles,   Ronald Swanstrom
October 1989   Peter K. Vogt

List of Contents

List of Contributors

(Their addresses can be found at the beginning of their respective chapters)

Retrovirus Phylogeny and Evolution

R. F. Doolittle, D. F. Feng, M. A. McClure, and M. S. Johnson

1 Introduction

During the past few years the nucleic sequences of a large number of retroviruses have been determined, making it possible to quantify how they are related to each other and to trace their evolutionary origins. There are two factors that complicate such studies, however. First, retroviruses, like other RNA viruses, mutate at a very rapid rate (HOLLAND et al. 1982) and as a consequence evolve very rapidly. Second, retroviruses can recombine with each other (see for example CLARK and MAK 1984; reviewed in LINIAL and BLAIR 1984), raising the possibility that simple phylogenies may be confounded by mosaic genomes.

These concerns notwithstanding, it has been possible to align and compare sequences from a broad range of retroviruses. Indeed, many working groups (WAIN-HOBSON et al. 1985; CHIU et al. 1985; ONO et al. 1986; GONDA et al. 1987; McCLURE et al. 1987, 1988; YOKOYAMA et al. 1988; DOOLITTLE et al. 1989) have published phylogenetic trees, based mostly on alignments of products from the *pol* gene, which includes the reverse transcriptase, ribonuclease H and endonuclease. These three gene products are among the slowest changing proteins of the

Department of Chemistry, Center for Molecular Genetics M-034, University of California, San Diego, La Jolla, CA 92093, USA

Current Topics in Microbiology and Immunology, Vol. 157
© Springer-Verlag Berlin·Heidelberg 1990

retrovirus and, for the most part, have yielded similar trees in all instances. There have been some minor differences in topology, however, and in this chapter we review the situation and attempt to resolve a few discrepancies. Our plan is to lay out the major subgroups of retroviruses as revealed by their sequences and then briefly to consider where and when the group as a whole arose. The evolutionary relationships of immunodeficiency viruses are considered in detail.

2 Methods

It is useful to review the methods employed in the construction of sequence-based phylogenies. Two fundamentally different approaches can be used, the more common being the matrix-based distance measure (FITCH and MARGOLIASH 1967). The alternative approach is a character-based parsimony method is which the amino acid or nucleotide positions are examined column-by-column for information about the relationships of the taxa under consideration (DAYHOFF et al. 1972). In either case, the alignment of sequences is all-important. In the studies reviewed here we have confined ourselves to the protein sequences of retroviruses and related entities, translated from available nucleic acid sequences.

Multiple sequence alignments are achieved in various ways, the most usual of which depend on attempts to optimize the entire ensemble so that the most similar residues are in the same columns. In our studies, however, including all the results presented in this chapter, we use a progressive alignment procedure that begins by aligning the most similar sequences and then adds in the next most similar sequence or set of sequences (FENG and DOOLITTLE 1987). These alignments, which adhere to the rule "once a gap, always a gap", are often significantly different from the "eyeball-optimized" alignments used by others.

Once the alignments are achieved, they can be analyzed by either the matrix or character-analysis methods. Matrix methods, which are based on a table of pairwise distances, yield both a branching order and quantitative branch lengths (FITCH and MARGOLIASH 1967). The values of the latter can be calculated by various procedures, but we have used a best fit of the pairwise distance data as determined by a least-squares calculation (KLOTZ and BLANKEN 1981). The trees obtained by these methods are "unrooted", although the root for any particular subset can be obtained by the inclusion of another "outgroup", a device we can readily take advantage of in the case of retroviruses.

That matrix methods can yield erroneous or ambiguous topologies is illustrated by the general observation that branches will occasionally shift positions when additional members are added to the tree or when particular members of the starting set, often far removed on the tree, are omitted. Also, branch lengths with "negative lengths" are occasionally obtained. Some investigators attempt to correct these shortcomings by empirically examining vast numbers of trees in an attempt to find the one with the most consistent set of

a   Origins of HIV and SIV.

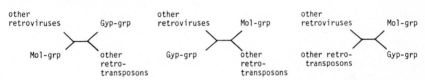

b   Phylogeny of Slow Viruses.

c   Origin of Vertebrate Retroviruses.

Fig. 1 a–c. Some ambiguous retrovirus relationships depicted in 4-taxa format. In panel **a**, the issue is whether or not SIV$_{agm}$ is a nearer neighbor to HIV-1 than is HIV-2. In panel **b**, the neighborliness of equine infectious anemia virus (EIAV) and visna relative to the immunodeficiency viruses is explored, and in panel **c** the relationship of the Moloney mouse group of retroviruses (*Mol-grp*) to a set of transposable elements (*Gyp-grp*) needs clarifying

branch lengths. In contrast, we now use an alternative character-based method to check all topologies (DOOLITTLE and FENG 1990). In its simplest form the method provides a tally of 4-taxa nearest neighbors (FITCH 1981). The approach has proved useful in defining ambiguities about origins and phylogenetic relationships, three of which are addressed in this chapter. These include the origin of immunodeficiency viruses, the internal relationship of slow viruses, and the relationship of a particular subgroup of retroviruses to a particular group of transposable elements (Fig. 1).

3 Definable Proteins

The coding portion of the retrovirus genome is divided roughly into three regions: *gag*, *pol*, and *env*. The initial polyproteins made from these sectors are cut into smaller polypeptides, including both enzymes and structural proteins. In addition, at least one of the final product proteins can be divided functionally into two different enzyme regions linked by a rather nondescript section we call a tether. Thus, one ca 550 residue protein contains both reverse transcriptase and ribonuclease H activities, the N-terminal 300 residues of which correspond to the transcriptase region and the C-terminal 150 residues to the ribonuclease H. Although this subdivision was originally proposed solely on the basis of sequence

Table 1. Ten definable coding regions of retrovirus genomes and their relative rates of evolutionary change

Original nomenclature	Standard nomenclature[a]	Other designations[b]	Rate of change[c]
Reverse transcriptase[d]	RT[d]	(p66, p80)[d]	1.00
Endonuclease	IN	p32, p46	1.4 ± 0.2
gag RNP	NC	p7, p10	1.5 ± 0.2
Ribonuclease H[d]	(RN)[d]	(p66, p80)[d]	1.6 ± 0.3
gag Core	CA	p25, p30	1.6 ± 0.3
Protease	PR	p12, p14	1.8 ± 0.3
Envelope (inside)	TM	g41, gp15E	1.9 ± 0.3
Tether[d]	(xx)[d]	—	2.2 ± 0.4
gag Amino	MA	p17, p15	2.4 ± 0.4
Envelope (outside)	SU	gp120, gp70	2.6 ± 0.5

[a] The suggested standardized nomenclature is from LEIS et al. (1988)
[b] Previous designations were often based on SDS-gel molecular weight estimations, many of which vary from virus to virus. The two values given here are from HIV-I and Mo-MLV only; p = protein and gp = glycoprotein
[c] In each case, rates of change were scaled relative to the reverse transcriptase
[d] The standardized nomenclature does not separate the reverse transcriptase and ribonuclease H activities, both of which occur in a single polypeptide chain

resemblances to similar nonretroviral proteins (JOHNSON et al. 1986), the validity of the proposal was subsequently demonstrated in a series of experiments by several different groups (HANSEN et al. 1988; TANESE and GOFF 1988).

All told, we divided the coding region of the retrovirus genome into 10 sectors. These included a 4-kilobase central region containing the four enzymes essential to retrovirus action: the protease, reverse transcriptase, ribonuclease H, and endonuclease (integrase). Also, as noted above, the reverse transcriptase and ribonuclease H are separated by a "tether" region. The other five sectors compared include two proteins generated from the initial *env* product and three from the *gag* region. Recently, an attempt was made to standardize the nomenclature for the various retrovirus coding regions (LEIS et al. 1988). We have attempted to adopt the new system (Table 1), although the new proposal does not distinguish between the reverse transcriptase and ribonuclease sequences.

In any event, we aligned each of the defined regions from a wide variety of retroviruses and constructed phylogenies from them (MCCLURE et al. 1988). Two important findings emerged from this study. First, we were able to compare the relative rates of change of each of these proteins (Table 1). Second, we pinpointed the occurrence of a major recombinational exchange of envelope genes between ancestors of two major groups.

4 The Major Groups of Retroviruses

Before the advent of sequence data, retroviruses were for the most part divided into groups on the basis of morphologic criteria as determined by electron microscopy (TEICH 1984). A-type particles, which are only found intracellularly, are 60–90 nm in diameter and double-shelled. B-type particles, on the other hand, are larger and more doughnut-shaped with surface spikes. C-type particles are usually associated with budding of the cell's plasma membrane, whereas D-type particles, which are found both inside and outside of cells, have shorter spikes and other morphologic features that distinguish them from B- and C-type particles. Recently, an attempt, was made to supplement the morphologic criteria with sequence data, a set of T-cell leukemia viruses being denoted type E (SAGATA et al. 1985).

At this point it seems more sensible to reclassify all retroviruses exclusively on the basis of their sequences and genome arrangement. Potential recombination problems can be minimized, we have found, by focussing on the more or less conservative 4-kilobase central section that includes the four retroviral enzymes. When such an approach is used, four major subgroups of retrovirus materialize (Figs. 2, 3). These are (a) a group of slow viruses, (b) a group of T-cell leukemia viruses, (c) a morphologically diverse group of exogenous and endogenous viruses and intercisternal particles, and (d) another "mixed group" that includes spumaviruses, various leukemia viruses, and several endogenous retroviruses. Among the viruses known to be in the last-named group that are not shown in

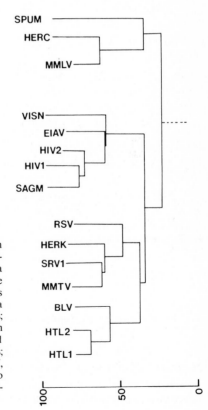

Fig. 2. Phylogeny of vertebrate retroviruses based on reverse transcriptase sequences. *HTL1, 2*, human T-cell leukemia virus I and II; *BLV*, bovine leukemia virus; *SRV1*, simian retrovirus I; *MMTV*, mouse mammary tumor virus; *HERK*, human endogenous retrovirus (K); *RSV*, Rous sarcoma virus; *VISN*, visna lentivirus; *EIAV*, equine infectious anemia virus; *SAGM*, simian immunodeficiency virus, African green monkey; *HIV1, 2*, human immunodeficiency virus 1 and 2; *MMLV*, Moloney mouse leukemia virus; *HERC*, human endogenous retrovirus (C), *SPUM*, human spumavirus. The Moloney mouse group also includes the feline leukemia virus, baboon endogenous virus, and avian reticuloendothelial virus

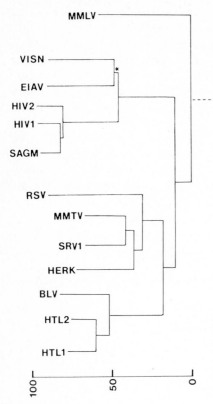

Fig. 3. Phylogeny of vertebrate retroviruses based on endonuclease sequences. Codes are given in legend to Fig. 2. (The endonuclease portion of the endogenous retrovirus denoted HERC is eroded to the point where its inclusion was not warranted.) Asterisk denotes position of a genomic segment relocation. (McClure et al. 1987)

Figs. 2 and 3 are feline leukemia virus, baboon endogenous virus, and the avian reticuloendotheliosis virus (McClure et al. 1988). (Previously, we had listed five groups, conferring separate status on the avian RSV. It is an arbitrary matter as to whether to keep it separate or to include it as a member of the MMTV group.)

As far as these major groups are concerned, the same trees emerge no matter which of the four enzyme sequences are used in the original alignment and regardless of whether a matrix or character-based method is used. The detailed relationships within a subgroup may vary slightly from one protein to another, and it is in these cases that careful scrutiny by both the matrix and character-based approaches can be helpful (Tables 2, 3).

4.1 Exogenous vs Endogenous Retroviruses

At this point we must digress from our main theme in order to show how sequence-based trees can be useful in understanding some more subtle aspects of retrovirus evolution. In particular, we are interested in the relationship between *exogenous* and *endogenous* retroviruses. Endogenous retroviruses are usually

Table 2. Nearest neighbor tally from residue-by-residue character state test based on alignment of 15 Reverse Transcriptases taken 4 at a time

	HTL1	HTL2	BLV	MMTV	HERV	SRV1	RSV	SAGM	HIV1	HIV2	EIAV	VISN	MoMLV	ERVH	SPUM
HTL1	—	78	66	18	19	16	21	9	9	11	12	14	33	35	23
HTL2		—	66	18	16	15	24	9	9	10	11	15	34	32	27
BLV			—	17	18	24	18	9	9	10	13	16	33	33	32
MMTV				—	66	78	55	8	13	15	20	15	13	13	15
HERV					—	66	56	8	15	17	21	19	14	14	15
SRV1						—	50	10	13	16	22	14	13	13	14
RSV							—	16	17	21	18	19	16	16	17
SAGM								—	77	66	55	45	15	17	20
HIV1									—	67	48	52	9	9	17
HIV2										—	50	51	10	9	11
EIAV											—	49	15	15	15
VISN												—	15	14	26
MoMLV													—	78	66
ERVH														—	66
SPUM															—

For abbreviations see Table 5. ERVH, Human Endogenous Retrovirus (C)

Table 3. Nearest neighbor tally from residue-by-residue analysis based on alignment of 12 endonuclease sequences taken 4 at a time

	HTL2	BLV	MMTV	SRV1	HERV	RSV	SAGM	HIV1	HIV2	EIAV	VISN	MMLV
HTL1	55	45	15	19	16	17	7	5	7	9	8	17
HTL2	—	45	16	18	17	17	7	7	8	6	7	17
BLV		—	14	19	17	20	7	8	9	9	7	20
MMTV			—	48	52	34	4	3	6	6	9	13
SRV1				—	45	28	6	5	6	6	7	13
HERV					—	33	4	3	5	7	7	14
RSV						—	6	7	8	13	21	16
SAGM							—	54	46	30	28	21
HIV1								—	45	34	28	21
HIV2									—	29	29	22
EIAV										—	47	24
VISN											—	22

For abbreviations, see Table 5

distinguished from exogenous viruses in that they are normally carried benignly in the germline, often in high numbers, many of which are likely defective. It is generally believed that exogenous retroviruses, because of their infectious nature and increased opportunities for reverse transcriptase-mediated life cycles, evolve much faster than their endogenous counterparts, some of which have been shown to be carried stably in the germline for periods greater than 5 million years (STEELE et al. 1986). The highly infectious immunodeficiency viruses, by contrast, have been found to be evolving into significantly different varieties within our own lifetimes (SMITH et al. 1988).

Certain endogenous retroviruses were initially identified by their ability to infect cells cocultured from a nonhost species (LEVY 1978). There is also good evidence that endogenous viruses can infect heterologous species in the wild as well (TODARO 1975). Since then, many endogenous retroviruses have been isolated on the basis of in vitro nucleic acid hybridization studies with material from related retroviruses (e.g., ONO et al. 1986; O'CONNELL et al. 1984).

The sequence-based classification of retroviruses does not distinguish endogenous from exogenous retroviruses, either with regard to their relative locations on the tree or the branch lengths leading to them (Fig. 2). We interpret this to mean that infectious retroviruses exist only for brief intervals in evolutionary time, after which they either become extinct or are integrated into their host's germline, which is to say, they become "endogenized". Presumably at some point the germline-infected host organism can become refractory to further somatic cell infection. The subsequent escape of some small fraction of endogenous viruses by infection of other species in which they are not resident in the germline maintains the cycle.

4.2 Phylogeny of the Slow Virus Group

When the retrovirus identified as the causative agent of AIDS was first isolated and sequenced, it was thought to be closely related to T-cell leukemia viruses and

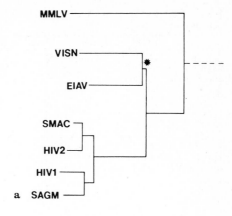

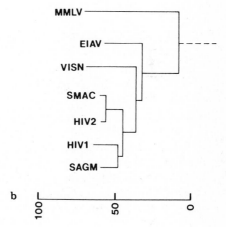

Fig. 4 a, b. Detailed relationship of slow retro-viruses. Tree denoted **a** is based on reverse transcriptase sequences. Tree denoted **b** is based on endonuclease sequences. Asterisk denotes the same genetic translocation event noted in Fig. 3. MMLV is used as an outlier for rooting

was thereby designated, at least by one group, HTLV-III (RATNER et al. 1985). Comparative sequence analysis, however, showed clearly that the virus was much more closely related to the lentivirus known as visna (CHIU et al. 1985). The lentivirus group ("slow viruses") includes visna, equine infectious anemia virus (EIAV), and the simian and human immunodeficiency viruses (SIV and HIV). The caprine arthritis encephalitis virus (CAEV) is a close relative of visna, but only a limited amount of sequence data is available at present. Similarly, scanty information has been published for a bovine immunodeficiency virus (BIV) (GONDA et al. 1987).

In the past, the relationship of a few of these viruses has proved problematic, and slightly different trees have emerged when different gene products have been used (GONDA et al. 1987; MCCLURE et al. 1987). The problem is that some of the HIV and EIAV sequences are just about equally distant from the corresponding sequences in other viruses. Thus, the branching order obtained for the reverse

Table 4. Nearest neighbor analysis of six slow viruses and Moloney mouse virus by 4-taxa character state method[a]

	SAGM	HIV1	SMAC	HIV2	EIAV	VISN	MMLV
SAGM	—	9	4	3	1	1	2
HIV1	10	—	3	3	3	1	1
SMAC	3	3	—	10	0	1	2
HIV2	3	3	10	—	1	1	2
EIAV	1	1	1	1	—	9	6
VISN	1	2	2	2	7	—	7
MMLV	2	1	1	1	9	6	—

[a] Lower left triangle = reverse transcriptase-based tally; upper right triangle = endonuclease-based. Numbers represent the number of times a given pair showed up as nearest neighbors in the most parsimonious tree for each set of four. SMAC, Simian, macaque; SAGM, Simian, African green monkey

transcriptase sequence is slightly different from that of endonuclease (Figs. 2–4).

Recently, we resolved the issue by resorting to a composite tree based on all four enzymes (McCLURE et al. 1988). We have now explored the problem utilizing residue-by-residue character analysis based on a 4-taxa provision and obtained the composite result (Table 4): To wit, EIAV is a nearer neighbor to visna (and CAEV) than are any of the immunodeficiency viruses. This is consistent with another character observed earlier, that visna and EIAV both have an extra segment between their ribonuclease H and endonuclease genes that is not found in immunodeficiency viruses or any other retroviruses examined so far (McCLURE et al. 1987). The simplest explanation is that the relocation event giving rise to the translocated segment occurred after the divergence of the visna-EIAV-CAEV line from the immunodeficiency and other viruses, as denoted by the asterisk * in Figs. 3. and 4.

5 The Simian-Human Connection

Uncovering the relationship of various simian retroviruses to HIVs has been beset with complications, some natural and others artifactual. For example, sequence studies revealed that one of the viruses that causes an immune deficiency-like state in monkeys is actually much more closely related to the well-known Mason-Pfizer monkey virus and to MMTV than to lentiviruses (POWER et al. 1986). This virus is now denoted SRV-1 (simian retrovirus) and another closely related one, SRV-2 (THAYER et al. 1987). The phylogenetic position of SRV-1 is shown in Figs. 2 and 3. The sequence of the simian equivalent to the human T-cell leukemia virus (HTLV-1) has also been published (WATANABE et al. 1985).

In 1985, a retrovirus causing immune deficiency was isolated from rhesus macaque monkeys housed in a primate center (DANIEL et al. 1985); the virus was called STLV-III, and its sequence was later reported by two different groups (FRANCHINI et al. 1987; CHAKRABARTI et al. 1987). Serological studies using antibodies to this virus led to reports (KANKI et al. 1986) that the same virus was widespread in a population of African green monkeys and also among Senagalese women, providing what appeared to be a definite link between simian and human retroviruses. Unfortunately, these conclusions were most likely incorrect, apparently because the green monkey and human cultures were contaminated by the original macaque virus isolate, which was being propagated in the same laboratory (KESTLER et al. 1988).

Almost simultaneous with this revelation, however, FUKASAWA et al. (1988) published the sequence of an authentic new retrovirus from feral African green monkeys, denoted SIV_{agm}. An unfortunate title appeared in an accompanying *Nature* News and Views article which did little to clarify the situation; it read: "Human AIDS Virus Not from Monkeys" (MULDER 1988). The News and Views article went on to note, "that the SIV_{agm} sequence is so remarkably different from the human AIDS viruses indicates that the human viruses cannot have originated from African green monkeys in recent times."

In fact, we would dispute that interpretation, as the relationship of the four viruses involved seems quite clear. To begin with, although the green monkey virus, SIV_{afg}, as pointed out by FUKASAWA et al. (1988), is almost equally distant from HIV-1 and -2, parsimony analysis indicates that it is significantly more closely related to HIV-1 than to HIV-2 (Tables 2, 3). Indeed, even the matrix methods put SIV_{afg} and HIV-1 in the same cluster (Fig. 3). Secondly, SMITH et al. (1988) have proposed, with good reason, that HIV-1 and -2 diverged as recently as 40 years ago. Similar conclusions have been reached by YOKAYAMA et al. (1988). Given Smith's timetable (SMITH et al. 1988) for the divergence, HIV-1 could easily have evolved from SIV_{afg} within the last half century.

At the same time, SIV_{mac} (formerly STLV-III) is extremely similar to HIV-2. It must be appreciated, however, that SIV_{mac} has only been isolated from monkeys in captivity, and then only in two particular primate centers in the USA. SIV_{afg}, on the other hand, appears to be endemic in certain central African monkey populations, the members of which are symptom-free with regard to immunodeficiency (FUKASAWA et al. 1988). The simplest coherent picture of all of these observations is that SIV_{afg}, widespread in the wild, may be undergoing "endogenization." As such, it could easily have spread to humans within the last half century, at which time the cross-infecting virus may also have acquired other attributes that makes it so fiercely pathogenic.

The sequence-based trees (Fig. 4) make it appear that HIV-2 was the earlier branch from the ancestral SIV_{afg} type. An alternative interpretation could be that the rate of evolution of HIV-1 has been slower than that of HIV-2, and that the true topology would have HIV-2 branching off after the divergence of SIV_{afg} and HIV-1. In this case, HIV-1 and HIV-2 populations would be the result of early "founder" groups seeding separate lines. Finally, without evidence to the contary, SIV_{mac} could conceivably be the result of inadvertent HIV-2 infection among colonized animals.

6 Evolutionary Origins of Retroviruses

Retroviruses are known to be widespread among mammals and birds, but their occurrence in other vertebrates—reptiles, amphibians, and fish—is very sporadic (TEICH 1984). Whether genuine infectious retroviruses are indigenous to invertebrate animals is doubtful, but many lower animals, plants, and fungi have transposable elements that strongly resemble endogenous retroviruses. Many

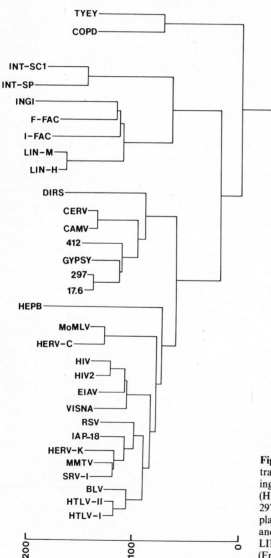

Fig. 5. Overall phylogeny of 31 reverse transcriptase-bearing entities, including 14 retroviruses, hepatitis B virus (HEPB), transposable element (17.6, 297, gypsy, 412, DIRS, COPD, TYEY), plant DNA viruses (CAMV, CERV), and elements related to LINEs (LIN-H, LIN-M, I-FAC, F-FAC, and INGI). (From DOOLITTLE et al. 1989)

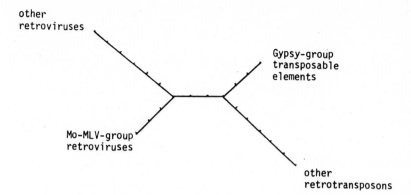

other
retroviruses

Gypsy-group
transposable
elements

Mo-MLV-group
retroviruses

other
retrotransposons

Fig. 6. Most likely explanation of the similarity of Gypsy group transposable element sequences (Fig. 5) to those of the Moloney mouse group of vertebrate retroviruses. The different limb lengths ("distances") are meant to imply slower or faster rates of evolution

transposable elements, for example, have the same four enzymes that typify retroviruses, and also RNA-binding and capsid structural proteins. Spliced envelope proteins appear to be uniformly absent, however. Although some of these transposable elements have been observed under the electron microscope and appear indistinguishable from retroviruses resident in the cytoplasm (ADAMS et al. 1987), there is no direct evidence that they ever escape the cell of their manufacture.

It seems quite reasonable to presume that infectious retroviruses evolved from transposable elements, perhaps at some point during the evolution of vertebrates, and possibly concomitant with the ability to generate a spliced envelope protein. Indeed, TEMIN (1980, 1985) has long held the view that retroviruses evolved from proretroviruses, and the elucidation of the first transposable element sequences showing similarities to retroviruses was regarded by him as confirmation of this view. In another article (DOOLITTLE et al. 1989), we have proposed a rather detailed scenario that might account for these events and presented sequence-based trees in accord with that view (Fig. 5).

There are some troubling aspects to the simple idea that retroviruses have evolved from transposable elements, however. In particular, there is the matter of whether the group of transposable elements we call the "Gypsy group" (named after the Gypsy transposable element of Drosophila) diverged before or after the emergence of genuine retroviruses (Fig. 5). There are several reasons to reflect on this particular relationship: First, the Moloney mouse virus and several of its close relatives have a single-domained NC unit, whereas virtually all other retrovirus groups have a double-domained unit (COVEY 1986). Even more to the point, a newly available spumavirus ("foamy virus") sequence (MAURER et al. 1988) and also the endogenous virus denoted HERC in Fig. 2 lack the characteristic RNP unit altogether (MAURER et al. 1988), an omission common to members of the Gypsy group also. Furthermore, the Gypsy group sequences are

Table 5. Nearest neighbor tally from residue-by-residue analysis of the same 31 reverse transcriptase sequences used in the phylogeny shown in Fig. 5[a]

	HTL2	BLV	SRV1	MMTV	HICP	HERV	RSV	HIV1	HIV2	EIAV	VISN	MMLV	ERVH	HEPB	176D	297D	GYPD	412D	CAMV	CERV	DIRS	HLIN	MLIN	IFAC	FE2D	INGI	C2IS	QXB1	COPD	TYEY
HTL1	406	378	215	250	208	241	226	161	166	162	152	194	200	106	70	63	76	57	78	62	80	57	43	68	47	60	53	58	53	70
HTL2		378	199	248	196	227	248	168	172	171	165	183	192	136	59	61	85	61	69	59	75	54	50	54	48	58	57	57	62	62
BLV			249	249	184	246	235	156	178	177	182	161	188	107	65	68	92	67	65	62	77	55	45	50	46	60	62	59	59	60
SRV1				406	376	353	321	192	208	212	189	145	188	96	59	59	67	59	54	59	77	31	45	50	36	60	62	49	59	47
MMTV					353	362	325	176	180	182	176	147	145	90	57	56	54	58	62	58	60	35	37	39	36	35	46	44	49	46
HICP						366	327	215	222	222	225	142	135	79	59	63	66	54	64	57	70	35	33	39	38	39	45	49	51	49
HERV							327	192	195	194	178	132	142	87	58	65	60	65	59	66	74	36	39	38	38	42	47	46	51	54
RSV								210	206	192	175	161	146	123	58	65	61	60	53	59	66	44	51	49	46	48	46	48	51	54
HIV1									406	356	373	136	143	108	77	105	68	79	77	84	65	44	51	46	54	49	67	64	70	65
HIV2										361	368	146	118	74	95	78	77	76	73	84	67	51	46	50	57	50	74	68	69	70
EIAV											352	169	142	103	76	71	78	77	83	83	77	67	46	49	57	60	70	68	71	65
VISN												137	119	116	77	93	72	81	78	83	77	94	79	68	55	60	74	64	66	75
MMLV													406	143	130	111	133	106	114	104	130	91	84	83	79	92	93	88	101	92
ERVH														131	126	102	177	128	130	119	126	85	84	83	88	97	87	87	95	98
HEPB															115	111	100	119	115	115	111	85	89	98	96	97	87	101	95	98
176D																406	360	369	300	300	272	197	193	173	173	175	190	214	219	206
297D																	378	351	300	299	255	197	193	173	173	190	107	104	113	103
GYPD																		406	303	297	279	99	100	102	106	108	107	109	115	98
412D																			303	299	241	85	81	107	107	97	107	104	128	98
CAMV																				406	277	104	100	102	106	107	108	109	115	96
CERV																					288	106	106	111	108	107	112	109	114	123
DIRS																						288	113	127	117	107	113	114	114	132
HLIN																							406	376	378	327	325	238	241	246
MLIN																								376	378	327	325	238	258	274

				349	326	272	254	239	230
IFAC	...	...	...	...	...	...	...	...	...
FE2D	...	...	...	380	278	279	233	233	
INGT	...	...	...	...	280	259	238	230	
C2IS	...	...	...	...	...	406	272	246	
QXB1	...	...	...	...	...	...	244	282	
COPD	...	...	...	...	...	...	...	406	

[a] The same branching order emerges from these data as from the matrix-method used in Fig. 5. For abbreviations, see caption to Fig. 2.

HTL1, Human T-cell Leukemia virus, type I; HTL2, Human T-cell Leukemia virus, type II; BLV, Bovine Leukemia Virus; SRV1, Simian Retrovirus, I; MMTV, Mouse Mammary Tumor virus; HICP, Hamster Intercisternal Particle (A-type); HERV, Human Endogenous Retrovirus (K); RSV, Rous Sarcoma Virus; HIV1, Human Immunodeficiency Virus 1; HIV2, Human Immunodeficiency Virus 2; EIAV, Equine Infectious Anemia Virus; VISN, Visna; MMLV, Mouse Moloney Leukemia Virus; ERVH, Human Endogenous Retrovirus (C); HEPB, Hepatitis B; 176D, Transposable Element 17.6, Drosophila; 297D, Transposable Element 297, Drosophila; GYPD, Transposable Element Gypsy, Drosophila; 412D, Transposable Element 412, Drosophila; CAMV, Cauliflower Mosaic Virus; CERV, Carnation Etched Ring Virus; DIRS, (Transposable element), Dictyostelium; HLIN, LINES (human); MLIN, LINES (mouse); IFAC, (Transposable element), I-factor, Drosophila; FE2D, (Transposable element), F-factor, Drosophila; INGT, (Transposable element), Ingi, Trypanosoma; C2IS, Intron in cytochrome oxidase, yeast mitochondria, S. Prombe; QCBI, Intron in cytochrome oxidase, yeast mitochondria, S. cerevisiae; COPD, (Transposable element), copia, Drosophila; TYEY, (Transposable element), I, Yeast;

clearly more similar to those of the Moloney mouse group than they are to other retrovirus sequences. Indeed, when various small subsets of sequences were aligned and phylogenies determined by the matrix method, occasionally Moloney mouse group members wandered into the Gypsy group. Given the intriguing question raised in the past (SHIBA and SAIGO 1983; FINNEGAN 1983) about the possibility of some transposable elements being the result of infection by vertebrate retroviruses, rather than vice versa, we again resorted to the four-taxa provision as an independent way of determining the topology.

As it happens, a full table of neighborliness (Table 5) gives the exact same branching order as our original matrix-derived tree (Fig. 5). Thus, the data still favor the more conservative notion that retroviruses have evolved from transposable elements rather than the other way around (Fig. 6).

7 Summary

The elucidation of complete genomic sequences from a wide variety of retroviruses and retrotransposons has allowed the construction of sequence-based phylogenies that reveal their evolutionary history. True retroviruses, whether exogenous or endogenous, tend to cluster into four major groups. Not only is there no distinction between exogenous and endogenous viruses, but their evolutionary limb lengths on the phylogenetic trees are comparable. This can be taken as evidence favoring a dynamic equilibrium balancing a constant invasion of germlines by infectious retroviruses on the one hand, with subsequent escape of endogenous viruses to alternative hosts on the other.

Retroviruses share a common ancestry with a wide variety of retrotransposons and other reverse transcriptase-bearing entities. One of these retrotransposon groups, the Gypsy group, resembles the Moloney mouse group of retroviruses much more closely than it does other retroviruses. The simplest explanation is that the evolutionary rate of the retrotransposon is much slower than the retrovirus rate and that among the retroviruses the Moloney mouse group has been evolving more slowly than the other three groups, leaving the two short-limbed taxa more similar (Fig. 6). The alternative explanation that these two groups actually shared a common ancestor more recently than has either with the other retrovirus groups is not supported by residue-by-residue character assessment.

References

Adams SE, Mellor J. Gull K, Sim RB, Tuite MF, Kingsman AJ (1987) The functions and relationships of Ty-VLP proteins in yeast reflect those of mammalian retroviral proteins. Cell 49: 111–119
Chiu I-M, Yaniv A, Dahlberg JE, Gazit A, Skuntz SF, Tronick ST, Aaronson SA (1985) Nucleotide

sequence evidence for relationship of AIDS retrovirus to lentiviruses. Nature 317: 366–368

Clark SP, Mak TW (1984) Fluidity of a retrovirus genome. J Virol 50: 759–765

Covey SN (1986) Amino acid sequence homology in *gag* region of reverse transcribing elements and the coat protein gene of cauliflower mosaic virus. Nucleic Acids Res 14: 623–633

Chakrabarti L, Guyader M, Alizon M, Daniel MD, Desrosiers RC, Tiollais P, Sonigo P (1987) Sequence of simian immunodeficiency virus from macaque and its relationship to other human and simian retroviruses. Nature 328: 543–547

Daniel MD, Letvin NL, King NW, Kannagi M, Sehgal PK, Hunt RD (1985) Isolation of T-cell tropic HTLV-III-like retrovirus from macaques. Science 228: 1201–1204

Dayhoff MO, Park CM, McLaughlin PJ (1972) Building a phylogenetic tree: cytochrome c. In: Dayhoff MO (ed) Atlas of protein sequence and structure, vol 5. National Biomedical Research Foundation, Washington DC pp 7–16

Doolittle RF, Feng D-F (1990) Nearest Neighbour Procedure for Relating Progressively Aligned Amino Acid Sequences. Methods Enzymol 183: 659–669

Doolittle RF, Feng D-F, Johnson MS, McClure MA (1989) Origins and evolutionary relationships of retroviruses. Q Rev Biol 64: 1–30

Feng D-F, Doolittle RF (1987) Progressive sequence alignment as a prerequisite to correct phylogenetic trees. J Mol Evol 25: 351–360

Finnegan DJ (1983) Retroviruses and transposable elements–which came first? Nature 302: 105–106

Fitch WM (1981) A non-sequential method for constructing trees and hierarchical classifications. J Mol Evol 18: 30–37

Fitch WM, Margoliash (1967) Construction of phylogenetic trees. Science 15: 279–284

Franchini G, Gurgo C, Guo H-G, Gallo RC, Collalti E, Fargnoli KA, Hall LF, Wong-Staal, Reitz Jr, MS (1987) Sequence of simian immunodeficiency virus and its relationship to the human immunodeficiency viruses. Nature 328: 539–543

Fukasawa M, Miura T, Hasegawa A, Morikawa S, Tsujimoto H, Miki K, Kitamura T, Hayami M (1988) Sequence of simian immunodeficiency virus from African green monkey, a new member of the HIV/SIV group. Nature 333: 457–461

Gonda MA, Braun MJ, Carter SG, Kost TA, Bess Jr, JW, Arthur LO, Van Der Maaten MJ (1987) Characterization and molecular cloning of a bovine lentivirus related to human immunodeficiency virus. Nature 330: 388–391

Hansen J, Schulze T, Mellert W, Moelling K (1988) Identification and characterization of HIV-specific RNase H by monoclonal antibody. EMBO J 7: 239–243

Holland J, Spindler K, Horodyski F, Grabau E, Nichol S, VandePol S (1982) Rapid evolution of RNA genomes. Science 215: 1577–1585

Johnson MS, McClure MA, Feng D-F, Gray J, Doolittle RF (1986) Computer analysis of retroviral pol genes: assignment of enzymatic functions to specific sequences and homologies with non-viral enzymes. Proc Natl Acad Sci USA 83: 7648–7652

Kanki PJ, Barin F, M'Boup S, Allan JS, Romet-Lemonne JL, Marlink R, McLane MF, Lee T-H, Arbeille B, Denis F, Essex M (1986) New human T-lymphotropic retrovirus related to simian T-lymphotropic virus type III (STLV-III$_{AGM}$). Science 232: 238–243

Kestler III, HW, Li Y, Naidu YM, Butler CV, Ochs MF, Jaenel G, King NW, Daniel MD, Desrosiers RC (1988) Comparison of simian immunodeficiency virus isolates. Nature 331: 619–622

Klotz LC, Blanken RL (1981) A practical method for calculating evolutionary trees from sequence data. J Theor Biol 91: 261–272

Leis J, Baltimore D, Bishop JM, Coffin J, Fleissner E, Goff SP, Oroszlan S, Robinson H, Skalka AM, Temin HM, Vogt V (1988) Standardized and simplified nomenclature for proteins common to all retroviruses. J Virol 62: 1808–1809

Levy JA (1978) Xenotropic Type C Viruses. Curr Top Microbiol Immunol 79: 111–118

Lineal M, Blair D (1984) Genetics of Retroviruses. In: Weiss R, Teich N, Varmus H, Coffin J (eds) Molecular Biology of Tumor Virus: RNA Tumor Viruses. Cold Spring Harbor Laboratory, Cold Spring Harbor, New York, pp. 649–783

Maurer B, Bannert H, Darai G, Flugel RM (1988) Analysis of the primary structure of the long terminal repeat and the *gag* and *pol* genes of the human spumaretrovirus. J Virol 62: 1590–1597

McClure MA, Johnson MS, Doolittle RF (1987) Relocation of a protease-like gene segment between two retroviruses. Proc Natl Acad Sci USA 84: 2693–2697

McClure MA, Johnson MS, Feng D-F, Doolittle RF (1988) Sequence comparisons of retroviral proteins: relative rate of change and general phylogeny. Proc Natl Acad Sci USA 85: 2469–2473

Mulder C (1988) Human AIDS virus not from monkeys. Nature 333: 396

O'Connell C, O'Brien S, Nash WG, Cohen M (1984) ERV3, a full-length human endogenous provirus: chromosomal localization and evolutionary relationships. Virol 138: 225–235

Ono M, Yasunaga T, Miyata T, Ushikubo H (1986) Nucleotide sequence of human endogenous retrovirus genome related to the mouse mammary tumor virus genome. J Virol 60: 589–598

Power MD, Marx PA, Bryant ML, Gardner MS, Barr PJ, Luciw PA (1986) Nucleotide sequence of SRV-I, a type D simian acquired immune deficiency syndrome retrovirus. Science 231: 1567–1572

Ratner L, Haseltine W, Patarca R, Livak KJ, Starcich B, Josephs SF, Doran ER, Rafalski JA, Whitehorn EA, Baumeister K, Ivanoff L, Retteway Jr, SR, Pearson ML, Lautenberger JA, Papas TS, Ghrayeb J, Chang NT, Gallo RC, Wong-Staal F (1985) Complete nucleotide sequence of the AIDS virus, HTLV-III. Nature 313: 277–283

Sagata N, Yasunaga T, Tsuzuku-Kawamura T, Ohishi K, Ogawa Y, Ikawa Y (1985) Complete Nucleotide sequence of the genome of Bovine Leukemia virus: its evolutionary relationship to other retroviruses. Proc Natl Acad Sci USA 82: 677–681

Shiba T, Saigo K (1983) Retrovirus-like particles containing RNA homologous to the transposable element copia in Drosophila melanogaster. Nature 302: 119–124

Smith TF, Srinivasan A, Schochetman G, Marcus M, Myers G (1988) The phylogenetic age of AIDS. Nature 333: 573–575

Steele PE, Martin MA, Rabson AB, Bryan T, O'Brien SJ (1986) Amplification and chromosomal dispersion of human endogenous retroviral sequences. J Virol 59: 545–550

Tanese N, Goff SP (1988) Domain structure of the Moloney Murine leukemia virus reverse transcriptase: mutational analysis and separate expression of the DNA polymerase and RNase H activities. Proc Natl Acad Sci USA 85: 1777–1781

Teich N (1984) Taxonomy of Retroviruses. In: Weiss R et al. (eds) RNA Tumor Viruses. 2nd edn. Cold Spring Harbor Laboratory, Cold Spring Harbor, pp 25–207

Temin H (1980) Origin of retroviruses from cellular moveable genetic elements. Cell 21: 599–600

Temin H (1985) Reverse transcription in the eukaryotic genome: retroviruses, pararetroviruses, retrotransposons and retrotranscripts. Mol Biol Evol 6: 455–468

Thayer RM, Power MD, Bryant M, Gardner MB, Barr PJ, Luciw PA (1987) Sequence relationships of type D retroviruses which cause simian acquired immunodeficiency syndrome. Virol 157: 317–329

Todaro GJ (1975) Evolution and modes of transmission of RNA tumor viruses. Am J Pathol 81: 590–605

Wain-Hobson S, Alizon M, Montagnier L (1985) Relationship of AIDS to other retroviruses. Nature 313: 743

Watanabe T, Seiki M, Tsujimoto H, Miyoshi I, Hayami M, Yoshida M (1985) Sequence homology of the simian retrovirus genome with human T-cell leukemia virus type I. Virol 144: 59–65

Yokoyama S, Gojobori T (1987) Molecular evolution and phylogeny of the Human AIDS viruses LAV, HTLV-III, and ARV. J Mol Evol 24: 330–336

Yokoyama S, Chung L, Gojobori T (1988) Molecular evolution of the human immunodeficiency and related viruses. Mol Biol Evol 5: 237–251

Integration of Retroviral DNA

P. O. Brown

1 Introduction

Integration of a DNA copy of the viral genome into host cellular DNA is an essential step in the life cycle of most, if not all, retroviruses (DONEHOWER and VARMUS 1984; SCHWARTZBERG et al. 1984a; PANGANIBAN and TEMIN 1984b; COLICELLI and GOFF 1985; HARRIS et al. 1984). Since retroviral DNA molecules are not ordinarily able to replicate autonomously as episomes, they depend upon integration for stable maintenance in dividing cells. Once integrated, the viral genome, or provirus, is transmitted as an integral element of the host genome. Integration appears moreover to be important, though perhaps not essential, for the transcription of viral DNA into new copies of the viral genome and messenger

Department of Pediatrics and Department of Biochemistry and Howard Hughes Medical Institute, Stanford University, Stanford CA 94305-5307, USA

RNAs that encode viral proteins. Thus, integration of a provirus defines the critical switch in the viral life cycle from mere subsistence to multiplication.

Beyond its importance to the reproduction of the virus itself, this distinctive feature of the retroviral life cycle accounts for many of the epiphenomena associated with retroviral infection, including insertional mutagenesis (VARMUS et al. 1981; JAENISCH et al. 1983; KING et al. 1985; FRANKEL et al. 1985; COPELAND et al. 1983; STOYE et al. 1988; STAVENHAGEN and ROBINS 1988), oncogenic transformation (BISHOP 1983; BISHOP and VARMUS 1985; VARMUS 1987), latency and persistence of infection (TEICH et al. 1982, 1985), and the usefulness of retroviruses as vectors for genetic engineering (SORIANO et al. 1989). These phenomena, as well as the general features of the retroviral life cycle, have recently been reviewed (WEISS et al. 1982, 1985; VARMUS and BROWN 1989; SORIANO et al. 1989). This article will therefore focus specifically on the mechanism of retroviral integration, emphasizing recent findings.

2 Working Model for Integration Reaction

We shall begin our discussion with a model for the integration mechanism. This will be followed by a detailed discussion of the individual steps and the experimental evidence that relates to each step. For the purposes of this review, I define the integration reaction as starting with the completion of viral DNA synthesis and terminating with the completion of covalent links joining each end of both viral DNA strands to host DNA. In our current view, based on in vitro experiments and in vivo observations, the reaction proceeds as follows (Fig. 1):

1. Early in a retroviral infection, a terminally redundant double-stranded DNA copy of the viral genome is synthesized in the cytoplasm by the viral reverse transcriptase. The terminal redundancies are called the long terminal repeats (LTRs). The viral DNA at the completion of its synthesis is most likely a blunt-ended linear molecule with termini determined by the primers for plus and minus strand DNA synthesis. Viral DNA is initially located in the cytoplasm of the infected cell and is held in a highly ordered nucleoprotein complex. This complex has properties that suggest a resemblance to the virion core particle. Among its components are the viral capsid protein (CA) and the viral IN protein.
2. Soon after completion of viral DNA synthesis, usually while still in the cytoplasm, the 3′-termini of the viral DNA are cleaved, eliminating the terminal one or two bases from each 3′ end and exposing the recessed 3′ OH groups that will define the boundaries of the integrated provirus. The viral IN protein is necessary and perhaps sufficient for this cleavage.
3. The viral nucleoprotein complex enters the nucleus, probably by an active translocation process.

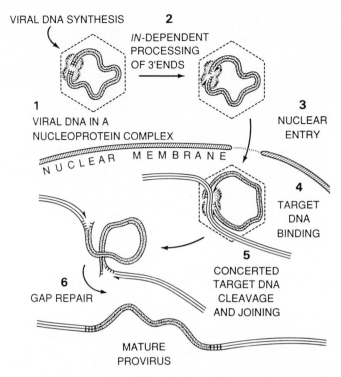

VIRAL DNA SYNTHESIS   **2**

IN-DEPENDENT
PROCESSING
OF 3'ENDS

1

VIRAL DNA IN A
NUCLEOPROTEIN COMPLEX

3

NUCLEAR
ENTRY

N U C L E A R   M E M B R A N E

4

TARGET
DNA
BINDING

5

CONCERTED
TARGET DNA
CLEAVAGE
AND JOINING

6

GAP REPAIR

MATURE
PROVIRUS

Fig. 1. A model of the retroviral integration process. The two strands of the viral DNA molecule are depicted here as *stippled ribbons* and the target DNA strands are shown as *white ribbons*. The terminal two base pairs of the viral DNA molecule are indicated by the *line segments perpendicular to the DNA axis*, as are the four base pairs of the target DNA molecule that are duplicated in the process of integration and flank the integrated provirus. The nucleoprotein complex that contains the viral DNA and the enzymatic machinery for integration is indicated here by the *open hexagon*. See the text for a detailed description of the steps depicted here

4. Upon entry into the nucleus the complex encounters the host DNA. Although specific target sequences are not required for integration, the entire genome is not equally accessible or attractive. In some cases, proteins bound to host DNA may be recognized by the viral integration machinery, directing integration to specific sites.

5. Binding of the viral nucleoprotein complex to host DNA is followed by a concerted reaction in which a staggered cut is made in the target sequence, and the energy of the broken phosphodiester bonds is used for formation of novel bonds joining the recessed viral 3' ends to the extended 5' ends produced by cleavage at the target site.

6. DNA synthesis, perhaps guided by viral proteins or carried out by the viral reverse transcriptase, extends from the host DNA 3' OH groups that flank the host-viral DNA junctions, filling in the gaps that flank the viral DNA and displacing the mismatched viral 5' ends. Following a ligation step, proviral

integration is complete. The further role, if any, of viral proteins that entered the cell in the infecting virion (e.g., in directing transcription factors to the provirus) is not known.

The structure of the integrated provirus is precisely defined and uniform for each viral strain (VARMUS 1983). The provirus is colinear with the unintegrated viral DNA molecule except for the loss of one or two bases from each end (SHIMOTONO et al. 1980; SHOEMAKER et al. 1980; MAJORS and VARMUS 1981; HUGHES et al. 1981). It consists of an internal coding region of about 6–8 kilobases (kb), flanked by LTRs that are generally a few hundred to a thousand base pairs in length. Three sections of the LTR, called U3, R, and U5, can be distinguished based on the locations of their counterparts in the RNA genome of the virion. Their order, from 5' to 3' along the proviral (+) strand, is U3-R-U5. The genetic structure of the provirus is discussed at length in WEISS et al. (1982, 1985) and VARMUS and BROWN (1989).

3 In Vitro Systems for Studying Integration

Methods have recently been developed for accurately reproducing the retroviral integration reaction in a cell-free system (BROWN et al. 1987, 1989; FUJIWARA and MIZUUCHI 1988; FUJIWARA and CRAIGIE 1989). The in vitro approach allows the reaction mechanism to be studied directly at the biochemical level. Products of the in vitro reaction can be recognized using either a genetic or a physical assay. The genetic assay provides superior sensitivity, while assays based on physical detection of reaction products allow direct examination of reaction intermediates.

The first assay exploits a powerful genetic selection in *Escherichia coli* to identify recombinants (Fig. 2). Bacteriophage λgtWES carries amber mutations in three genes required for lytic growth. Consequently, it is unable to make plaques on a lawn of wild-type (sup°) *E. coli* but makes plaques with normal efficiency if the *supF* amber suppressor allele is present. MLV *supF* is a replication competent derivative of the Moloney strain of murine leukemia virus (MLV) that carries the *E. coli supF* gene (LOBEL and GOFF 1984). The principle of the assay is that integration of an MLV *supF* provirus into a non-essential region of λgtWES produces a recombinant lambda genome able to suppress its own amber mutations and thus to make plaques on a non-suppressor strain of *E. coli*.

Extracts made from cells acutely infected with the MLV*supF* virus provide unintegrated MLV*supF* DNA precursors and the enzymatic machinery required for their integration. Following incubation of λgtWES DNA with crude or fractionated cellular extracts, the DNA is recovered and packaged into bacteriophage particles in vitro. Overall recovery of the target DNA is determined by plating on a *supF E. coli* strain. To score for integration of the MLV*supF* provirus, the phages are plated on a sup° strain of *E. coli* that restricts growth of

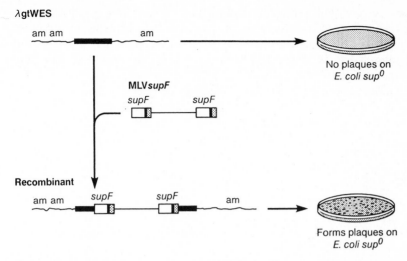

Fig. 2. In vitro assay for MLV integration. λgtWES carries amber mutations in three essential genes and is thus unable to make plaques on a sup° *E. coli* host. The amber mutations can be suppressed by integration of an MLV provirus containing the *supF* amber suppressor gene, allowing the recombinants to make plaques on the sup° lawn. The portion of the λgtWES genome dispensable for lytic growth is indicated by the *thick line*. See the text for a detailed description of the assay

λgtWES but allows the recombinants (having acquired the *supF* gene) to make plaques (Fig. 2). The proviruses integrated in vitro are structurally indistinguishable from normal proviruses, affirming the authenticity of the in vitro reaction. This assay is widely applicable to the study of nonhomologous intermolecular recombination reactions. It has now been used successfully to detect integration of RSV (LEE and COFFIN, unpublished results) and the yeast Ty1 element (EICHINGER and BOEKE 1988) in vitro.

While the genetic assay is highly sensitive and allows facile molecular cloning of the proviruses integrated in vitro, it requires that the retrovirus being investigated carry a bacterial genetic marker, and it does not allow direct examination of intermediates in the reaction. Physical methods have therefore been developed that enable one to detect and characterize these intermediates (FUJIWARA and MIZUUCHI 1988; BROWN et al. 1989). Because of their lower sensitivity, these methods typically require a higher reaction yield (on the order of 1% of the viral DNA integrated into the target) to be useful.

In one such assay, gel electrophoresis is used to separate the products of the integration reaction from unintegrated viral DNA molecules. The separated reaction products are then detected by Southern blotting followed by hybridization with a labelled probe for viral DNA sequences. As this assay does not require the construction of a specially-marked virus, it can be applied directly to available viral strains. For example, it has been used for biochemical studies of HIV integration (P. BROWN, unpublished results). The yield of the reaction followed in this manner is similar to that calculated using the genetic assay.

Reaction products and intermediates separated by gel electrophoresis can be isolated and subjected to further physical analysis. For example, as discussed later in this chapter, the structure of the junction between viral and target DNA in an early intermediate in MLV integration has been so elucidated (FUJIWARA and MIZUUCHI 1988; BROWN et al. 1989).

A powerful alternative approach to studying integration uses a genetically-marked, cloned model viral DNA substrate in place of the viral DNA isolated from infected cells (FUJIWARA and CRAIGIE 1989). Proteins isolated from virions or from virally-infected cells are used to carry out integration of this substrate into lambda DNA. The recombinants are detected after in vitro packaging into phage particles, by plating and genetic selection on *E. coli*. The efficiency with which these model substrates are integrated has thus far been many orders of magnitude lower than the efficiency seen in the assays previously described. Nevertheless, this system represents an important advance, as it allows independent manipulation of the DNA substrates and the proteins required for its integration.

The conditions that allow MLV integration in vitro are summarized below (BROWN et al. 1987). Remarkably similar conditions have recently been defined as optimal for in vitro integration of HIV (P. BROWN, unpublished results), and the yeast Ty1 element (EICHINGER and BOEKE 1988). EDTA abolishes activity, implying that a divalent cation is essential—Mg^{2+}, Ca^{2+}, Zn^{2+}, putrescine, or Mn^{2+} is acceptable. The optimal KCl concentration is about 150 mM, and activity is markedly inhibited by concentrations above 300mM. The pH range for activity is broad, extending at least from pH 6.6 to 8.6. The optimal temperature range for incubation is 15°–43°C; no detectable integration occurs at 0°. Pretreatment of the integrative precursors with SDS and proteinase K or with 5 mM N-ethylmaleimide abolishes activity, whereas pretreatment with RNAse A does not. Neither ATP nor any other rNTP or dNTP is required for integration in vitro (BROWN et al. 1987).

4 Structure and State of Unintegrated Viral DNA

The predicted linear product of reverse transcription is a largely double-stranded molecule with blunt ends defined by the 5'-ends of plus and minus strand strong stop DNA (reviewed in VARMUS and SWANSTROM 1982, 1985). This structure is inferred from what we know of viral DNA synthesis (VARMUS and SWANSTROM 1982, 1985), from the sequence of the ends of the single unintegrated linear molecule cloned to date (SCOTT et al. 1981), and from the sequence of a circular form of viral DNA that is presumed to result from blunt ligation of the ends of the linear molecule (SHOEMAKER et al. 1980). Recent studies have shown that some of the unintegrated viral DNA molecules found in MLV-infected cells do indeed have this structure (FUJIWARA and MIZUUCHI 1988; BROWN et al. 1989).

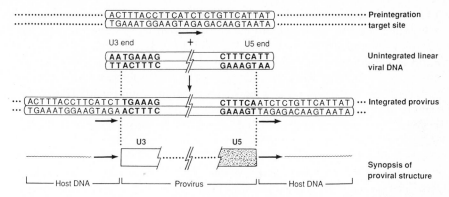

Fig. 3. Structure of the integrated MLV provirus and its unintegrated precursor. The upper strand of the viral and target DNA molecules in this illustration read from 5' to 3'. Reverse transcription of the viral genome results in a blunt-ended linear viral DNA molecule as shown here. This structure is therefore a likely precursor to the integrated provirus, but, as discussed in Sect. 5, it undergoes a specific processing step before being joined to the target DNA molecule. Note that in the integrated provirus, the terminal 2 base pairs of the blunt-ended linear molecule have been lost. A 4 base pair sequence, present in a single copy in the DNA target, is duplicated upon MLV integration and flanks the integrated provirus. In this illustration the duplicated target sequence is *underlined by an arrow*. The specific sequence that is duplicated upon MLV integration is variable, but its length is consistently 4 base pairs

However, the majority of unintegrated viral DNA molecules found in the infected cell are not blunt ended but have termini with 3'-ends that are recessed by two bases relative to the 5'-ends (FUJIWARA and MIZUUCHI 1988; BROWN et al. 1989). As discussed further below, it is likely that these molecules represent a later intermediate in the integration reaction pathway, generated by removal of the terminal two bases from each 3'-end of a blunt-ended precursor.

Figure 3 illustrates the relationship between the sequences at the ends of an integrated provirus and the corresponding sequences in the predicted blunt-ended product of reverse transcription. The integrated provirus is exactly colinear with the unintegrated linear precursor, except that the terminal 2 bp from each end of the precursor are lost upon integration (SHOEMAKER et al. 1980; SHIMOTONO et al. 1980; HUGHES et al. 1981; VARMUS 1982). HIV is a rare exception to this rule in that the ends of the putative linear precursor extend only 1 rather than 2 bp beyond the ends of the integrated HIV provirus (RATNER et al. 1985).

4.1 Viral DNA Is in a Nucleoprotein Complex

A variety of data suggests that viral DNA cannot serve as a substrate for normal retroviral integration unless its presence in the cell is established by infection. For example, molecular clones of viral DNA or naked viral DNA isolated from infected cells can be stably introduced with low efficiency into a target cell's genome by transfection, yielding an active provirus, but the junctions between the transfected provirus and host DNA have an erratic structure quite unlike that of a normally integrated provirus (COPELAND et al. 1981; LUCIW et al. 1984) Thus, in the absence of the viral proteins normally associated with the viral DNA, proviral insertions occur by the poorly understood DNA transfection pathway rather than by the normal integration process. This apparent confinement of integration activity to authentic viral reverse transcripts is consistent with a model in which subviral structures maintain a high degree of order during replication. Indeed, most of the unintegrated viral DNA produced by reverse transcription in MLV-infected cells can be isolated in stable $160S$ nucleoprotein complexes that also contain virally encoded proteins (BOWERMAN et al. 1989). These complexes, when separated from the bulk of cellular constituents by rate-zonal sedimentation, gel-exclusion chromatography or equilibrium density gradient centrifugation, retain the full integration activity present in crude cellular extracts in an in vitro integration assay (BROWN et al. 1987; BOWERMAN et al. 1989). The integration activity of the isolated complexes is not appreciably enhanced by supplementation with extracts from infected cells, implying that all the components necessary for integration are intrinsic to the nucleoprotein complex. Moreover, naked viral DNA is ordinarily not a competent substrate for integration when it is added to extracts from infected cells (BROWN et al. 1987), implying that the integrative complex, though it is capable of assembling onto an exogenous DNA substrate, does so with low efficiency (FUJIWARA and CRAIGIE 1989). Thus, it appears that reverse transcription of the retroviral genome takes place within a subviral core structure, and that the complexes active in integration are derived from this structure.

The idea that the complexes are a metamorphic derivative of the virion core receives support from the observation that the MLV nucleoprotein complexes competent for integration in vitro can be immunoprecipitated efficiently with antisera specific for the CA protein, $p30^{gag}$ (BOWERMAN et al. 1989). Thus, this protein, which forms the icosahedral shell of the virion core particle, is also a component of the MLV integrative complex. Since CA probably does not bind directly to DNA, perhaps it maintains its association with the viral DNA by containing the DNA in a shell. The sedimentation coefficient of the complex is close to that expected for such a structure (for example $\phi \times 174$ virions have an $s_{20,w}$ of $108S$, SV40 virions have a sedimentation coefficient of $240S$, while the nucleocapsid of the RSV virion sediments at about $130S$). When the nucleoprotein complexes are treated with restriction enzymes, the viral DNA can be cleaved, implying that the structure is quite permeable, yet the sedimentation of the complexes is not altered by the cleavage, and all the resulting DNA fragments remain associated with the $160S$ complex. Thus, the protein-DNA interactions maintaining the integrity of the complex are not strictly local ones (e.g., like those in an SV40 minichromosome) but hold together distant portions of the viral DNA molecule, as expected for a model in which the DNA is kept inside a (permeable) protein shell. Further purification and characterization of the integrative complex using the in vitro integration assay should allow the complete identification of its protein constituents and determination of its structure.

Integration ultimately requires exposure of the provirus ends to the target DNA substrate. Whether complete or partial exposure of the DNA in the complex occur concomitantly with DNA synthesis or is closely coupled to the integration process (e.g., induced by recognition of target DNA) requires investigation.

5 Recognition and Cleavage of 3'-Ends of Viral DNA Molecules

5.1 Defining Viral Sequences Required in *cis* for Integration

Integrated proviruses are colinear with unintegrated linear viral DNA and are joined to host DNA at the edges of their LTRs (HUGHES et al. 1978, 1981; DHAR et al. 1980; SHIMOTONO et al. 1980; MAJORS and VARMUS 1981). The existence of normally integrated proviruses with extensive internal deletions or substitutions but intact LTRs points to the LTRs as the viral sequences required in *cis* for integration. The viral sequences at the joint are precise and invariant for each virus species (VARMUS 1983) and always correspond to sites 1 or 2 bp from the ends of the unintegrated linear viral DNA molecules. These observations suggest that the terminal sequences of the LTRs might define the viral *att* sites, required in *cis* for integration. To investigate this hypothesis, the effect on integration of mutations in the sequences at the edges of the LTRs has been investigated for MLV, spleen necrosis virus (SNV), and avian sarcoma and leukosis viruses (ASLV) (PANGANIBAN and TEMIN 1983; COLICELLI and GOFF 1985, 1988a; COBRINIK et al. 1987).

As is evident from Fig. 4, the terminal sequences of the retroviral DNA molecule are typically inverted repeats. These vary from long perfect palindromes with substantial potential for forming alternative secondary structures (e.g., MLV) to hyphenated (e.g., ASLV) or very short (e.g., HIV, HTLV-I) repeats with little or no apparent ability to form stable cruciform structures (LILLEY 1983). It is therefore unlikely that such alternative secondary structures are of general importance to the integration mechanism. Instead, the presence of terminal inverted repeats points to the likelihood that the juxtaposed ends of the LTRs are recognized by a multimeric protein with a twofold axis of symmetry, perhaps a homodimer.

MLV can provide the viral functions required in *trans* for integration of a large group of closely related retroviral genomes (members of the MLV-MSV family), among which the 13 bp inverted repeats are the only completely conserved portions of the LTR termini (Fig. 4). Moreover, deletions extending distally toward either end, up to the 13-bp inverted repeat sequence, fail to prevent integration of MLV (J. MURPHY and S. GOFF, personal communication).

```
                      U5              ↓         ↓          U3
    RSV    CACCTGCATGAAGCAGAAGGCTTCATT    AATGTAGTCTTATGCAATACTCTTGTAG
    MLV    ACTACCCGTCAGCGGGGGTCTTTCATT    AATGAAAGACCCCACCTGTAGGTTTGGC
    SNV    GAATCCGTAGTACTTCGGTACAACATT    AATGTGGGAGGGAGCTCTGGGGGGAATA
    MMTV   ACCCTCAGGTCAGCCGACTGCGGCATT    AATGCCGCGCCTGCAGCAGAAATGGTTG
    HIV    TAGTCAGTGTGGAAAATCTCTAGCAG      CTGGAAGGGCTAATTTGGTCCCAAAGA
a   HTLV-II ATTGTCTTCCCGGGGAAGACAAACAAT    GATGACAATGGCGACTAGCCTCCCGAGC
```

```
                  U5                          U3            strain
    ACTACCCGTCAGCGGGGGTCTTTCATT    AATGAAAGACCCCACCTGTAGGTTTGGC    MO-MLV
    ACTACCCGTCTC-GGGGGTCTTTCATT    AATGAAAGACCCCACCTGTAGGTTTAGC    FR-MLV
    ACTACCCGTTAGTGGGGGTCTTTCATT    AATGAAAGACCCCACCTGTAGGTTTGGC    HA-MSV
    ACTACCCA-CGACGGGGGTCTTTCATT    AATGAAAGACCCCACCCGTAGG--TGGC    MO-MSV
    ACTACCCG-CCTCGGGGGTCTTTCATT    AATGAAAGACCC-ACCATCAGGTTTAGC    CAS-BR-E
    ACTGCCCAGCCT-GGGGGTCTTTCATT    AATGAAAGACCCCTTCCTAAGGCTTAGT    FBJ
    ACTGCCCAGCCT-GGGGGTCTTTCATT    AATGAAAGACCCCTTCATAAGGCTTAGC    FBR
    ACTGCCCA-CCTCGGGGGTCTTTCATT    AATGAAAGACCCCACCAAGTTGCTTAGC    SFFV
    ACTACCCGTCAGCGGGGGTCTTTCATT    AATGAAAGACCCCACCAAGTTGCTTAGC    AB-MLV
    ACTGCCCAGCCT-GGGGGTCTTTCATT    AATGAAAGACCCCTTCATAAGGCTTAGC    AKV
                                   AATGAAAGACCCCACCATAAGGCTTAGC    MCF-247
    ACCTACCTAGTTCGGGGGTCTTTCATT    AATGAAAGACCCCACCCCAAAATTTAGC    FeLV-GA
```

```
                                         CT
    ACTACCCGTCAGCGGGGGTCTTTCATT    AATGAAAGACCCCACC    mutant    integration
                                                      wt            +
    ACTACCCGTCAGCGGGGGTCTTTCATA    AATGAAAGACCCCACC    sub594       ↓↓
    ACTACCCGTCAGCGGGGGTCTTTCAT-    AATGAAAGACCCCACC    dl594        ↓
    ACTACCCGTCAGCGGGGGTCTTTCA--    AATGAAAGACCCCACC    dl593        0
    ACTACCCGTCAGCGGGGGTCTTTCATATA  AATGAAAGACCCCACC    in594-2      ↓↓
    ACTACCCGTCAGCGGGGGTCTTTCATATT  AATGAAAGACCCCACC    in594-2R     ↓
    ACTACCCGTCAGCGGGGGTCTTTCAG-    AATGAAAGACCCCACC    in592-R2     ↓
    ACTACCCGTCAGCGGGGGT--------    AATGAAAGACCCCACC    dl587        0
    GCGGGGGTCTTTCACTGGAATTCCAG-    AATGAAAGACCCCACC    in592-12     ↓↓↓
    GCGGGGGTCTTTCACTGGAATTACAG-    AATGAAAGACCCCACC    in592-12R1   ↓
    CCAAACCTACAGGTGGGGTCTTTCATT    AATGAAAGACCCCACC    U3-U3        (+)
b   aCtaccc------gggGGtcTTtCAtt    aATGAAAGACCCcacc    CONSENSUS
```

```
               U5                          U3        mutant  integration
    GAATCCGTAGTACTTCGGTACAACATT    AATGTGGGAGGGAGCTCTGGGG    wt        +
    GTAGTCAAGCGGAATTCCGACAACATT    AATGTGGGAGGGAGCTCTGGGG    183       +
    CCTTTTCTACATGACTGAGGATACATT    AATGTGGGAGGGAGCTCTGGGG    233       ↓
    GGGCGCAGGGATCCGGACGACAACATT    AATGTGGGAGGGAGCTCTGGGG    211       +
    CTGGGTGGGCGCAGGGATCCGGACATT    AATGTGGGAGGGAGCTCTGGGG    206       −
    CTGGGCGCAGGGATCCGGACTGAATCC    AATGTGGGAGGGAGCTCTGGGG    207       −
    GAATCCGTAGTACTTCGGTACAACATT    AATGTGGGAGGGGGGGAATAGT    121       +
    GAATCCGTAGTACTTCGGTACAACATT    AATGTGGGAGGGAGCTTTCTGT    144       (+)
    GAATCCGTAGTACTTCGGTACAACATT    AATGGGGGGAATAGTGCTGGC     150       −
    GAATCCGTAGTACTTCGGTACAACATT    TCTGTACACATGCT*           147       −
c   -------------------acaACAT     AATGTGGGAGGG----------   CONSENSUS
```

(Fig. 4. Continued)

```
            U5                                    U3                      strain
ACGAGCACCTGCATGAAGCAGAAGGCTTCATT    AATGTAGTCTTATGCAATACTCTTGTAGTC    SRA
GCGAACACCTGAATGAAGCTGAAGGCTTCATT    AATGTAGTCTTAATCGTAGGTTAACATGTA    AMV
GCGAACACCTGAATGAAGCAGAAGGCTTCATT    AATGTAGTCTTATGCAATACTCCTGTAGTC    PRC
ACGAACACCTAAATGAAGCGGAAGGCTTCATT    AATGTAGTCTTATGCAATACTCTTATGTAA    UR2
ACGAGCACCTGAATGAAGCAGAAGGCTTCATT    AATGTAGTCTTATGCAATACTCTTATGTAA    Y73
GCGAACACCTGAATGAAGCGGAAGGCTTCATT    GATGTTGCCAGTTAGTCATCATTGCCACTT    FSV
GCGAACACCTGAATGAAGCAGAAGGCTTCATT    AATGTAGTCAAATAGAGCCAGAGGCAACCT    RAV0
ACGCGAACCTGAATGAAGCAGAAGGCTTCATT    ------------------------------    MC29
------------------------------      AATGTAGCCTTACACAATAGCCTTACACAA    MH2
```

```
                                                      mutant  integration
ACGAGCACCTGCATGAAGCAGAAGGCTTCATT    AATGTAGTCTTATGCAATA    SRA        +
GATTGCACATGCATGAAGCAGAAGGCTTCATT    AATGTAGTCTTATGCAATA    Δ15       ↓↓
ACCGTTGATTGCATGAAGCAGAAGGCTTCATT    AATGTAGTCTTATGCAATA    Δ21        ↓
TGGCCGGACCGTTGATTGCAGAAGGCTTCATT    AATGTAGTCTTATGCAATA    Δ28        0
d aCgagcaccTgaATGAAGCAGAAGGCTTCATT    aATGtaGtCttataca      CONSENSUS
```

Fig. 4a–d. Viral sequences required in *cis* for integration. In each example, the plus strand sequence is shown from 5′ to 3′. The U5 and U3 sequences are shown juxtaposed, as they presumably are during integration. Abbreviations: MO-MLV, Moloney murine leukemia virus; FR-MLV, Friend murine leukemia virus; HA-MSV, Harvey murine sarcoma virus; MO-MSV, Moloney murine sarcoma virus; CAS-BR-E, Lake Casitas neurotropic wild mouse virus; FBJ, FBJ murine osteogenic sarcoma virus; FBR, FBR murine osteogenic sarcoma virus; SFFV, Friend spleen focus forming virus; AB-MLV, Abelson murine leukemia virus; AKV, AKR murine leukemia virus; MCF-247, AKR mink cell focus forming virus MCF-247; FeLV-GA, Gardner–Arnstein strain of feline leukemia virus; SRA, Schmidt–Ruppin A strain of RSV; AMV, avian myeloblastosis virus; PRC, Prague C strain of RSV; UR2, avian sarcoma virus UR2; Y73, avian sarcoma virus Y73; FSV, Fujinami sarcoma virus; RAV0 Rous associated virus 0; MC29, avian myelocytomatosis virus MC29; MH2, avian carcinoma virus MH2. Except where noted, sequences shown in this figure were from VAN BEVEREN et al. 1985. **a.** Wild type long terminal repeat sequences differ markedly among retroviruses, *Vertical arrows* indicate the sites at which the integrated proviral DNA is joined to host DNA. *Horizontal arrows* indicate inverted repeats. **b.** *att* site of MLV. *Upper panel* shows the U5 and U3 ends of several strains of the MLV group. *Lower panel* shows mutations in the U5 ends that were tested for their effects on integration of MO-MLV in vivo (COLICELLI and GOFF 1985, 1988a, b). (+) indicates wild type levels of integration, *downward arrows* indicate reduced integration activity, and 0 indicates completely defective integration. The bases that differ from MO-MLV are *underlined*. The consensus sequence shown in this panel and in panels C and D reflect bases conserved among integration-competent mutants and the wild type strains shown. In the consensus sequence, completely conserved bases are shown in *upper case*; the bases shown in *lower case* are less well conserved; and *dashes* indicate positions for which no strong nucleotide preference is apparent. Since the sample size on which the consensus is based is small, the apparent conservation at many positions may not be functionally significant. **c.** Putative *att* site mutants of SNV. The effects of the mutations on integration are indicated as in **b**. The bases that differ from wild-type SNV are *underlined*. *Asterisk* indicates that the remainder of the sequence of mutant 147 cannot be discerned from the published data (PANGANIBAN and TEMIN 1983). **d.** *att* site of ASLV. *Top panel* shows the U5 and U3 ends of several members of the ASLV group of viruses. *Bottom panel* depicts the putative *att* sites of three RSV mutants with deletions extending toward the U5 end. The effects of the mutations on viral replication (not necessarily in integration per se) are indicated as in **b**. The bases that differ from the wild-type Schmidt–Ruppin A strain of RSV are indicated

Thus, the sequences required in *cis* for integration are confined to the inverted repeat at the outer edges of the LTR. The dispensibility of the U5 sequences outside of the inverted repeat is further emphasized by the identification of an MLV provirus that apparently integrated using two copies of the U3 terminus in inverted orientation (COLICELLI and GOFF 1988b). Within the inverted terminal repeat of MLV, sequences can also be altered substantially without preventing integration (COLICELLI and GOFF 1985, 1988a). Genetic analysis of this region is not yet sufficiently complete to allow definition of the sequence features essential for recognition by the integration apparatus. However, it is clear from this work that the potential of the inverted repeat sequence to form a cruciform structure by base pairing between the copies at the U3 and U5 ends appears not to be essential for MLV integration, as mutations that would destabilize such a structure (e.g., in592-12R1, Fig. 4) do not abolish integration.

The actual site on the proviral DNA that is covalently joined to the target DNA is almost always a 5′.......CA 3′ (VARMUS 1983). The CA dinucleotide is conserved at each end of the provirus, even in otherwise divergent retroviruses and retrotransposons. In almost all cases this dinucleotide is situated exactly 2 bp from each end of the putative linear precursor, and typically the terminal 4 bp in the precursor are 5′.....CATT 3′. However, genetic analysis has shown that at least for MLV the spacing of the CA dinucleotides from the ends of the linear precursor is flexible within a few base pairs; from 1 to at least 4 bp are tolerated distal to the CA at the U5 edge. Moreover, the identity of the bases distal to the joining site is not precisely specified for MLV, although the wild-type dinucleotide TT appears to be preferred (COLICELLI and GOFF 1988a).

The terminal inverted repeat of SNV is substantially shorter than that of MLV, 5 vs 13 bp (Fig. 4). Genetic deletion analysis of SNV indicates that the sequences required for *att* site function are confined to the terminal 5–12 bp of U3 and the terminal 6–8 bp of U5 (Fig. 4; PANGANIBAN and TEMIN 1983).

In viruses of the ASLV group, deletion experiments indicate that viral replication requires specific sequences in the terminal 17–23 bp of U5, presumably for integration (COBRINIK et al. 1987), and except for the 13th position from the U5 terminus, these sequences are highly conserved (Fig. 4). The extent of the U3 terminal sequences required for ASLV *att* site function in vivo has not been investigated by deletion analysis. These sequences are generally much less well conserved than the sequences at the U5 terminus, but it is worth noting that the terminal 5–9 bp of U3 are the most highly conserved. Approximately the same sequences whose importance in replication is implied by sequence conservation and deletion analysis—the terminal 18–22 bp of U5, together with the terminal 5–8 bp of U3—are required for in vitro circle junction cleavage by the IN protein of ASLV (see below), providing circumstantial evidence for the role of this activity in integration (COBRINIK et al. 1987).

Recognition of the viral *att* site cannot simply involve specificity for each of the individual LTR terminal sequences, as these same sequences are present at the internal as well as the external edge of the LTR. Perhaps the proximity of these sequences to the end of a DNA molecule is important for recognition as an *att* site. Alternatively, juxtaposition of the sequences at the U3 and U5 ends of the linear precursor may be required for recognition. The IN protein of MLV has recently been shown to bind with high specificity to a model DNA substrate with ends mimicking those of the blunt-ended linear MLV DNA precursor (S. BASU, personal communication). This result suggests that the IN protein may determine the site specificity of the integration machinery for the viral *att* site and provides an experimental approach to defining the determinants of that specificity.

5.2 Cleavage of 3′-Ends of Viral DNA

Two working groups have determined the structures of the ends of unintegrated viral DNA molecules from MLV-infected cells (FUJIWARA and MIZUUCHI 1988; BROWN et al. 1989). A minority of these molecules were found to have the blunt-ended structure that had been predicted for the primary product of viral DNA synthesis. The majority (usually more than 80%) differed from this blunt-ended molecule in that the 3′-ends were recessed by 2 bp, terminating with free 3′ OH groups (Fig. 5). These 3′ ends therefore precisely match the boundaries of the integrated provirus.

What is the ontogeny of this recessed 3′-end? One possibility is that viral DNA synthesis stops 2 bases short of the end of the template. Alternatively, DNA synthesis could continue unimpeded to the end of the template, producing a flush-ended molecule from which the 3′ terminal dinucleotide is subsequently removed. Two lines of evidence favor the latter hypothesis.

First, when the distribution of 3′-ends from the viral right end in a purified preparation of full-length linear viral DNA molecules is compared with that in an unfractionated population of viral DNA molecules from an infected cell cytoplasm, it is apparent that the 2-base-recessed ends are proportionally more abundant in the purified full-length linear molecules (BROWN et al. 1989). Although the structures of the other DNA molecules in the unfractionated population are not known in detail, they are presumed to be intermediates in viral DNA synthesis. The fact that, compared with its precursors, the ultimate product of viral DNA synthesis is enriched for the 2-base-recessed 3′-end implies that the recessed end is the result of a late processing event. Second, enzymological analyses of the IN protein from ASLV, discussed below, have demonstrated an endonuclease activity whose properties could account for such a processing event.

That the IN protein plays an essential role in integration has been established genetically for SNV, ALV and MLV. Viruses carrying mutations in the region of the *pol* gene that encodes IN are capable of carrying out the early steps of the viral life cycle, from transcription of the provirus through viral DNA synthesis, nuclear entry, and circularization, but integration of the mutant viruses is markedly impaired, and viral replication is blocked (DONEHOWER and VARMUS 1984; SCHWARTZBERG et al. 1984a; PANGANIBAN and TEMIN 1984b). Structural analysis of rare MLV proviruses that manage to insert into the target genome in the

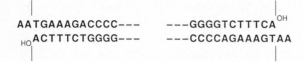

Fig. 5. Structure of the ends of unintegrated MLV DNA molecules. In cells infected with wild-type MLV, most of the unintegrated linear DNA molecules have the structure shown. The top strand is in the 5' to 3' orientation. The 5'-ends extend 2 bases beyond the boundaries of the integrated provirus (indicated by the *vertical lines*). The 3'-ends are recessed by two bases, terminating precisely at the 3' OH group that is joined to target DNA in the integrated provirus

absence of a normal IN protein demonstrated that, as with transfected viral DNA, their junctions with the host sequences were not produced by the standard retroviral integration mechanism (HAGINO-YAMAGISHI et al. 1987; DONEHOWER 1988). Thus, the IN protein is required specifically for normal integration.

Recent work has provided direct evidence for the participation of the IN protein in determining the 3'-end of the viral DNA molecule (BROWN et al. 1989). Unintegrated viral DNA molecules in cells infected with an MLV derivative, SF2 (DONEHOWER and VARMUS 1984), that carries a frameshift mutation in IN were shown uniformly to lack the recessed 3'-end characteristic of the viral DNA molecules in cells infected with wild-type MLV. Thus, the IN protein is required for formation of the recessed 3'-end, most likely by cleavage of a blunt-ended precursor. (An alternative possibility is that the IN protein might direct the termination of viral DNA synthesis.) This role in processing the viral 3'-end is sufficient to explain why IN is required for integration, though it is possible that IN also plays an essential role in later steps, such as joining viral DNA to its DNA target.

The genetic approach that led to the identification of IN as an essential function for integration cannot readily be extended to investigate the possibility that other virally encoded proteins, such as CA, NC (nucleocapsid), or RT (reverse transcriptase), might be required for integration. This is because unlike those affecting IN, mutations in other viral genes typically interfere with earlier steps in the transposition cycle, thus obscuring their possible direct effects on integration (CRAWFORD and GOFF 1984; GOFF 1984; SCHWARTZBERG et al. 1984b; HSU et al. 1985).

Studies of the IN protein (sometimes referred to as p32^{pol}) and the $\alpha\beta$ and $\beta\beta$ forms of reverse transcriptase (the C-terminal domain of the β subunit is identical to IN) from ASLV have identified an endonuclease activity whose properties are consistent with a direct role in processing the viral 3'-end (GRANDGENETT et al. 1978, 1986; GOLOMB and GRANDGENETT 1979; GOLOMB et al. 1981; DUYK et al. 1983, 1985; LEIS et al. 1983; GRANDGENETT and VORA 1985; COBRINIK et al. 1987). In the presence of a divalent cation, either Mg^{2+} or Mn^{2+}, the enzyme cleaves on the 3' side of a phosphodiester bond, producing ends terminated by a 3' OH and a 5' phosphate (LEIS et al. 1983). Neither of the ends produced by the cleavage is covalently linked to a protein, as they might be if cleavage resulted from an abortive topoisomerase or recombinase reaction (REED and GRINDLEY 1981; WANG 1985). The enzyme is more active on single-stranded than on double-stranded DNA but will cut double-stranded DNA, especially when the DNA is negatively supercoiled. The ends of unintegrated linear viral DNA have not been investigated as substrates, but the inverted repeat sequence of a cloned circle junction is indeed a preferred site for cleavage by both the $\alpha\beta$ and p32^{pol} forms of the ALV endonuclease (DUYK et al. 1983, 1985; GRANDGENETT and VORA 1985; GRANDGENETT et al. 1986; COBRINIK et al. 1987). Under most conditions, the preference is only a modest one, and the precise sites at which this sequence is cut in the in vitro reaction are offset by 1 base from the actual sites of integrative recombination. However, recent work has defined conditions under which the preferred site for cleavage by the purified p32 endonuclease, in a cloned double-stranded RSV circle junction, corresponds exactly to the site of integrative recombination (GRANDGENETT and VORA 1985; GRANDGENETT et al. 1986). Moreover, there is a rough correlation between the sequence requirements for (inaccurate) in vitro cleavage of a circle junction DNA fragment and the sequences required at the ends of the LTR for normal integration in vivo (COBRINIK et al. 1987).

The MLV IN protein isolated from virus particles has not been shown convincingly to have intrinsic endonuclease activity (PANET and BALTIMORE 1987). Because of the technical obstacles to obtaining large quantities of IN directly from virions, several workers have used bacterial or yeast expression systems to produce the protein (ROTH et al. 1988; S. BASU, personal communication). However, since no enzymatic activity has been defined for the natural protein, it is difficult to establish that the IN protein isolated from these expression systems is in native form. Extensive efforts to detect a nuclease activity in the protein produced by expression of the MLV IN coding region in *E. coli* have been fruitless, though the resulting protein does have an apparently nonspecific DNA binding activity (ROTH et al. 1988). MLV IN protein produced in *Saccharomyces cerevisiae* shows specific binding to the ends of MLV DNA in a model substrate; however, no endonuclease activity has yet been detected (S. BASU, personal communication).

The IN coding domain from SNV has also been expressed in *E. coli*. The resulting protein has no detectable endonuclease activity but, like its ASLV and MLV cousins, binds to single- and double-stranded DNA. Ordinary DNA binding by SNV IN protein shows no discernable sequence specificity. However, formation of DNA aggregates held together non-covalently by the SNV IN protein—a mysterious reaction that occurs only at a very high temperature (65°)—seems to require sequences specific to U5 (LUK et al. 1987).

In summary, while the extent and the precise details of the role of the IN protein in integration remain to be established, the evidence suggests that like the gene A protein of bacteriophage Mu (MIZUUCHI and CRAIGIE 1986; CRAIGIE and MIZUUCHI 1987) it acts to prepare the viral DNA ends for integration by endonucleolytic cleavage of the 3'-ends of the proviral DNA precursor. It is likely that faithful in vitro duplication of the native activity of the IN protein will require that it be assembled in a complex with other viral, and perhaps host, components.

6 Entry into the Nucleus

Viral DNA must enter the nucleus of the infected cell to gain access to its DNA target. In the nucleus, unintegrated viral DNA molecules are found in a large (160S) nucleoprotein complex, indistinguishable from that found in the cytoplasm. It seems improbable that such a large structure could diffuse passively through the nuclear pores (BONNER 1975). Perhaps the complexes enter the nucleus via the same active transport system used by cellular proteins that are localized to the nucleus (DINGWALL and LASKEY 1986). Such a transport process would depend on interactions between viral and cellular components and thus be susceptible to inhibition by viral mutations. To date no such mutants have been identified, perhaps because they have not been sought directly. One viral protein, the IN protein of ALV, has been shown to carry a signal for nuclear localization, but the role that it plays in the normal life cycle of the virus, if any, remains to be established (MORRIS-VASIOS et al. 1988). As an alternative to passage through nuclear pores, it is conceivable that the complex could enter the nucleus when the nuclear membrane is transiently disassembled during mitosis. This critical step in the viral life cycle is a fertile and unexplored area for investigation.

7 Recognition and Binding of Target DNA
by the Integration Complex

Since naked, linear (relaxed) DNA can serve as a target for integration in vitro, the DNA target for integration need not be supercoiled or assembled into chromatin (BROWN et al. 1987). It remains possible, however, that a supercoiled or otherwise modified DNA molecule might be a preferred target for integration.

The lack of a requirement for dNTPs or rNTPs implies that neither transcription nor DNA synthesis per se are required for target DNA function. Clearly, generation of the flanking repeat requires DNA synthesis, but formation of the initial covalent linkage between provirus and target DNA does not (see Sect. 7 and Fig. 7). Experiments in vivo show that integration occurs at least preferentially in cells that are actively replicating their DNA (VARMUS et al. 1977; HUMPHRIES et al. 1981). Perhaps, in the cell, replication physically exposes the DNA to the integration machinery; this would be unnecessary when naked DNA

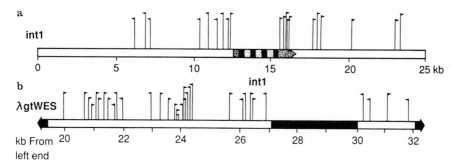

Fig. 6 a, b. Many DNA sites can function as integration targets. *Flags* indicating the position and orientation of the provirus point from 5' to 3' relative to the viral (+) strand. **a** MMTV proviral integration sites near the mouse *int1* locus in mammary tumors. Each *flag* corresponds to the site of proviral integration from an individual tumor. *Shaded arrow* indicates the approximate extent of the normal *int1* transcript. *Closed boxes* indicate coding domains, introns are *lightly stippled*, and non-coding portions of exons are marked by *heavy stippling*. Note that there are multiple MMTV insertion sites throughout the vicinity of the gene, including some that abut but none that interrupt the coding region or the 5' untranslated portion of the transcript (VAN OOYEN and NUSSE 1984). **b** In vitro MLV proviral integration sites in *λ*gtWES DNA. Each *flag* marks the site of the integrated provirus in a single recombinant clone arising from an in vitro integration event (BROWN et al. 1987). The regions of the lambda genome required for growth on a *rec*A-host are indicated in *black*

is used as target in the in vitro reaction. Alternatively, these data could reflect a role for cellular functions related to DNA replication, or incidentally expressed during S phase, in maturing the viral DNA precursor for integration (RICHTER et al. 1984).

Comparison of numerous sequenced integration sites for individual host/virus pairs has not revealed any sequence motif that predisposes a host DNA site for integration (SHOEMAKER et al. 1981; VARMUS 1983; BROWN et al. 1987). Even when integration events restricted by subsequent selection to a limited DNA region are examined, they are typically scattered at many sites in the region (HAYWARD et al. 1981; PAYNE et al. 1982; VAN OOYEN and NUSSE 1984; BROWN et al. 1987) (Fig. 6). However, there is considerable evidence that not all sites in the target genome are equally favored for integration in vivo. For example, integration sites are found near transcribed regions and DNase1-hypersensitive sites at a frequency much greater than expected (VIJAYA et al. 1986; ROHDEWOHLD et al. 1987), perhaps accounting for the observation that proviruses introduced into cells by natural integration are generally transcribed at a higher level than proviruses introduced by transfection (HWANG and GILBOA 1984). Moreover, integration of MLV into the HPRT gene in F9 mouse cells occurs about 100-fold less frequently than would be expected if there were no bias (KING et al. 1985).

The best evidence for preferred integration sites is provided by the recent work of SHIH et al. (1988). They searched specifically for integration "hot spots" by cloning thousands of independent integration sites and probing the entire collection with individual, randomly selected members, looking for sites present in more than one independent clone in the collection. They found clear evidence for such hot spots, estimating that there are on the order of 500 such sites in the chicken genome and that about 20% of all RSV integrations occur at a hot spot. The hot spots are not simply preferred regions for integration but are precise to the nucleotide. A typical hot spot is used for about 1/3000 integrations, or about 10^6 fold more frequently than expected for a random site. No common sequences or potential secondary structure motifs are discernable within several hundred base pairs on either side of the two such sites that have been sequenced (SHIH et al. 1988). Furthermore, cloned DNA fragments containing a hot spot are not preferred integration targets when tested as naked DNA molecules in vitro, nor are integrations into these fragments directed preferentially to the same precise sites favored in vivo (SHIH et al., personal communication). These results imply that the local DNA sequence per se cannot account for the favored status of the hot spots. The tropism of proviruses for transcriptionally active targets is consistent with the idea that physical accessibility plays a major role in target site selection, but it is unlikely that this can account for the acute site specificity of RSV integration into hot spots. Surprisingly, most of the hot spots for RSV integration that have been examined to date are neither transcriptionally active nor in proximity to DNase hypersensitive site (SHIH et al., personal communication). Perhaps cellular proteins that can interact with integrative complexes serve as targets to direct integration to specific sites. Proteins that bind to target DNA molecules or to specific target DNA sequences play a critical role in the efficient integration of bacteriophage λ (THOMPSON and LANDY 1989), bacteriophage Mu (PATO 1989), and the transposable element Tn7 (CRAIG 1989). Identification of proteins bound in the vicinity of the hot spots, examination of the physical state of the DNA at these sites, and determining whether the preferential use of integration hot spots is cell-type-specific or virus-specific should provide important insights into the selection of integration target sites.

8 Target DNA Cleavage and the Joining Reaction

Upon integration, a small sequence (4–6 bp) of host DNA is duplicated flanking the integrated provirus (SHOEMAKER et al. 1980; SHIMOTONO et al. 1980; MAJORS and VARMUS 1981; HUGHES et al. 1981; VAN BEVEREN et al. 1982; VARMUS 1983). The target sequences are otherwise not modified or rearranged. With rare exceptions (COLICELLI and GOFF 1988a), the length of the duplicated region is uniform for a given viral species, whereas the species of the host cell appears not to influence the repeat length (VARMUS 1983). Since the length of the flanking repeat is presumed to reflect the spacing between the cleavages in the two strands of the target DNA molecule (SHAPIRO 1979), it is likely that a virally encoded function participates in target site cleavage. As discussed below, target DNA cleavage appears to be coupled to the joining of viral and target DNA molecules. A viral function is thus also implicated in the joining reaction.

When linear viral DNA molecules enter the nucleus, some of them are circularized by covalently joining their ends to produce molecules called 2-LTR circles. The novel sequence created at the site of this ligation is commonly called the circle junction. Both the linear molecule and the 2-LTR circle are reasonable candidates for the ultimate precursor to the integrated provirus. Is circularization of the viral DNA molecule required for integration?

In one experiment, the circle junction sequence of SNV, when inserted at an internal site in the SNV genome, appeared able to serve as the viral attachment site for integration (PANGANIBAN and TEMIN 1984a). This result pointed to the 2-LTR circle as the ultimate precursor in SNV integration. However, the results of an analogous experiment with MLV do not support the 2-LTR circle as the proximal precursor to the integrated MLV provirus (LOBEL et al. 1989). In vitro, the cytoplasmic linear form of unintegrated viral DNA can serve as a precursor to the integrated provirus (BROWN et al. 1987, 1989; FUJIWARA and MIZUUCHI 1988). It does not necessarily follow, however, that the linear molecule is the direct precursor to the integrated provirus, since the circularization reaction could, in principle, occur in vitro prior to integration. That the direct precursor to the integrated provirus is indeed a linear molecule has recently been established by an approach that depends on a precise relationship between the topology of the precursor and the structure of integration intermediates (Fig. 7).

One can outline a plausible reaction pathway invoking either the linear viral DNA molecule or the 2-LTR circular form as the proximal precursor to the integrated provirus (Fig. 7). (SHOEMAKER et al. 1980; BROWN et al. 1987). In pathway A the proximal precursor is the 2-LTR circle (1A), formed by ligation of the ends of the linear molecule. In pathway B the linear viral DNA (1B) is itself the substrate for integration. In the DNA breakage and joining step, viral and target DNA strands are broken at the sites marked by the arrowheads. The 3' OH ends of the viral DNA are then joined to the corresponding 5' P ends of the target DNA. The cuts in the viral and target DNA molecules do not need to occur in concert, but the joining reaction is probably coupled to cleavage of the target DNA, for reasons discussed below. In the resulting intermediate (2A or 2B), the provirus is flanked by short gaps that are the precursors to the flanking repeats in the final product. DNA synthesis primed by the 3' OH on the target side of the gap can initiate repair of the gap to yield the mature integrated provirus.

In the gapped initial product of the integration reaction, the expected structure of the free viral DNA end differs depending on whether the ultimate precursor is linear or a 2-LTR circle (Fig. 7, structures 2A and 2B). In pathway A, this free viral DNA end is longer by two bases than the corresponding end of the linear precursor. These two extra bases are covalently joined to the end in the circularization step, and left attached when the viral DNA is cleaved two bases to one side of the circle junction. In pathway B, the free viral DNA end in the gapped intermediate is identical to the corresponding end of the linear precursor, having never been covalently modified. Given the strict dependence of the structure of this intermediate on the topology of its precursor, it is possible to deduce the topology of the precursor by comparing the free viral DNA ends in the gapped intermediate with their counterparts in the unintegrated linear DNA molecule.

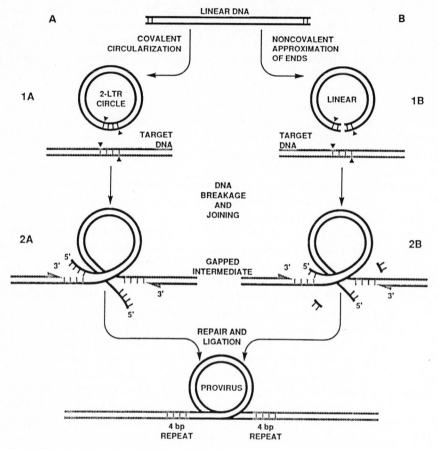

Fig. 7. Two possible pathways for integration of linear retroviral DNA. The steps illustrated here are described in the text. Target DNA is indicated by the *gray line*, viral DNA by the *black line*. The 4 base pairs of viral DNA that are ultimately lost upon integration (two from each end of the linear molecule) and the 4 base pair target sequence that is duplicated upon integration of MLV DNA are indicated by the *line segments perpendicular to the DNA strands*

Two groups have used gel electrophoresis to purify the gapped integration intermediate in an in vitro MLV integration reaction (FUJIWARA and MIZUUCHI 1988; BROWN et al. 1989). In the recovered intermediate, the 3′-end of the viral DNA molecule was found to be joined to the target DNA molecule, while the viral DNA 5′-end was free, and this 5′-end was identical to that of the linear precursor. This structure precisely matches that predicted for direct integration of a linear precursor (Fig. 7, structure 2B). Thus, circularization does not appear to play a role in MLV integration. This conclusion contrasts with the deduction by PANGANIBAN and TEMIN (1984a) that the 2-LTR circle is a precursor in SNV integration. This apparent inconsistency might be reconciled in any of several ways. It is conceivable that integration of a 2-LTR circle, accompanied or followed by absolutely efficient and precise removal of the terminal 2 bases from the viral 5'-end, could account for the observed structure of the MLV integration intermediate, but such a processing reaction appears gratuitous and therefore implausible. Alternatively, the two viruses might differ in the preferred topology of the integrative precursor, just as they differ in the primary structure of their attachment sites. However, since the evidence for a circular intermediate even in SNV integration is equivocal (A. PANGANIBAN, personal communication), and there is no compelling mechanistic purpose for the circularization step, the hypothesis that both viruses ordinarily integrate via a linear precursor appears the most plausible.

Like many previously characterized specialized DNA recombination reactions (HOWE and BERG 1989), MLV integration can occur in vitro without an extrinsic energy source (BROWN et al. 1987). The DNA breakage and joining reactions are therefore probably coupled. There are many precedents for such energy conservation occurring via a transient high-energy covalent protein-DNA phosphodiester bond (e.g., REED and GRINDLEY 1981; WANG 1985), and this is a plausible mechanism in the integration reaction (Fig. 8a). In all previously defined mechanisms of this kind, the joining reaction uses a terminal OH group as the acceptor for the activated phosphoryl end in the enzyme-DNA intermediate. Our evidence suggests that it is the viral DNA that contributes the 3' OH group to the initial viral-target DNA bond. An alternative solution to the energy coupling problem (CRAIGIE and MIZUUCHI 1987) calls for an enzyme-catalyzed nucleophilic attack by the viral 3' OH terminus on a phosphodiester bond in the target DNA, resulting in an essentially isoenergetic transesterification, much like that which occurs in RNA splicing (PADGETT et al. 1986) (Fig. 8b). A third possible model for formation of the new bonds in the recombinant is that rather than conserving the energy released by cleavage of donor or target DNA the complex carries an energy charge that is used in forming the new bonds (for example, it could carry an adenylated ligase activity).

The viral 3'-ends that are joined to target DNA in the initial covalent joining reaction determine the boundaries of the integrated provirus. Accordingly, to account for both the observed structure of the gapped intermediate and the structure of the integrated provirus by any model, the viral 3'-end that is joined to the target DNA needs to be recessed by 2 bases from the 5'-end. Since most viral DNA molecules have this structure even before they enter the nucleus (FUJIWARA and MIZUUCHI 1988; BROWN et al. 1989), cleavage of the viral 3'-end must not generally be coupled to the joining reaction. Thus, it is likely that the joining reaction is energetically coupled to target DNA cleavage. If the exigencies of energy conservation therefore cannot account for the cleavage of the viral 3'-ends, why is a recessed 3'-end used for integration rather than a flush 3'-end, presumably at the cost of an additional step in the integration mechanism? Perhaps the 5' extension that distinguishes the two structures is important for an effective interaction with the integration machinery. However, genetic analysis of the effect on integration of mutations in the MLV DNA ends indicates a

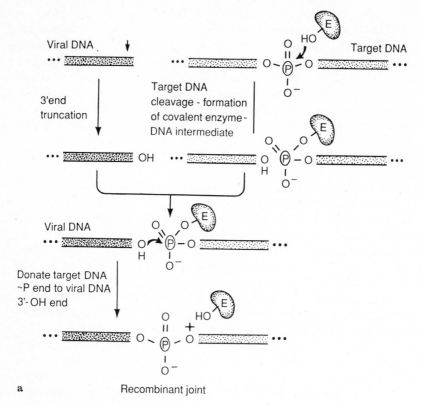

a   Recombinant joint

Fig. 8a (*Continued*)

considerable flexibility in the sequence and even the length of the 5′ overhang (COLICELLI and GOFF 1988a; Sect. 5.1).

Although processing of the 3′-end of the unintegrated DNA molecule appears to be a conserved feature of the retroviral integration reaction, it may not be conserved among all members of the large family of retrovirus-like transposable elements. The position of the putative primer binding site in the nucleotide sequence of the yeast retrotransposon Ty1 (CLARE and FARABAUGH 1985) predicts that the ends of unintegrated Ty1 DNA molecules should be identical to the ends of the integrated element. Thus, for this retrovirus-like element, integration probably does not require processing of the 3′-ends. Nevertheless, the integration step in Ty1 transposition has been shown to require sequences homologous to the retroviral IN gene (EICHINGER and BOEKE 1988). This observation suggests that the IN protein probably plays a role other than in 3′-end processing in the integration of Ty1 and thus perhaps in retroviral integration as well. Perhaps, like the Mu gene A protein in bacteriophage Mu transposition, the IN protein is responsible not only for viral DNA cleavage but also for target DNA cleavage and the joining reaction. However, the spatial and temporal separation of the cleavage of the viral 3′-ends from their joining to

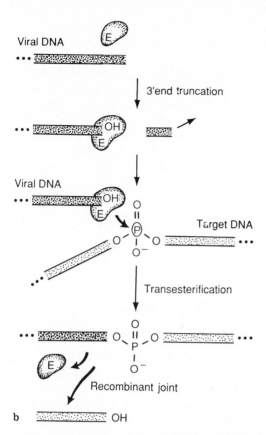

Viral DNA

3'end truncation

Viral DNA

Target DNA

Transesterification

Recombinant joint

b

Fig. 8 a, b. The DNA breakage and joining reaction. For simplicity, this figure depicts events affecting only one DNA strand, although it is likely that breakage and joining events on the two strands actually occur in a coordinated fashion. **a** Topoisomerase model. Target DNA molecule is cleaved by exchange of a DNA backbone phosphodiester bond for a high-energy protein DNA phosphodiester bond. Terminal 3'OH group of the viral DNA molecule then serves as the acceptor for formation of a new phosphodiester bond joining viral and target DNA, using energy stored in the protein-DNA bond. **b** Transesterification. Terminal 3'OH group of the viral DNA molecule is used as the attacking group in a direct, enzyme-catalyzed, nucleophilic attack on a phosphodiester bond in the target DNA molecule. This results in an essentially isoenergetic phosphodiester bond exchange that joins the viral to target DNA, displacing a target DNA 3' OH group. In this illustration, the same enzyme is depicted as catalyzing both the cleavage of the viral 3'-end and the transesterification step, although this is not a necessary feature of the model

target DNA raises the possibility that these steps might be carried out by different proteins. Whether or not the same protein is responsible for both reactions, it will be interesting to determine if these activities can be separated genetically or by using specific inhibitors, and if different active sites are involved in the two activities. The sequence-sensitive interaction of the integration apparatus with the viral DNA ends and the apparently-insensitive recognition of the DNA target for integration are in any case likely to be mediated by different DNA binding domains, if not different proteins.

9 Maturation

The initial joining step in integration yields a viral genome joined to host DNA by only one strand of the double helix at each end. To complete the process leading to a mature provirus the gaps flanking the viral DNA must be filled in by extending the free 3′-end of the target DNA, the mismatched viral 5′-end must be trimmed, and the resulting 3′- and 5′-ends must be ligated. This maturation process remains completely unexplored. Does the virus, after completing the numerous steps leading up to establishment of a provirus, leave this ultimate step in the integration process to chance? The cell has the enzymatic wherewithal to carry out this maturation process without the participation of viral functions. It is nevetherless conceivable that viraly encoded proteins might direct the necessary cellular enzymes to this substrate or even act directly to repair the gaps.

10 Influence of Host Cellular Proteins on Integration

The properties of hot spots of RSV integration (SHIH et al. 1988) and the tropism of proviruses for transcriptionally active regions suggest that host proteins might influence the efficiency and target site specificity of the reaction through an interaction with the target DNA. Other cellular components might also influence integration through more direct interactions with the viral integrative complex.

For example, replication of certain strains of MLV is inhibited in strains of mice or cell lines that carry particular alleles of the Fv-1 gene (JOLICOEUR 1979). The Fv-1 gene serves an unkown cellular function in the absence of infection. The two well-characterized alleles of this gene, Fv-1^n and Fv-1^b, determine the ability of alternative MLV strains to establish a provirus upon infection of a mouse cell. MLV strains are designated as either N-tropic, B-tropic, or NB-tropic depending on their ability to replicate in cells of different Fv-1 genotypes: Cells carrying the Fv-1^n allele do not allow establishment of a provirus by B-tropic MLV strains; cells carrying the Fv-1^b allele restrict N-tropic MLV strains; cells carrying both Fv-1 alleles restrict both N- and B-tropic viruses. NB-tropic MLV strains are not restricted by either Fv-1 allele, while phenotypically mixed viruses carrying both determinants are restricted by both alleles. Viral N/B tropism has been mapped to the CA coding region of the gag gene (BOONE et al. 1983; OU et al. 1983). A simple interpretation of the Fv-1 restriction phenomenon is that the host Fv-1 gene product interacts adversely with the cognate CA protein of an infecting subviral particle. However, while they tend to corroborate the in vitro evidence suggesting that CA is an essential part of the MLV integration complex, in vivo studies of Fv-1 restriction do not specifically implicate integration as the target for the inhibitory action of the Fv-1 product (YANG et al. 1980; JOLICOEUR and RASSART 1980, 1981). The in vitro integration system (BROWN et al. 1987) provides a way of explore directly the effects on integration of the Fv-1 gene product and other host cellular components, e.g., functions involved in cellular DNA synthesis (CHINSKY and SOEIRO 1982; RICHTER et al. 1984) or those induced by interferons (AVERY et al. 1980).

11 Prospects

Substantial progess has been made recently toward an understanding of the molecular basis of retroviral integration. Indeed, integration is now probably the best understood recombination reaction in higher eukaryotes. Yet fundamental questions remain to be answered, and the molecular biology of retroviral integration is likely to be a fertile problem for many years to come. Nothing is known regarding the mechanism for entry of the viral DNA and its associated proteins into the nucleus of the infected cell. The constituents of the integration complex remain to be defined—are they entirely viral in origin or do cellular proteins play a role? What is the 3-dimensional structure of the integration complex—does it indeed resemble the viral core particle? Is this large nucleoprotein complex actually essential for integration activity or can one or a few proteins catalyze the reaction? How does the integration machinery recognize its viral and target DNA substrates? How are target sites for integration selected—why are certain sites highly preferred? Where are the catalytic sites for viral DNA cleavage, target DNA cleavage, and the joining reaction? How is catalysis achieved, and what is the source of energy for the formation of the new phosphodiester bond joining viral and target DNA?

The availability of a cell-free system that faithfully duplicates the integration reaction has opened up the possibility of a complete molecular characterization of retroviral integration. Ultimately, the detailed biochemistry can best be illuminated by using defined, purified components to reconstruct the complete integration reaction and its individual steps. Stages of the integration reaction that might usefully be studied in isolation include viral DNA binding and cleavage, target DNA binding and cleavage, and the joining reaction itself. Reconstitution of these activites using purified proteins and DNA components is thus a principal goal of current research.

There are important practical reasons for studying retroviral integration. With the rapid growth in our understanding of the genetic basis of human disease, the prospects for rational therapeutic intervention directed at underlying genetic causes appear promising. Retroviruses are now widely used as vectors for genetic engineering in higher eukaryotes, and they are likely to be the first vectors used in gene replacement therapy for human genetic diseases, owing to their natural aptitude for introducing foreign genes into cellular chromosomes. Progress in understanding the means by which they do so may lead to the development of still more powerful tools for molecular medicine. Moreover, since integration of a provirus is fundamentally important to the replication of retroviruses, requires the active participation of viral proteins, and has no recognized counterpart essential to the economy of a normal cell, this reaction is an appealing target for inhibitors that might be useful in treating HIV infection. The growing impact of AIDS on public health worldwide thus provides added incentive and urgency to work aimed at understanding retroviral integration.

References

Avery RJ, Norton JD, Jones JS, Burke DC, Morris AG (1980) Interferon inhibits transformation by murine sarcoma viruses before integration of provirus. Nature 288: 93–95

Bishop JM (1983) Cellular oncogenes and retroviruses. Annu Rev Biochem 52: 301–354

Bishop JM, Varmus HE (1985) Functions and origins of transforming genes. In: Weiss R, Teich N, Varmus HE, Coffin J (eds) RNA tumor viruses, vol 2. Cold Spring Harbor Laboratory, Cold Spring Harbor, pp 999–1108

Bonner WM (1975) Protein migration into nuclei. I. Frog oocyte nuclei in vivo accumulate microinjected histones, allow entry to small proteins, and exclude large proteins. J Cell Biol 64: 421–430

Boone LR, Myer FE, Yang DM, Ou C-Y, Koh MCK, Roberson LE, Tennant RW, Yang WK (1983) Reversal of *Fv-1* host range by in vitro restriction endonuclease fragment exchange between molecular clones of N-tropic and B-tropic murine leukemia virus genomes. J Virol 48: 110–119

Bowerman B, Brown PO, Bishop JM, Varmus HE (1989) A nucleoprotein complex mediates the integration of retroviral DNA. Genes Development 3: 469–478

Brown PO, Bowerman B, Varmus HE, Bishop JM (1987) Correct integration of retroviral DNA in vitro. Cell 49: 347

Brown PO, Bowerman B, Varmus HE, Bishop JM (1989) Retroviral integration: structure of the initial covalent product and its precursor, and a role for the viral IN protein. Proc Natl Acad Sci USA 86: 2525–2529

Chinsky J, Soeiro R (1982) Studies with aphidicolin on the Fv-1 host restriction of Friend murine leukemia virus. J Virol 43: 182–190

Chinsky J, Soeiro R, Kopchick J (1984) Fv-1 host cell restriction of Friend leukemia virus: microinjection of unintegrated viral DNA. J Virol 50: 271–274

Clare J and Farabaugh P (1985) Nucleotide sequence of a yeast Ty element: evidence for an unusual mechanism of gene expression. Proc Natl Acad Sci USA 82: 2829–2833

Cobrinik D, Katz R, Terry R, Skalka AM, Leis J (1987) Avian sarcoma and leukosis virus *pol*-endonuclease recognition of the tandem long termina repeat junction: minimum site required for cleavage is also required for viral growth. J Virol 61: 1999–2008

Colicelli J, Goff SP (1985) Mutants and pseudo revertants of Moloney murine leukemia virus with alterations at the integration site. Cell 42: 573–580

Colicelli J, Goff SP (1988a) Sequence and spacing requirements of a retrovirus integration site. J Mol Biol 199: 47–59

Colicelli J, Goff SP (1988b) Isolation of an integrated provirus of Moloney murine leukemia virus with LTRs in inverted orientation: integration utilizing two U3 sequences. J Virol 62: 633–636

Copeland NG, Jenkins NA, Cooper GM (1981) Integration of Rous sarcoma virus DNA during transfection. Cell 23: 51–60

Craig NL (1989) Transposon Tn7. In: Howe M, Berg D (eds) Mobile DNA, ASM Press, Washington DC, pp 211–226

Craigie R, Mizuuchi K (1986) Role of DNA topology in Mu transposition: Mechanism of sensing the relative orientation of two DNA segments. Cell 45: 793–800

Craigie R, Mizuuchi K (1987) Transposition of Mu DNA: joining of Mu to target DNA can be uncoupled from cleavage at the ends of Mu. Cell 51: 493–501

Crawford S, Goff SP (1984) Mutations in gag proteins P12 and P15 of Moloney murine leukemia virus block early stages of infection. J Virol 49: 909–917

DesGroseillers L, Jolicoeur P (1983) Physical mapping of the Fv-1 tropism host range determinant of BALB/c murine leukemia viruses. J Virol 48: 685–696

Dhar R, McClements WL, Enquist LW, Vande Woude GF (1980) Nucleotide sequences of integrated Maloney sarcoma provirus long terminal repeats and their host and viral junctions. Proc Natl Acad Sci USA 77: 3937–3941

Dingwall C, Laskey RA (1986) Protein import into the cell nucleus. Annu Rev Cell Biol 2: 367–390

Donehower LA (1988) Analysis of mutant Moloney murine leukemia viruses containing linker insertion mutations in the 3′ region of pol. J Virol 62: 3958–3964

Donehower LA, Varmus HE (1984) A mutant murine leukemia virus with a single missense codon in pol is defective in a function affecting integration. Proc Natl Acad Sci USA 81: 6461–6465

Duyk G, Leis J, Longiaru M, Skalka AM (1983) Selective cleavage on the avian retroviral long terminal repeat sequence by the endonucleases associated with the form of avian reverse transcriptase. Proc Natl Acad Sci USA 80: 6745–6749

Duyk G, Longiaru M, Cobrinik D, Kowal R, deHaseth P, Skalka AM, Leis J (1985) Circles with two tandem long terminal repeats are specifically cleaved by pol gene-associated endonuclease from avian sarcoma and leukosis viruses: nucleotide sequences required for site-specific cleavage. J Virol 56: 589–599

Eichinger DJ, Boeke JD (1988) The DNA intermediate in yeast Ty1 element transposition copurifies with virus-like particles: cell-free Ty1 transposition. Cell 54: 955–966

Frankel W, Potter TA, Rosenberg N, Lenz J, Rajan TJ (1985) Retroviral insertional mutagenesis of a target allele in a heterozygous murine cell line. Proc Natl Acad Sci USA 82: 6600–6604

Fujiwara T, Craigie R (1989) Integration of mini-retroviral DNA: A cell-free reaction for biochemical analysis of retroviral integration. Proc Natl Acad Sci USA 86: 3065–3069

Fujiwara T, Mizuuchi K (1988) Retroviral DNA integration: structure of an integration intermediate. Cell 54: 497–504

Goff SP (1984) The genetics of murine leukemia viruses. Curr Top Microbiol Immunol 112: 45–69

Golomb M, Grandgenett DP (1979) Endonuclease activity of purified RNA directed DNA polymerase from AMV. J Biol Chem 254: 1606–1613

Golomb M, Grandgenett DP (1981) Virus-coded DNA endonuclease from avian retrovirus. J Virol 38: 548–555

Grandgenett DP, Vora AC (1985) Site-specific nicking at the avian retrovirus LTR circle junction by the viral pp32 DNA endonuclease. Nucleic Acids Res 13: 6205–6221

Grandgenett DP, Vora AC, Schiff RD (1978) A 32,000-dalton nucleic acid-binding protein from avian retrovirus cores possesses DNA endonuclease activity. Virology 89: 119–132

Grandgenett DP, Vora AC, Swanstrom R, Olsen JC (1986) Nuclease mechanism of the avian retrovirus pp32 endonuclease. J Virol 58: 970–974

Hagino-Yamagishi K, Donehower LA, Varmus HE (1987) Retroviral DNA integrated during infection by an integration-deficient mutant of murine leukemia virus is oligomeric. J Virol 61: 1964–1971

Harris JD, Blum H, Scott J, Traynor B, Ventura P, Hasse A (1984) Slow virus visna: reproduction in vitro of virus from extrachromosomal DNA. Proc Natl Acad Sci USA 81: 7212–7215

Hayward WS, Neel BG, Astrin SM (1981) Activation of a cellular onc gene by promoter insertion in ALV-induced lymphoid leukosis. Nature 290: 475–480

Howe M, Berg D (eds) (1989) Mobile DNA. ASM Press, Washington DC

Hsu HW, Schwartzberg P, Goff SP (1985) Point mutations in the p30 domain of the gag gene of Moloney murine leukemia virus. Virology 142: 211–214

Hughes SH, Mutschler A, Bishop JM, Varmus HE (1981) A Rous sarcoma virus provirus is flanked by short direct repeats of a cellular DNA sequence present in only one copy prior to integration. Proc Natl Acad Sci USA 78: 4299–4303

Hughes SH, Shank PR, Spector DH, Kung HJ, Bishop JM, Varmus HE, Vogt PK, Breitman ML (1978) Proviruses of avian sarcoma virus are terminally redundant, co-extensive with unintegrated linear DNA and integrated at many sites. Cell 15: 1397–1410

Humphries EH, Glover C, Reichmann ME (1981) Rous sarcoma virus infection of synchronized cells establishes provirus integration during S phase DNA synthesis prior to cell division. Proc Natl Acad Sci USA 78: 2601–2605

Hwang JV, Gilboa E (1974) Expression of genes introduced into cells by retroviral infection is more effective than that of gene introduced into cells by DNA transfection. J Virol 50: 417–424

Jaenisch R, Harbers K, Schnicke A, Lohler J, Chumakov I, Jahner D, Grotkopp D, Hoffmann E (1983) Germ line integration of Moloney murine leukemia virus at the Mov13 locus leads to recessive lethal mutation and early embryonic death. Cell 32: 209–216

Jenkins JA, Copeland NG, Taylor BA, Lee BK (1981) Dilute (d) coat colour mutation of DBA/2J mice is associated with the site of integration of an ecotropic MuLV genome. Nature 293: 370–374

Jolicoeur P (1979) The Fv-1 gene of the mouse and its control of murine leukemia virus replication. Curr Top Microbiol Immunol 86: 67–122

Jolicoeur P, Rassart E (1980) Effect of Fv-1 gene on synthesis of linear and supercoiled viral DNA in cells infected with murine leukemia virus. J Virol 33: 183–195

Jolicoeur P, Rassart E (1981) Fate of unintegrated viral DNA in Fv-1 permissive and resistant mouse cells infected with murine leukemia virus. J Virol 37: 609–619

King W, Patel MD, Lobel LI, Goff SP, Nguyen-Huu MC (1985) Insertion mutagenesis of embryonal carcinoma cells by retroviruses. Science 228: 554–558

Leis J, Duyk G, Johnson S, Longiaru M, Skalka A (1983) Mechanism of action of the endonuclease associated with $\alpha\beta$ and $\beta\beta$ forms of avian RNA tumor virus reverse transcriptase. J Virol 45: 727–739

Leis J, Baltimore D, Bishop JM, Coffin J, Fleissner E, Goff P, Oroszlan S, Robinson H, Skalka AM, Temin HM, Vogt V (1988) A standardized and simplified nomenclature for proteins common to all retroviruses. J Virol 62: 1808–1809

Lilley DMJ (1983) Dynamic, sequence-dependent DNA structures as exemplified by cruciform extrusion from inverted repeats in negatively supercoiled DNA. CSHSQB 47: 101–112

Lobel LI, Goff SP (1984) Construction of mutants of Moloney murine leukemia virus by suppressor-linker insertional mutagenesis: Positions of viable insertion. Proc Natl Acad Sci USA 81: 4149–4153

Lobel LI, Murphy J, Goff, SP (1989) The palindromic LTR-LTR junction is not an efficient substrate for proviral integration. J Virol 63: 2629–2637

Luciw PA, Oppermann H, Bishop JM, Varmus HE (1984) Integration and expression of several forms of Rous sarcoma virus DNA used for transfection of mouse cells. Mol Cell Biol 4: 1260–1269

Luk KC, Gilmore TD, Panganiban AT (1987) The spleen necrosis virus *int* gene product expressed in *Escherichia coli* has DNA binding activity and mediates *att* and U5-specific DNA multimer formation in vitro. Virology 157: 127–136

Majors J, Varmus HE (1981) Nucleotide sequences at host-proviral junctions for mouse mammary tumor virus. Nature 289: 253–258

Mizuuchi K, Craigie R (1986) Mechanism of bacteriophage Mu transposition. Annu Rev Genet 20: 385–429

Morris-Vasios C, Kochan JP, Skalka AM (1989) Avian sarcoma-leukosis virus pol-endo proteins expressed independently in mammalian cells accumulate in the nucleus but can be directed to other cellular compartments. J Virol 62: 349–353

Ou C-Y, Boone, LR, Koh C-K, Tennant RW, Yang WK (1983) Nucleotide sequence of *gag-pol* regions that determine the Fv-1 host range property jof BALB/c N-tropic and B-tropic murine leukemia viruses. J Virol 48: 779–784

Padgett RA, Grabowski PJ, Konarska MM, Seiler S, Sharp PA (1986) Splicing of messenger RNA precursors. Annu Rev Biochem 55: 1119–1150

Panet A, Baltimore D (1987) Characterization of endonuclease activities in Moloney murine leukemia virus and its replication-defective mutants. J Virol 61: 1756–1760

Panganiban AT, Temin HM (1983) The terminal nucleotides of retrovirus DNA are required for integration but not virus production. Nature 306: 155–160

Panganiban AT, Temin HM (1984a) Circles with two tandem LTRs are precursors to integrated retrovirus DNA. Cell 36: 673–679

Panganiban AT, Temin HM (1984b) The retrovirus pol gene encodes a product required for DNA integration: Identification of a retrovirus int locus. Proc Natl Acad Sci USA 81: 7885–7889

Pato ML (1989) Bacteriophage Mu. In: Howe M, Berg D (eds) Mobile DNA. ASM Press, Washington DC, pp 23–52

Payne GS, Bishop JM, Varmus HE (1982) Multiple arrangements of viral DNA and an activated host oncogene in bursal lymphomas. Nature 295: 209–213

Ratner et al (1985) Complete nucleotide of the AIDS virus, HTLV-III. Nature 313: 277–284

Reed RR, Grindley NDF (1981) Transposon-mediated site-specific recombination in vitro: DNA cleavage and protein-DNA linkage at the recombination site. Cell 25: 721–728

Richter A, Ozer HL, DesGroseillers L, Jolicoeur P (1984) An X-linked gene affecting mouse cell DNA synthesis also affects production of unintegrated linear and supercoiled DNA of murine leukemia virus. Mol Cell Biol 4: 151–159

Rohdewohld H, Weiher H, Reik W, Jaenisch R, Breindl M (1987) Retrovirus integration and chromatin structure: Moloney murine leukemia virus gene expression. Proc Natl Acad Sci USA 84: 4919–4923

Roth MJ, Tanese N, Schwartzberg P, Goff SP (1988) Gene product of Moloney murine leukemia virus required for proviral integration is a DNA binding protein. J Mol Biol 203: 131–140

Schwartzberg P, Colicelli J, Goff SP (1984a) Construction and analysis of deletion mutants in the pol gene of Moloney murine leukemia virus: a new viral function required for establishment of the integrated provirus. Cell 37: 1043–1052

Schwartzberg P, Colicelli J, Gordon ML, Goff SP (1984b) Mutation in the *gag* gene of Moloney murine leukemia virus: effects on production of various and reverse transcriptase. J Virol 49: 918–924

Scott ML, McKeregan K, Kaplan HS, Fry KE (1981) Molecular cloning and partion characterization of unintegrated linear DNA from gibbon ape leukemia virus. Proc Natl Acad Sci 78: 4213–4217

Shapiro JA (1979) Molecular model for the transposition and replication of bacteriophage Mu and other transposable elements. Proc Natl Acad Sci USA 76: 1933–1937

Shih C-C, Stoye JF, Coffin JM (1988) Highly preferred targets for retrovirus integration. Cell 53: 531–538

Shimotono K, Mizutani S, Temin HM (1980) Sequence of retrovirus provirus resembles that of bacterial transposable elements. Nature 285: 550–554

Shinnick T, Lerner R, Sutcliffe JG (1980) Nucleotide sequence of Moloney murine leukemia virus. Nature 293: 543–548

Shoemaker C, Goff S, Gilboa E, Pasking M, Mitra SW, Baltimore D (1980) Structure of a cloned circular Moloney murine leukemia virus molecule containing an inverted segment: implications for retrovirus integration. Proc Natl Acad Sci USA 77: 3932–3936

Shoemaker C, Hoffmann J, Goff SP, Baltimore D (1981) Intramolecular integration within Moloney murine leukemia virus DNA. J Virol 40: 164–172

Soriano P, Gridley T and Jaenisch R (1989) Retroviral tagging in mammalian development and genetics. In: Howe M, Berg D (eds) Mobile DNA. ASM Press, Washington DC, pp 927–938

Stavenhagen JB, Robins DM (1988) An ancient provirus has imposed androgen regulation on the adjacent mouse sex-limited protein gene. Cell 55: 247–254

Stoye JP, Fenner S, Greenoak GE, Moran C, and Coffin JM (1988) Role of endogenous retroviruses as mutagens: the hairless mutation of mice. Cell 54: 383–391

Surette MG, Buch SJ, Chaconas G (1987) Transpososomes: stable protein-DNA complexes involved in the in vitro transposition of bacteriophage Mu DNA. Cell 49: 253–262

Swanstrom R, DeLorbe WJ, Bishop JM, Varmus HE (1981) Nucleotide sequence of cloned unintegrated avian sarcoma virus DNA: viral DNA contains direct and inverted repeats similar to those in transposable elements. Proc Natl Acad Sci USA 78: 124–128

Teich N, Wyke J, Mak T, Bernstein A, Hardy W (1982) Pathogenesis of retrovirus-induced disease. In: Weiss R, Teich N, Varmus H, Coffin J (eds) RNA tumor viruses, Cold Spring Harbor Laboratory, Cold Spring Harbor, pp 785–998

Teich N, Wyke J, Kaplan P (1985) Pathogenesis of retrovirus-induced disease, In: Weiss R, Teich N, Varmus H, Coffin J (eds) RNA tumor viruses, Cold Spring Harbor Laboratory, Cold Spring Harbor, pp 187–248

Thompson JF, Landy A (1989) Regulation of bacteriophage lambda site-specific recombination. In: Howe M, Berg D (eds) Mobile DNA. ASM Press, Washington DC, pp 1–22

van Beveren C, Coffin J, Hughes S (1985) Appendices. In: Weiss R, Teich N, Varmus H, Coffin J (eds) RNA tumor viruses, Cold Spring Harbor Laboratory, NY, pp 559–1221

van Beveren C, Rands E, Chattopadhyay SK, Lowy DR, Verma IM (1982) Long terminal repeat of murine retroviral DNAs: sequence analysis, host-proviral junctions and preintegration site. J Virol 41: 542–556

van Ooyen A, Nusse R (1984) Structure and nucleotide sequence of the putative mammary oncogene int-1: proviral insertions leave the protein-encoding domain intact. Cell 39: 233–240

Varmus HE (1982) Form and function of retroviral proviruses. Science 216: 812–820

Varmus HE (1983) Retroviruses: In: Shapiro J (ed) Mobile genetic elements. Academic, New York, pp 411–503

Varmus HE (1987) Cellular and viral oncogenes. In: Stamatoyannopoulos G, Nienhuis AW, Leder P, Majerus PW (eds) Molecular Basis of Blood Diseases. Saunders, Philadelphia, pp 271–346

Varmus HE, Brown P (1989) Retroviruses. In: Howe M, Berg D (eds) Mobile DNA. ASM Press, Washington DC pp 53–109

Varmus HE, Swanstrom R (1982) Replication of retroviruses, In: Weiss R, Teich N, Varmus H, Coffin J (eds) RNA tumor viruses. Cold Spring Harbor Laboratory, NY, pp 369–512

Varmus HE, Swanstrom R (1985) Replication of retroviruses. In: Weiss R, Teich N, Varmus H, Coffins J (eds) RNA tumor viruses. Cold Spring Harbor Laboratory, Cold Spring Harbor, pp. 75–134

Varmus HE, Padgett T, Heasley S, Simon G, Bishop JM (1977) Cellular functions are required for the synthesis and integration of avian sarcoma virus-specific DNA. Cell 11: 307–319

Varmus HE, Quintrell N, Ortiz S (1981) Retroviruses as mutagens: insertion and excision of a non-transforming provirus alters expression of a resident transforming provirus. Cell 25: 23–26

Vijaya S, Steffen DL, Robinson HL (1986) Acceptor sites for retroviral integrations map near DNase I-hypersensitive sites in chromatin. J Virol 60: 683–692

Wang JC (1985) DNA topoisomerase. Ann Rev Biochem 54: 665–697

Weiner AM, Deininger PL, Efstratiadis A (1987) Nonviral transposons: Genes, pseudogenes, and transposable elements generated by the reverse flow of genetic information. Annu Rev Biochem 55: 631–662

Weiss R, Teich N, Varmus H, Coffin J (eds) (1982, 1985) RNA tumor viruses, Cold Spring Harbor Loboratory, NY

Yang WK, Kiggens JO, Yang D-M, Ou C-Y, Tennant RW, Brown A, Bassin RH (1980) Synthesis and circularization of N- and B-tropic retroviral DNA in FV-1 premissive and restrictive mouse cells. Proc Natl Acad Sci USA 77: 2994–2998

The Structure and Function of Retroviral Long Terminal Repeats

J. MAJORS

Department of Biochemistry and Molecular Biophysics, Washington University School of Medicine,
660 South Euclid, St. Louis, MO 63110, USA

Current Topics in Microbiology and Immunology, Vol. 157
© Springer-Verlag Berlin·Heidelberg 1990

1 Introduction

During the natural course of reverse transcription, sequences from the 5′ (R-U5) and 3′ (U3-R) ends of retroviral genomic RNA are fused through the direct repeat sequence, R, and duplicated to form a linear duplex molecule with long terminal repeats (LTRs). Subsequent insertion of this molecule into a site within the chromosomal DNA of an infected host cell allows the viral DNA to function as a template for the transcription of new viral RNA molecules. Synthesis of these molecules is catalyzed by the host RNA polymerase II and initiates at the U3-R border. The 3′-ends of these molecules are generated by cleavage and polyA addition at the R-U5 boundary. A direct consequence of this pathway is that sequences immediately upstream from the transcription start are virus-coded and derive from the 3′-end of viral RNA. By analogy with the structures of cellular pol II promoters, elements which instruct the host polymerase when and where to initiate viral RNA synthesis should lie within these upstream sequences. The central role in viral replication of this host-dependent transcription step and the broad spectrum of host cell-specific transcription patterns mean that many biological properties of retroviruses will be determined by sequences within the LTR.

The role played by transcriptional control mechanisms in fundamental problems in biological regulation is clear. Rapid advances in understanding these mechanisms has been made possible by the introduction of simple procedures for genetic manipulation in vitro and for analysis of the consequences of these manipulations on function in vivo. These procedures permit straightforward definition of sequence elements responsible for directing transcription of cellular and viral genes. Accompanying these genetic advances have been improved biochemical procedures for isolating sequence-specific DNA binding proteins which recognize these elements and provide molecular instructions to the polymerase. In this chapter, I will describe recent results which derive from the application of these procedures to the study of retrovirus biology.

Systematic characterization of selected viral and cellular gene promoters shows that their capacity to promote transcription is generated by arrays of short sequence elements. Included among these are (a) the TATA element, located between 20 and 30 bp upstream from the transcription start site, which determines both the site of initiation and also affects the efficiency of initiation; (b) more distal promoter elements, generally within the first 100–150 bp upstream from the start site; and (c) enhancer-like sequences, which often lie quite far from the promoter region in either an upstream or downstream location. Patterns of tissue-specific viral or cellular gene expression are generally associated with linkage to element arrays which behave as tissue-specific enhancers when tested in heterologous promoter assays. The LTRs of each of the retroviruses discussed in this chapter have TATA elements, distal promoter elements, and sequences which score in enhancer assays. In succeeding sections I will explore the identity of these elements and will discuss their role in the biology of the viruses.

I will confine the discussion to questions addressed by study of five different retroviral families: the avian sarcoma/leukosis viruses, the mouse mammary tumor virus, murine leukemia viruses, the human T-lymphotropic viruses HTLV-1 and HTLV-2, and the human immunodeficiency viruses HIV-1 and HIV-2. For each of these families I will focus on issues which are of particular interest to those studying that particular family. Problems to be explored include: (a) The role of host-specific proteins in promoting viral RNA synthesis, especially for LTRs which respond to small molecule inducers or which are expressed in tissue-specific ways. (b) The role of virus-coded gene products in both controlling patterns of viral RNA synthesis and generating altered patterns of cellular gene expression. (c) The contribution of these cellular and viral regulators to the pathogenic behavior of individual members of these different virus classes.

2 Avian Leukosis/Sarcoma Viruses

The avian leukosis/sarcoma viruses make up a large family of rapidly oncogenic, slowly oncogenic, and nononcogenic retroviruses. The LTRs of the oncogenic members must promote expression of viral RNA levels which ensure efficient virus propagation and appropriate levels of oncogene expression. The latter may result from expression of oncogene sequences directly incorporated into the viral genome, or from expression of cellular sequences placed under the influence of nearby proviral regulatory elements.

2.1 Structure of the Long Terminal Repeat

The isolated RSV LTR functions as a potent transcriptional promoter both in vitro and after being introduced into cultured cell lines (Gorman et al. 1982). Although its ability to promote the synthesis of linked sequences is most effective in avian cells (relative to other strong promoters), the universal observation is that its promoter shows little specificity with respect either to cell type or to the conditions under which the cells are grown. In fact, it finds frequent use as a control promoter in studies of regulated promoters. Analyses of RSV LTR functions address several general issues related to the use of LTR structures to promote retroviral RNA synthesis.

Comparative analysis of the individual members of the family shows identity or near identity of their cis-acting control elements. Within the LTR their R and U5 elements show little variation. Significantly more variation exists in U3, especially in sequences which have been shown to be important for enhancer function. Figure 1 compares the U3 sequences of several of these viruses. Readily identifiable elements include a polyadenylation signal AATAAA located immediately upstream of the transcription start site (from -2 to -7) and a TATA-like sequence, TATTTAA, at an appropriate position (-25 to -31). Sequence

```
       INT          C/EBP        C/EBP      C/EBP           ?            ?
RAV1   AATGTAGTCTTATGCAATACTCTAATGCAATATCTTGCAACATGCTTATGTAACGATGAGTTAGCAACATG
RAV2   ....................T      GTAG     ...........................
SRA2   ....................T      GTAG     ...........          ...........
PRC    ...................        GTAG     ....................          ....T...
UR2    ......................               ............AAC.....A...
Y73    .....................               ............AAC.....T...
PRCII  ...........CA......              ...T  .............AC.....T...
MC29   ...........CA.....A.    TGTAGA        ...........AAC.....T.C.
E26    ......C...CA.....      GCCTTACACAATAATG      ...........T.. C....GT...
MH2    ......C...CA..:...     GCCTTACACAATTATG      .............  AAC.....T.C.
RPV    ......A..GG   ....C.TGC         TTAT          .....................
CT10   .....          212 BASE PAIRS              .......CA......CAC.....T...
```

```
          CArG                          CCAAT          Enhancer Core
RAV1   CCTTATAAGGAGAGAAAAGGCACCGTGCATGACGATTGGTGGGAGTAAGGTGGTATGATCGTGGTATGA
RAV2   ...............A...........C...........................
SRA2   .....C.........A...........C...........A...........        C..
PRC    .....C...A.................C...........T...........        C..
UR2    .........G..A..G.....  T..A....TT.......A...  ...................C..
Y73    ...........TA........TA.A....TT.......A...              ...
PRCII  ...........G..T...........T.......A..C...A.....          ...
MC29   .............T...........T.......A.....                  C..
E26    ..A.......GA..G..G.A....ACA.....T.......A.....A.....     ...
MH2    ...........G..T...........T.......A.....                 CC.
RPV    ...........A......A...........C.......A.............[....X2...]
CT10   ...........A.A...  .....T..A.C.TT.........A...........
```

```
          CArG               ?          CCAAT               ?
RAV1   CGTGCCTTATTAGGAAGGCAACAGACGGGTCTAACACGGATTGGACGAACCACCGAATTCCGCATTGC
RAV2   T.......G...........................................T...........
SRA2   T............................G...T...........................
PRC    T............T.T.............T.........................C..
UR2    T.........................G........TA....C..T.G...........
Y73    T.A........T...........T........TC..T.T...........
PRCII  T............T...........T........T.TC..AG.C......A.T
MC29   T............T...........T........T.T...TG.......A.T
E26    T............T.T.......:.C..CG.........AG......T.G.......A.T
MH2    T..C............TAT.......C..CA.:.......TAG...G..T.G.......A.T
RPV    .........................................T............
CT10   ........................G...T........T.TC.TT.G...........
```

```
       TATA              PolyA
RAV1   AGAGATATTGTATTTAAGTGCCTAGCTCGATACAATAAAGGC
RAV2   ...............................C..
SRA2   ...............................C..
PRC    ...............................C..
UR2    .A....A.........A...G...T:..GT.....C..
Y73    ......A.A.................T..........C..
PRCII  ...A..G..........AG......T..........C..
MC29   ...A..G.................TA.........C..
E26    ......G.....C..........G...T..C.T......C..
MH2    ......G..........AG......T...........C..
RPV    .........C.......................C..
CT10   ......G..................CT...........C..
```

scanning (see below) reveals elements which resemble those found in other transcriptional control regions, and direct tests for functional elements have begun to reveal the structure of the LTR.

Sequences from the 5'-end of the LTR activate expression from heterologous promoters; that is, they have the properties of a transcriptional enhancer (LUCIW et al. 1983; LAIMINS et al. 1984b). Enhancer activity of a 3' LTR distributes over an extended region upstream of − 150 and even extends beyond the LTR into unique sequences flanked by *src* and the polypurine tract (LUCIW et al. 1983; LAIMINS et al. 1984b). This extended region could be divided into three sequence blocks, the 65 bp immediately adjacent and 5' to the LTR, 100 bp at the 3'-end of the LTR, and 86 bp from − 53 to − 140. The middle segment in combination with either of the flanking segments, or multimers of the middle segment, were sufficient to enhance expression from an SV40 promoter in chick cells (LAIMINS et al. 1984b). None of the isolated segments provided enhancer function. Analysis of 5' deletions of the LTR confirmed the role of the 5'-most 100 bp as removal of these sequences decreases promoter function from 20- to 200-fold in different assays (NORTON and COFFIN 1987; CULLEN et al. 1985b; GOWDA et al. 1988). (These and other early studies of LTR function are reviewed in JU and SKALKA 1985.) A high resolution map of sequence elements within the LTR which provide either the enhancer activity or promoter function is not yet available. However, combined results from protein-binding studies, directed mutagenesis, and comparisons with other promoter/enhancer regions make possible the construction of a plausible structure for the LTR.

2.2   Protein Binding to the Long Terminal Repeat

Several protein factors present in crude extracts from avian cell nuclei interact with specific sequences within the RSV LTR (SEALEY and CHALKLEY 1987; RUDDELL et al. 1988; GOODWIN 1988). Prominent among them is a heat-stable factor which recognizes multiple copies of the sequence GCAATA near the 5'-end of the LTR. These elements lie within the region of the LTR which has enhancer activity. The factor, called EFII (SEALEY and CHALKLEY 1987) or FIII (GOODWIN 1988) is probably similar to C/EBP (for CCAAT/enhancer binding protein), characterized by MCKNIGHT and colleagues (LANDSCHULZ et al. 1988). Purified

◄ ───

Fig. 1. *U3 sequences of members of the avian sarcoma/leukosis virus family.* The sequences extend from the AATG sequence at the 5'-end of the long terminal repeat to the transcription start point. Shown are sequences from the following viruses: RAV-1 (HODGSON et al. 1987); RAV-2 (WESTAWAY et al. 1984); Schmidt-Ruppin A (SRA) (SWANSTROM et al. 1981); Prague C (PrC) (SCHWARTZ et al. 1983); MC29 (REDDY et al. 1983); E26 (NUNN et al. 1984); MH2 (KAN et al. 1984); UR2 (NECKAMEYER and WANG 1985); Y73 (KITAMURA et al. 1982); PRCII (HUANG et al. 1984); ringneck pheasant virus (RPV) (SMITH et al. 1985); and CT10 (MAYER et al. 1988). Indicated *above* aligned sequences are regions of apparent conserved sequence. Elements demonstrated to be targets for known DNA binding proteins and elements whose sequences are similar to identified control elements are identified. Apparent conserved elements not in either of these classes are marked by a *question mark.* *INT* denotes sequences important for reverse transcription and integration

C/EPB covers the same sequences as EFII and FIII and has multiple binding sites within all of the avian sarcoma/leukosis virus LTRs (RYDEN and BEEMON 1989). A similar activity also binds to sequences within an internal *gag* enhancer (KARNITZ et al. 1989; see below). A second factor, termed EFI (SEALEY and CHALKLEY 1987) or FII (GOODWIN 1988), binds to a CCAAT motif located at − 130. Disruption of that sequence results in a 20-fold decrease in promoter activity and prevents EFI binding (B. GREUEL, unpublished data). A similar factor, purified from rat liver nuclei (MAITY et al. 1988), acts as a heterodimer and behaves in a fashion similar to CBP-1 of HeLa cells (CHODOSH et al. 1988). Although not yet documented, other conserved elements within the LTRs of this family should be targets for protein binding. Included among these are CArG elements (see Fig. 1) which bind several cellular proteins including the serum response factor (TREISMAN 1987; PRYWES and ROEDER 1987; GUSTAFSON et al. 1988; WALSH 1989), and enhancer core sequences, which also are likely targets for multiple DNA binding proteins (reviewed in JONES et al. 1988b).

2.3 Involvement of the LTR in Oncogenesis and Communication Between LTRs

Replication-competent, slowly transforming retroviruses generally contribute to tumor formation by acting as insertional mutagens. For such viruses a necessary step in the path toward malignancy is the occasional insertion of viral DNA in the vicinity of one or more of a set of cellular genes whose subsequent misexpression results in altered cell growth properties (reviewed in VARMUS 1987). Although inserted viral DNAs may alter patterns of neighboring gene expression by several pathways, most will do so at least in part through the provision of powerful *cis*-acting transcriptional control elements.

Induction of bursal lymphomas by avian leukosis viruses (ALV) is a well-characterized example of this phenomenon. Most ALV-induced tumors have proviral DNA inserted into the c-*myc* locus in a configuration which results in hybrid U5/c-*myc* transcripts that initiate in the 3′ LTR (HAYWARD et al. 1981). Associated with these 3′ LTR-promoted transcripts are, first, deletions in the proviral sequences, which generally remove large regions from the 5′-end of the LTR, and second, an absence of expression from the upstream LTR (PAYNE et al. 1981; GOODENOW and HAYWARD 1987). Attempts to account for these results have led investigators to look more closely at patterns of LTR-promoted RNA synthesis from randomly inserted proviruses.

The 5′ and 3′ LTRs of a provirus are identical in sequences, and each functions equally well in short-term promoter activity assays. The same may not be true for integrated LTRs; stable transcripts which initiate in the 5′ LTR of randomly integrated ALV proviruses are at least 50 times more abundant than those which initiate in the 3′ LTR (HERMAN and COFFIN 1986). Cellular sequences flanking the 3′ LTR are expressed but as read-through transcripts which initiate in the 5′ LTR. The failure of the 3′ LTR to generate stable transcripts may be transcriptional or posttranscriptional. One way to account for this result is the promoter interference model in which passage of 5' LTR-initiated polymerases through the U3 region of the 3' LTR inhibits its enhancer/promoter activity. An experimental test of this model showed that the presence of an upstream LTR represses downstream LTR activity three- to fourfold using a plasmid-mediated short-term expression assay (CULLEN et al. 1984).

An alternative explanation for differential activation of the 5' LTR arises from the discovery of a complex enhancer element in *gag* (ARRIGO et al. 1987; STOLTZFUS et al. 1987; CARLBERG et al. 1988). Contained within both the *gag* and LTR enhancers are binding sites for the protein factor C/EBP (CARLBERG et al. 1988; RYDEN and BEEMON 1989; KARNITZ et al. 1989). Interactions between the two enhancer elements may dictate LTR selection (CARLBERG et al. 1988), but experimental support for this model is not yet available. A related phenomenon has been noted by investigators attempting to make retroviral vectors with multiple promoters, where selection for expression of one promoter generally leads to inactivation of the second promoter (EMERMAN and TEMIN 1984).

A role for the LTR in viral oncogenicity is supported by studies which show a direct correlation between the ability of a virus to induce bursal lymphomas and the ability of its U3 sequences to function in enhancer assays (CULLEN et al. 1985a). U3 sequences of nononcogenic RAV-0 have little if any enhancer activity when measured in typical assays and differ significantly from those presented in Fig. 1. Although RAV-0 replicates to a significant titer in infected animals, substitution of its LTR with that of the oncogenic RAV-1 strain results in a virus which both replicates better and has significant oncogenic capacity (ROBINSON et al. 1982, 1985; BROWN et al. 1988). Regions outside the LTR are also influential (ROBINSON et al. 1985).

The capacity of an LTR to promote tumorigenesis is also affected by the host environment. LTR-initiated transcription in bursal lymphoma tumor cell lines is sensitive to protein synthesis inhibitors; transcription in infected fibroblasts or T cells is unaffected by similar treatments (LINIAL et al. 1985). Paralleling the inhibitor-induced decreased transcription rate is a loss of nuclease hypersensitive sites within the LTR. In a similar fashion, LTR-promoted transcription in infected lymphocytes from chicken lines sensitive to bursal transformation by ALV is sensitive to protein synthesis inhibitors; transcription in lymphocytes from nonsusceptible lines is resistant to the inhibitors (RUDDELL et al. 1988). Directly correlating with these patterns of RNA synthesis are nuclear proteins which bind to LTR U3 sequences; their presence is also sensitive to protein synthesis inhibitors (RUDDELL et al. 1988). The manner in which this unusual property of the enhancer binding proteins permits bursal infection and transformation is not yet understood. A suggested possibility is that temporary relief of c-*myc* activation allows putative bursal stem cells, previously driven to proliferate by elevated expression of c-*myc*, to home to the bursa and differentiate. Subsequent reactivation of c-*myc* would lead first to transformed bursal follicles and eventually to a tumor (RUDDELL et al. 1988).

2.4 Activity of the LTR in Nonavian Cells

The RSV LTR functions as an efficient promoter in most cell types when tested in short-term transfection assays. Curiously, the same is not true when the LTR is introduced into cells in the context of an integrated provirus. In this form, the LTR is extremely active in avian cells but almost inactive in mammalian cells. When rat fibroblast cells are infected with RSV, fewer than 1 in 1000 infected cells express high v-*src* levels and are transformed (reviewed in GREEN and WYKE 1988). The remaining infected cells express little if any viral RNA and are not transformed. A majority of proviruses in singly infected, transformed cell clones show unusual rearrangements of the viral DNA at their 5'-ends (GREEN et al. 1986). These rearrangements generally result in placement of regions of the viral *gag* and v-*src* genes upstream of what should be the 5' LTR. How these rearrangements promote expression from normally silent LTRs is not known. Explanations put forward include that the viral sequences provide a buffer which separates the LTR from chromosomal silencer elements, and that the viral sequences provide additional enhancer elements which only function in mammalian cells when placed upstream of an LTR. The active proviruses in many transformed cell clones are made transcriptionally silent after fusion with normal cells, supporting the existence of factors in normal cells which suppress LTR activity (DYSON et al. 1985). These factors may work through sequences in flanking cellular DNA, as the sequences retain their capacity to affect proviral expression in genomic gene transfer experiments (AKROYD et al. 1987). Whether these effects are specific to proviral structures is not clear. Isolated LTRs can be used in gene transfer experiments to express selectable marker genes efficiently in cultured cells (GORMAN et al. 1982), and to express the CAT gene in transgenic mice (OVERBEEK et al. 1986). In the latter case high level expression was confined largely to tissue rich in tendon, bone, and muscle.

3 Mouse Mammary Tumor Virus

MMTV is an effective agent for inducing mammary carcinomas in susceptible mice. Expression of viral RNA in infected mice is largely confined to the lactating mammary gland, and expression of viral RNA in infected cells in culture is regulated at the transcriptional level by steroid hormones. Studies of MMTV have been directed toward a complete understanding first, of the role of the MMTV LTR in tissue-specific expression and hormonal regulation and second, of the ways in which these properties contribute to tumor induction.

3.1 Structure of the Long Terminal Repeat

Figure 2 shows the structure of the LTR. It is unique among the retroviral LTRs because of its length, 1332 bp. Much of this length is taken up by protein-coding

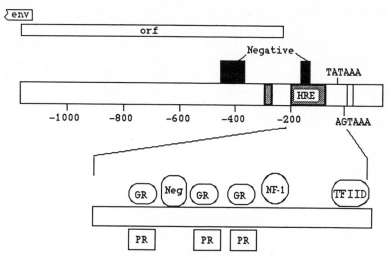

Fig. 2. *Structure of the mouse mammary tumor virus long terminal repeat (MMTV LTR).* U3, R, and U5 are 1197, 15, and 120 base pairs long, respectively. Important features of the MMTV LTR which are discussed in the text are shown: Regions coding for the C-terminus of the *env* gene and for the 960-bp LTR open reading frame (*orf*); two sites implicated in *negative* regulation of LTR promoter activity; target sites for glucocorticoid receptor binding (shown as the *crosshatched region*) within and upstream of the hormone response element (*HRE*); and the location of the TATA element (*TATAAA*) and the poly A addition signal (*AGTAAA*). Shown in greater detail are binding sites for proteins within the 200-bp sequence immediately upstream from the transcription start point. These proteins include the glucocorticoid (*GR*) and progesterone (*PR*) receptors, nuclear factor 1 (*NF-1*), *TFIID*, and a factor (*neg*) which inhibits transcription in vitro

sequences. The 5'-end of the LTR codes, in overlapping reading frames, for both the C-terminus of the *env* gene and for the N-terminus of the 36 K LTR orf protein.

3.2 Early Studies of Hormone Regulation

The observation that expression of MMTV RNA in virus-infected cells could be induced many-fold by the addition of glucocorticoid hormone to the culture medium, and the subsequent demonstration that this regulation was effected at the level of transcription initiation, led to the use of the MMTV LTR as a model substrate for analyzing control of inducible transcription by polymerase II. This work has been described in many reviews (RINGOLD 1985; YAMAMOTO 1985). Early studies using fragments of molecularly cloned MMTV DNA showed that an isolated LTR, fused to non-MMTV sequences, promotes expression of the heterologous DNA in a hormone-dependent fashion (LEE et al. 1981; HUANG et al. 1981). Characterization of the sequences in the LTR responsible for this regulation came both from biochemical studies with partially or wholly purified receptor protein and from expression studies which explored the ability of fragments of the LTR to function as hormone response elements. Straightforward deletion analysis showed that glucocorticoid regulation was conferred by a truncated LTR containing only 200 bp 5′ to the transcription start site (to − 200); shorter fragments (to − 140) were defective (MAJORS and VARMUS 1983a; HYNES et al. 1983). More striking was the observation that fragments of DNA harboring this region of the LTR, when placed adjacent to heterologous promoters, would render them hormone inducible, in a manner which was relatively independent of the position or orientation of the MMTV sequences (CHANDLER et al. 1983; PONTA et al. 1985). These observations led to the view that this small region of the LTR was a glucocorticoid response element (GRE) and that it functioned as a hormone-inducible enhancer (CHANDLER et al. 1983). Parallel biochemical studies showed that this same region of the LTR harbored multiple binding sites for the glucocorticoid receptor protein (PAYVAR et al. 1983; SCHEIDEREIT et al. 1983). DNAse I footprint studies revealed multiple independent binding sites, shown in Fig. 2, within each of which is a core recognition element 5′-TGTTCT-3′. These studies also revealed receptor binding sites which lay outside the genetically defined GRE, both within the LTR and at multiple sites within protein-coding sequences outside the LTR (PAYVAR et al. 1983). The role of these elements in MMTV biology is not understood.

3.3 Activation of the LTR by Other Steroid Hormones

The role of glucocorticoid regulation of MMTV LTR promoter function in the relatively specific expression of MMTV RNA in lactating mammary glands is unclear. Glucocorticoid receptors are ubiquitously distributed, and there is no clear biological rationale for their involvement in MMTV RNA synthesis. The first indication that hormone regulation of the LTR was more complex came from the demonstration that partially purified progesterone receptor protein bound to sequences within the LTR which were similar if not identical to those bound by glucocorticoid receptor (VON DER AHE et al. 1985). Sequences within the chick lysozyme gene promoter region also bound both proteins. Subsequent work showed that the same region of the LTR which conferred glucocorticoid inducibility in gene transfer studies permitted induction not only by progesterone (CATO et al. 1986) but also by androgens (CATO et al. 1987; DARBRE et al. 1986) and mineralocorticoids (CATO and WEINMANN 1988). Regulation simply depnds on target cells harboring the appropriate steroid receptor. This has led to the general designation HRE (for hormone response element) for the region of the LTR between − 60 and − 200. Estrogens have no effect, and the estrogen receptor recognizes a sequence, GGTCANNNTGACC, which, though related, is clearly different from that seen by the glucocorticoid/progesterone receptor, GGTACANNNTGTTCT (KLOCK et al. 1987).

3.4 Fine-Structure Analysis of the HRE and the MMTV Promoter

The biochemical data showing multiple binding sites for steroid receptor proteins within the HRE suggest that regulation might be complex. Fine-structure genetic analysis supports this view. Several groups analyzed the effects on expression of systematically altering the sequence of short regions of the HRE (KUHNEL et al. 1986; BUETTI and KUHNEL 1986; MIKSICEK et al. 1987; CATO et al. 1988; CHALEPAKIS et al. 1988; HAM et al. 1988).

Glucocorticoid Regulation. In two studies using mammary cell lines, mutations which separately interrupt each of the four receptor binding sites (the TGTTCT elements at − 175, − 119, − 98, and − 83) all led to significantly decreased levels of expression (CATO et al. 1988; CHALEPAKIS et al. 1988). In a third study disruption of the -98 and -83 elements had little effect, possibly reflecting the use of fibroblasts in the assay (BUETTI and KUHNEL 1986). None of these disruptions affected the ability of the receptor to form complexes in vitro with other sites on HRE-containing fragments, suggesting that binding of receptor to the multiple sites is not cooperative. Activation probably requires a functional interaction between the receptors bound to the different elements, either with each other or with other components of the transcription initiation complex. Full activity also requires sequences centered around -69 which permit binding of the nuclear factor 1 (NF-1) protein (MIKSICEK 1987; BUETTI and KUHNEL 1986; CATO et al. 1988; CHALEPAKIS et al. 1988; KUO et al. 1988). NF-1, also known as the TGGCA protein and CTF, is a ubiquitous nuclear protein which functions both as a transcription activator protein and as a component of the adenovirus replication origin complex (JONES et al. 1988b). Regulation by androgens is similarly affected (CATO et al. 1988).

Progesterone Regulation. Interruption of each of the consensus receptor elements also decreases progesterone-induced expression (CATO et al. 1988; CHALEPAKIS et al. 1988). However, disruption of sequences in other regions distinguishes the responses of the two harmones. In particular, the NF-1 site has little effect on induction by progesterone (CATO et al. 1988; CHALEPAKIS et al. 1988). A perhaps more interesting observation results from varying the spacing between the promoter proximal receptor binding sites (those at − 83, − 98, and − 119) and the distal site (at − 175). Increasing the separation by more than 60 bp significantly inhibits expression under all hormonal regimes. Insertion of 5 bp increased inducibility by glucocorticoids twofold but decreased progesterone inducibility, consistent with the view that progestins may be the most important regulator of MMTV LTR activity in the infected mouse (CHALEPAKIS et al. 1988).

3.5 Mechanism of Steroid Receptor-Mediated Transcription Activation

The means by which transcriptional activator proteins like those of the steroid receptor family alter rates of transcription initiation is only beginning to be understood. The recent isolation of molecular clones of the genes which code for the receptor proteins has greatly facilitated their biochemical and genetic analysis (reviewed in EVANS 1988). The glucocorticoid receptor can be divided into three domains; an N-terminal domain which is antigenic and contributes to the ability of the protein to activate transcription; a central domain which is sufficient for DNA binding and which alone can inefficiently activate transcription; and a C-terminal domain which harbors the ligand-binding determinants (EVANS 1988). The central DNA-binding domain is highly conserved among the different members of the receptor family, and domain exchange experiments show that the specificity of DNA binding resides within a short region of the domain which is thought to form a zinc finger structural motif (EVANS 1988). The ability to manipulate the structure of the protein should hasten progress towards understanding the biochemistry of activation.

For reasons which are not clearly understood, efforts to demonstrate regulated expression from the MMTV LTR in vitro with isolated protein have not succeeded. The presence of repressor-like factors within these crude cellular extracts may be partly responsible (LANGER and OSTROWSKI 1988). The best picture of the biochemical consequences of hormone activation comes from experiments which analyze the patterns of protein binding to the LTR on nuclear chromatin. An immediate consequence of hormone activation is the formation of a DNAse I hypersensitive region within the GRE, whose presence depends on the continued presence of hormone (ZARET and YAMAMOTO 1984; PETERSON 1985). High resolution analysis of this event, using an ExoIII/S1 mapping procedure, showed that hormone activation leads to disruption of a phased nucleosome structure over the HRE/promoter region (RICHARD-FOY and HAGER 1987), accompanied by the induced binding of protein to the NF-1 site and to the TATA region (CORDINGLEY and HAGER 1987). Proteins found in crude nuclear extracts will bind efficiently to these sequences on naked DNA (CORDINGLEY and HAGER 1988), suggesting that in this case, the receptor may promote access of the NF-1 and TATA proteins to their target sites. Whether the receptor also affects rates of initiation at other steps in the assembly of a transcription initiation complex is not known. A better understanding awaits successful reconstruction of the activation process. One step along this path is the recent demonstration that a DNA fragment from the MMTV HRE/promoter region, formed into a nucleosome with the same phase as that detected in vivo, will form a ternary complex with purified glucocorticoid receptor in vitro (PERLMANN and WRANGE 1988).

3.6 Mechanism of Mammary Tissue-Specific Expression and Oncogenesis

An isolated MMTV LTR promotes expression in cultured cells derived from many tissue types, and many vectors engineered to allow inducible expression of foreign gene products in cells in culture employ an MMTV LTR. Nonetheless, virus replication is generally confined to the mammary and salivary glands of female mice and to the accessory genital glands and salivary glands of male mice (TSUBURA et al. 1986). Lymphoid tissue may be inefficiently infected (LIEGLER and BLAIR 1986). Infection of the mammary glands leads to transformation of mammary tissue through the integration of viral DNA in the neighborhood of several cellular genes, the best characterized of which are *int*-1 and *int*-2 (NUSSE et al. 1984; DICKSON et al. 1984). MMTV activation of *int*-1 or *int*-2 expression generally results from proviral DNA insertion upstream of the activated gene in a transcriptionally divergent direction, or downstream of the gene such that viral and cellular gene transcription is oriented in the same direction (NUSSE et al. 1984; DICKSON et al. 1984). For each of these cases the cellular *int*-1 or *int*-2 promoters could be activated by putative MMTV LTR mammary gland tissue-specific enhancer elements. Direct support for the existence of such elements comes mostly from studies with transgenic mice. Transgenic mice generated by injecting an *env*/LTR fragment fused to either a c-*myc* or v-Ha-*ras* gene show expression primarily in tissue of the salivary and mammary glands with occasional expression in the spleen, thymus, lung, seminal vesicle, and Harderian gland (STEWART et al. 1984; SINN et al. 1987). Those generated by fusing a GR strain MMTV LTR/*pol* fusion fragment to the HSV *tk* showed expression both in the lactating mammary gland and in the testes (ROSS and SOLTER 1985). Surprisingly, mice injected with a nearly full length C3H strain LTR fused to the SV40 early region show a broader range of expression in the epithelial tissue of many organs, including lung, prostate, salivary, mammary glands, and lymphoid cells (CHOI et al. 1987). A single study of the abilities of specific LTR fragments to promote these same patterns of expression suggested that sequences from the 5'-end of the LTR, when separated from the HRE and fused to a basal promoter fragment, were sufficient to generate a normal pattern of non-mammary tissue-specific expression, although their role in mammary tissue-specific expression was not addressed (STEWART et al. 1988).

Support for the presence of a tissue-specific element in the 5'-end of the LTR comes from studies of MMTV-activated *int*-2 expression in the RAC mammary tumor cell line. RAC cells, which have MMTV DNA integrated upstream of the *int*-2 gene, show multiple cellular phenotypes with related patterns of MMTV and *int*-2 regulation (SONNENBERG et al. 1987). Polygonal RAC cells resemble epithelial cells and efficiently express *int*-2 and MMTV in a hormone-independent manner; cuboidal and elongated RAC cells resemble fibroblasts, fail to express *int*-2, and express MMTV in a strictly hormone-dependent fashion (SONNENBERG et al. 1987). Analysis of the chromatin structure of the MMTV LTR in these cells shows that a specific nucleosome at the 5'-end of the LTR (nucleosome F in RICHARD-FOY and HAGER 1987) is displaced in the polygonal RAC cells (G. HAGER, personal communication). Sequences in the region of the displaced nucleosome are logical candidates for a mammary or epithelial cell-specific enhancer element.

Further clues to the role of the LTR in tissue-specific expression come from studies of the association of variant MMTVs with non-mammary tumors. Before discussing those variants we first need to address the problem of the LTR protein-coding ORF.

3.7 The MMTV LTR ORF Protein

Initial evidence for the presence of a potential protein-coding ORF within the extended MMTV LTR came from cell-free translation studies of LTR-specific RNA, which showed that LTR sequences could be translated into a 36K protein (DICKSON et al. 1981). Subsequent DNA sequence analyses of cloned DNA fragments confirmed this observation, showing the presence of an uninterrupted protein coding sequence extending 960 bases in from the 5'-end of the LTR (DONEHOWER et al. 1983; MAJORS and VARMUS 1983b; FASEL et al. 1982). The first 50 bases of this sequence codes, in a different frame, for the C-terminal end of the *env* gene (REDMOND and DICKSON 1982; MAJORS and VARMUS 1983). The role of the putative LTR protein in virus biology remains a mystery. Candidate mRNAs for its expression have been detected in certain mouse strains, but clear evidence for an association of these RNAs with the normal course of MMTV infection is not available (WHEELER et al. 1983; VAN OOYEN et al. 1984; GRAHAM et al. 1984).

Antibodies raised against synthetic peptides have been used to precipitate cell-free translation products of hybrid-selected cellular mRNA; unfortunately, they fail to detect similar proteins in extracts from cells from which the mRNA was isolated (RACEVSKIS and PRAKASH 1984). Curiously, similar antibodies react with several species of protein from partially purified intracytoplasmic A particles, an immature, intracellular form of MMTV (SMITH et al. 1987). A better understanding of the role of the ORF protein will probably come from genetic studies of the virus, made possible by the recent isolation of infectious molecular clones of the virus (SALMONS et al. 1985; SHACKLEFORD and VARMUS 1988; MORRIS et al. 1989).

3.8 MMTVs with Truncated LTRs Have Altered Tissue Specificity

Although the principal site of MMTV-induced tumorigenesis is the mammary gland, the virus has also been associated with thymic lymphomas and renal carcinomas. Molecular characterization of viral DNAs associated with these non-mammary tumors has without exception revealed characteristic sequence rearrangements within the LTR. The rearranged LTRs in the thymic lymphomas typically result from deletions which remove the C-terminal 100–103 aa of the ORF protein and may extend part way through the GRE (to -133 in one case) (KWON and WEISSMAN 1984; MICHALIDES et al. 1985; MICHALIDES and WAGENAAR 1986; LEE et al. 1987; BALL et al. 1988; HSU et al. 1988). Small duplications of sequences flanking the deletion end points are also seen. The LTR associated with renal carcinoma shows a smaller deletion, removing only 33 aa of ORF, with the insertion of 91 bp of a foreign sequence (WELLINGER et al. 1986).

Although most of the thymic lymphomas fail to yield infectious virus, a leukemogenic virus stock, DMBA-LV, was isolated from a chemically induced thymoma (BALL and McCCARTER 1971). Neither that virus nor the one associated with renal carcinomas will induce mammary tumors (BALL et al. 1985; CLAUDE 1967), suggesting that the tissue specificity of the viruses has been altered. Proposals to explain the altered specificity and tumorigenicity of these viruses include: (a) Loss of ORF protein function; (b) generation of novel enhancer elements at the deletion junctions (MICHALIDES et al. 1985; MICHALIDES and WAGENAAR 1986); (c) loss of a negative regulatory element located 5' to the GRE (between -364 and -455) which is deleted in all of the altered LTRs (HSU et al. 1988); (d) alteration of the GRE. The contribution of these different effects to the unique tissue specificities of the variant viruses is not known, but none affects the region of the LTR harboring the putative mammary tissue-specific element described above. These variant viruses should provide useful reagents for exploring the role of the LTR in the biological properties of MMTV.

4 Murine Leukemia Viruses

Relication-competent MuLVs show a broad disease spectrum. Included among them are viruses which are nonpathogenic, those which normally induce T-cell leukemias, and those which induce erythroid leukemias. Early studies used recombinant viruses to show that important determinants of disease specificity mapped to the viral LTRs (CHATIS et al. 1983, 1984; DESGROSEILLERS et al. 1983; DESGROSEILLERS and JOLICOUER 1984). Subsequent efforts have focussed on a better understanding of the role of the LTR in disease induction and on identification of disease-specific elements within the LTR.

4.1 Structure of the Long Terminal Repeat

MuLV LTRs have the basic structure shown in Fig. 3. The LTRs are about 600 bp long; R and U5 are generally 68 and 77 bp in length, respectively, and U3 is of variable length. Most of our attention will be focussed on U3 sequences. Figure 4 presents the U3 sequences of several representative MuLV strains, and that of the closely related FeLV strain. As was the case with the ASLV family, there are regions of conserved sequence, interspersed with relatively nonconserved regions. Most of the conserved regions have been implicated in LTR function and will be discussed below. Easily recognized elements, noted in Fig. 4, include an A/T-rich TATA element between -23 and -30 and a CCAAT element at -78. These elements, which flank repeated CGCTT motifs, contribute to basal promoter activity (GRAVES et al. 1985a, b). Near the 5'-end of the LTR is a short region of conserved sequence which harbors a negative upstream control element (UCR)

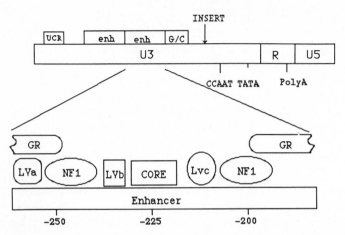

Fig. 3. *Schematic structure of the Moloney murine leukemia virus long terminal repeat (LTR)* U3, R, and U5 are 449, 68, and 77 base pairs long, respectively. Noted are the negative-acting upstream control region (*UCR*), the 75-base pair direct repeats which have enhancer activity (*enh*), a *G/C*-rich region required for maximal enhancer activity, the position of a 190-base pair *insert* found in LTRs of endogenous proviral elements with a polytropic host range, canonical promoter elements, and the signal for polyadenylation (*Poly A*). Also shown in expanded form is the pattern of cellular protein binding sites within the 75-base pair direct repeat enhancer region (SPECK and BALTIMORE 1987)

that, in the appropriate context, inhibits LTR promoter activity (FLANAGAN et al. 1989). Further upstream in the Moloney (Mo) MuLV U3 is a G/C-rich region and a sequence of about 75 bp which is present as a tandem repeat. The repeats have enhancer activity when appended to heterologous promoters (LAIMONS et al. 1984a) and are required along with the G/C-rich region for maximal LTR activity (LAIMONS et al. 1984a; GRAVES et al. 1985a). As will be discussed shortly, the repeats are largely responsible for the disease spectra and patterns of tissue-specific expression exhibited by different MuLV strains. Biochemically, they constitute complex arrays of protein binding sites.

Fig. 4. U3 sequences of representative members of the murine leukemia virus family. Sequences include that of Moloney murine leukemia virus, MOL (SHINNICK et al. 1981); the CAS BR (CHATTOPADHYAY et al. 1989); the endogenous ecotropic Akv virus, AKV (VAN BEVEREN et al. 1982); the NFS xenotropic virus, XENO (KHAN and MARTIN 1983); the MCF 247 virus, MCF (KELLEY et al. 1983); a representative endogenous polytropic proviral element, ENDO (KHAN and MARTIN 1983); and the SM-FeSV virus, FELV (GUILHOT et al. 1987). Noted are the following conserved elements and/or targets for DNA binding proteins: *INTEGRATION*, sequences at the 5'-end of the long terminal repeat (LTR) which promote integration; *NEGATIVE UCR*, sequences which negatively regulate LTR activity (FLANAGAN et al. 1989); *LVb, CORE, LVc, NF1, GRE*, binding sites for proteins detected in crude nuclear extracts of murine cells (SPECK and BALTIMORE 1987); *CCAAT, CGCTT, TATA*, sequence elements responsible for basal promoter activity (GRAVES et al. 1985b). For clarity of presentation sequences present as direct repeats in most of these viruses are shown with only a single copy. These repeats, which significantly increase LTR enhancer activity and which are required for efficient tumorigenicity, generally include the LVb, CORE, LVc, NF1, and GRE elements. For the endogenous ENDO sequence, short direct repeat insertions are shown *below* the primary sequence, and the site of a 190-base pair insertion is marked with an *asterisk*

INTEGRATION   NEGATIVE UCR

```
MOL     AATGAAAGACCCCACCTGTAGGTTTGGCAAGCTAGCTT  AAGTAACGCCATTT    TGCAAGGCATGGAAAAATAC
CASBR   .............ATC. ....A.........   ...   ........ATTT........C...........
AKV     ............TTCATA...C..A..C.....A..GC   ...   ........    ...........G........
XENO    ...............ATA..C..A..A.........GC   ...   ........    ...............A....G...
MCF     ...............ATA..C..A.........GC      ...   ........    ...........A....G...
ENDO    ............AC.G.AAG.XTTAGCGGGXXXXXXXXXXXXXX   ........    ...........A....G...
FELV    .............C..CACCCCAAAACTT...C....ACTGC.ATG.T.......   CA..............T...
```

```
MOL     ATAA CTGAGAATAG      AGAAGTTCAGATCAAGGTCAG     GAACAGATG  GAACAG  CTGA ATAT
CASBR   CG.. ..........      G..........   .......AA   ....   .... .GT.
AKV     CAG.G....TGT.CTCAGAAA.C....A ACA.GG...TA...   A..   GGCTG...AGTA .C.GG.CTA
XENO    CAG.G.....TT.TC      .A.....ACA.AA...T.T.GTTAAA...T.AGG.TG ..T.ATA...GG.C.G
MCF     CAG.G....ATTCTC      .A....CACA.GG...T.T..TTAAA...T.AGGCTG ....AAA...GG.C.G
ENDO    CAG.G...G.TTCTC      .A.....ACA.GG,..T....TTATA..TT.AGGCTG ..T..CA...GG.C.G
                                              ...TTAAA..T..A
FELV    CC..G.ATG TTCCCATGAGATATAAGGAAGTTAG...C              ..  .....
```

LVb   CORE   LVc   NF1   GRE

```
MOL     GGGGCCAAACAGGATATCTG TGGT AAGCAGTTCCTGCCCCGGCTCAGGGCCAAGAACAGATGGTCCCCAGATGC
CASBR   ....................      .........T.G.....C.GA..............AT
AKV     ....................      ....C.....C.AGG ........C...................AAT
MCF     ....................      ...CG....CC.GG ...................A.T....AA
XENO    G...................      ...CG....CC.GG ...................A.T....AA
ENDO    .....G..............      ...G....CG....CC.GG .................T.T.....AA
FELV        G............      C...T..C..CC.GG .................CT.AAG..T.G...CT
```

```
MOL     GGTCCAGCCCTCAGCAGTTTCTAGAGAACCA        TCAGAT GTTTCCAGGGTGCCCCA AGGACCTG AAAT
CASBR   ..C...AT.................G..C...        ...... ....T....C........ .A....... ..G.
AKV     A.CTA.AA.AA..A.......A....C...        GA.AC. ..C. ..A...T....G.T....G.GG.TC
XENO    A.CGG.A..AG..A.......GA.A..GTC        CCACCTCA.....A..TT .....A.T....A. G..A
MCF     A.CGA.A.TAG..A.......G..A.GT.C        CACCTC A......A.T. ......A....G. G..A
ENDO    A.CGG.A..AG..A...ACA.AGA.. C..CGATAGACGTCAG. ...*T.. TT. .....A.T....G.G..G.
FELV    A.CTG.AA.AG...A......A..GCC..TG        C...CA ..C......CTC...AG TT....A. .GT.
```

CCAAT   CGCTT

```
MOL     GACCCTGT GCCTTATTTGAACTAACCAATCAGTTCGCTTCTCGCTTCTGTTCGCGCGCTTC TGCTC
CASBR   ........ ...................C.............G...T......... .....
AKV     A....CAA ....C....A.............C.................A.C.......AT....
XENO    T....CAA ....C...................C.................A.C.......TT....
MCF     A....CAA .........A............................AC.......TA.....
ENDO    AC...AAA .....C............C..C...............ATAC.......TT.....
FELV    C.A...TCC .....C....A.............CCCA...C.............A.........TC...
```

TATA

```
MOL     CCCGAGCTCAATAAAA GAGCCCACAACCCCTCACTCGG .
CASBR   .........T...... ...:.A.................
AKV     G..C.....T...... AG.GTA.G......A........
XENO    ... ...C.T...... AG.GTA.G...T..A....G..
        ... ...
MCF     ... ...C.T...... AG.GTA.A......A........
ENDO    ... ...C.T...... AG.GTACA...T..A........
          T ...C.
FELV         T......C.....ATGC.G.......CG..
```

4.2 Patterns of Protein Binding

Attempts to characterize patterns of protein binding to the LTRs of different MuLV strains are still in their early stages. Mobility shift analysis of proteins bound to the Mo-MuLV LTR reveals a complex set of at least six proteins present in nuclear extracts of murine tissue culture cells, which bind specifically to sequences within the U3 direct repeats (SPECK and BALTIMORE 1987). Included among these proteins, diagrammed in Fig. 3, are NF-1, an enhancer core binding protein (to the sequence GGTGTATG), and a factor which binds to the same sequence as the glucocorticoid receptor (and may be the glucocorticoid receptor). Also detected were three additional factors (termed LVa, b and c, for *leukemia virus* factors) whose relationship to previously characterized factors is not known. As shown in Fig. 4, several of these factors bind to sequences which are conserved in all MuLV LTRs and are probably required for LTR function in all contexts. Notable among these is the LVb factor which covers an EcoRV site (GATATC) found in all MuLV LTRs and whose disruption disrupts enhancer function (MIKSICEK et al. 1986). The functional role of these proteins in MuLV expression is also not yet established, and several of the sites overlap. For example, although the in vitro assays demonstrate binding of a glucocorticoid receptor-like protein, the Mo-MuLV LTR is not responsive to glucocorticoid hormones (OVERHAUSER and FAN 1985). However, the LTRs of the related viruses Moloney murine sarcoma virus (Mo-MSV), Akv, and SL3-3 are responsive to glucocorticoids (DEFRANCO and YAMAMOTO 1986; MIKSICEK et al. 1986; CELANDER and HASELTINE 1987; CELANDER et al. 1988) and also contain multiple binding sites for the glucocorticoid receptor protein (DEFRANCO and YAMAMOTO 1986; CELANDER et al. 1988).

4.3 Role of the LTR in Patterns of Oncogenesis

Strains of MuLV show distinct patterns of disease induction. Included among these are: (a) the nonleukemogenic Akv; (b) T-lymphomagenic viruses derived from Akv, SL3-3, Gross passage A, and recombinant Mink Cell Focūs-Forming Virūses (MCFs); (c) T-lymphomagenic Mo-MuLV; and (d) the erythroleukemogenic Friend MuLV. Tumor induction requires not only that the virus replicate well in appropriate target tissue but also that it act, in its role as an insertional mutagen, to induce levels of expression of cellular oncogenes sufficient to induce transformation. A popular approach to the problem of mapping viral determinants of disease specificity has been to manipulate the LTR sequences, either by mutation or by making appropriate fusions between molecular clones of different viruses and then to assess the biological properties of the novel recombinants. Without exception, these studies implicate LTR sequences as important determinants in patterns of pathogenesis and demonstrate the complex nature of the interactions between viral and host *cis-* and *trans*-acting factors which are responsible for these patterns. Included among these studies are the following.

Leukemogenicity of Mo-MuLV. Mo-MuLV induces thymic T-cell lymphomas with a latency of several months when injected into newborn mice of the appropriate strain. This induction is thought to occur by a two-step mechanism, with the first step characterized by mild splenomegaly and general hematopoietic hyperplasia and the second step, by secondary infection of hyperplastic lymphoid stem cells after their migration to the thymus (DAVIS et al. 1987a). The second infection results in proto-oncogene activation and tumor formation (CUYPERS et al. 1984; GRAHAM et al. 1985; LI et al. 1984; SELTEN et al. 1984; STEFFEN 1984). Mutant Moloney viruses with altered LTRs display different biological properties. Viruses with LTRs deleted of the enhancer region, of the G/C-rich region, or of the region harboring the CCAAT and CGCTT elements replicate poorly (HANECAK et al. 1986; FAN et al. 1986). Insertion of SV40 enhancer sequences between the Moloney enchancer and promoter results in a virus with normal leukemogenic properties, while substitution of the Moloney enhancer element with that of SV40 yields a virus which induces primarily B-cell tumors (HANECAK et al. 1988). While insertion of polyoma enhancer sequences upstream of the Moloney enhancer yields a virus with nearly normal leukemogenic properties, the properties of viruses generated from insertion of polyoma sequences downstream of the Moloney enchancer vary greatly with small differences in the polyoma sequence. Insertion of wild-type polyoma enhancer sequences at that position produces a virus that behaves much like normal Mo-MuLV (FAN et al. 1988); insertion of mutant polyoma enhancers which function better in embryonic carcinoma (EC) cells are either nonleukemogenic because they fail to induce hematopoietic hyperplasia (DAVIS et al. 1987a) or leukemogenic but activate a different spectrum of proto-oncogenes (FAN et al. 1988).

Moloney MuLV vs. Friend MuLV. The Friend strain of MuLV fails to induce thymic lymphomas but induces erythroleukemias over a similar time course. Elements within the LTRs of the two viruses are the principal determinants of this disease specificity (CHATIS et al. 1983, 1984). Initial studies mapped the determinants to the region of the LTR harboring the direct repeat enhancer elements and the G/C-rich element (LI et al. 1987; ISHIMOTO et al. 1987; THIESEN et al. 1988). Fine-structure analysis shows that multiple elements within this region cooperate in some fashion to account for the disease specificities of the two viruses. Although the sequences of the two enhancer regions are similar, recombinants with hybrid enhancers harboring elements from both of the viruses show intermediate patterns of specificity (THIESEN et al. 1988; GOLEMIS et al. 1989). Comparative protein binding studies suggest complex differences in patterns of protein binding (cited in GOLEMIS et al. 1989).

Leukemogenicity of Gross A MuLV. The enhancer element within the LTR of Gross A virus significantly increases the oncogenic potential of a weakly oncogenic BALB/c MuLV (DESGROSEILLERS and JOLICOUER 1984). The principal difference between the Gross A enhancer region and its nonleukemogenic Akv parent is the insertion of a 36-bp sequence within the enhancer region and the transition of a C to a T within the enhancer core sequence element TGTGGTCAAG (see Fig. 4) (VILLEMUR et al. 1983).

SL3-3 vs Akv. Like the Gross A virus, SL3-3 is a T-lymphomagenic virus derived from the endogenous ecotropic Akv virus of the AKR mouse strain. SL3-3 virus efficiently induces T lymphomas after introduction into several strains of mice while the Akv virus is nonleukemogenic. Recombinants between the two with only an SL3-3 LTR are leukemogenic (LENZ et al. 1984) and replicate well in thymocytes (ROSEN et al. 1985a). Studies to examine the abilities of the Akv and SL3-3 LTRs to promote expression of CAT activity in different cell types showed that the SL3-3 LTR is preferentially active after introduction into T-cell-derived lines; in fibroblast cell lines, the Akv LTR is more active (CELANDER and HASELTINE 1984; SHORT et al. 1987). The sequences of the two LTRs are essentially identical in the region outside the U3 enhancer. Within the enhancer, SL3-3 virus has two and one-half copies of a 72-bp sequence while the Akv virus has two copies of a related 99-bp sequence. Further investigations showed that a significant fraction of the T-cell specificity of the SL3-3 enhancer region is determined by a sequence element GTGGTTAA, present twice within the SL3-3 LTR (BORAL et al. 1989; HALLBERG and GRUNDSTROM 1988). Protein binding studies detect a factor(s) termed S-CBF (BORAL et al. 1989) or SEF-1 (THORNELL et al. 1988) which recognizes this sequence. The related sequence TGTGGTCAA, present twice within the Akv LTR, neither promotes T-cell-specific expression nor binds the factor(s).

MCFs Isolated from AKR Thymomas. Although the Akv virus isolated from AKR mice is itself nonleukemogenic, AKR mice develop thymic tumors after a long latency. The proximal cause of these tumors is probably a virus (called MCF virus) derived from two recombination events. The first substitutes the 5' *env* sequences of the Akv virus with those of a family of endogenous elements with extended host range (See HUNTER and SWANSTROM, this volume). The LTRs of these endogenous elements contain characteristic 190-bp insertions (KHAN and MARTIN 1983) (see Figs. 3 and 4), and they still function as promoters (LEVY et al. 1987). Their biological properties are not well understood. A second recombination substitutes the LTR and part of p15E of the Akv virus by sequences from an endogenous virus of xenotropic host range (KHAN and MARTIN 1983; QUINT et al. 1984). Figure 4 compares the U3 sequences of an MCF with those of Akv and Mo-MuLV. Recovered leukemogenic MCFs have tandem copies of sequences present once in the endogenous xenotropic LTR (KHAN and MARTIN 1983). Although LTRs harboring single copies of these sequences replicate efficiently and are thymotropic, only those with the repeats are oncogenic (HOLLAND et al. 1989).

4.4 Expression in Cells of Embryonic Origin

Retroviruses are effective agents for the efficient introduction of new genetic material into cells. Successful implementation of this strategy requires not only that the virus efficiently integrate into the host DNA but also that the newly introduced genetic material be expressed. The Mo-MuLV LTR is active in most cell types, but attempts to infect and obtain viral protein expression in early embryonic cells were unsuccessful. Molecular analysis of this phenomenon showed that the virus could enter embryonic cells, be reverse transcribed and integrated, but proviral transcription was blocked (JAHNER et al. 1982). The nonexpressing proviral DNA was eventually methylated, becoming permanently silent. A similar block to expression results after infection of embryonal carcinoma (EC) cell lines, which provide in vitro systems for studying expression in embryonal stem cells (STEWART et al 1982). In a similar way, isolated MuLV LTRs fail to function as effective promoters in EC cells in short-term expression assays (LINNEY et al. 1984). The reason for this decreased activity is not fully understood. Experimental data support both the presence of a repressor activity (GORMAN et al. 1985; FLAMANT et al. 1987) and the absence of an activator activity (LOH et al. 1987) in EC cells. The profound inability of the LTR to promote transcription in these cells is supported by analysis of active proviruses detected in EC cells, which show that their ability to express a selectable marker is strictly integration site dependent (BARKLIS et al. 1986; TAKETA and TANAKA 1987). Proviral DNA isolated from these cells is active only when linked to flanking cellular sequences, which presumably harbor EC cell-specific enhancer elements (BARKLIS et al. 1986; TAKETA and TANAKA 1987). These elements either activate the normal MuLV promoter or cause marker gene expression by read-through transcription from a cellular promoter.

The same experiment implicates a second region near the tRNA primer binding site in the block to provirus expression in EC cells. An active provirus was found to have undergone a single base alteration within the tRNA primer binding site, which significantly increased its activity after subsequent introduction into the embryonal cells (BARKLIS et al. 1986). Deletion of the wild-type sequences increases expression in EC cells, and competition experiments support their role as a target for a *trans*-acting EC-specific inhibitor factor (LOH et al. 1987, 1988).

Additional support for the presence of two inhibitory elements comes from the properties of a variant Mo-MuSV, myeloproliferative sarcoma virus (MPSV). MPSV is efficiently expressed in the EC cell line, F9 (FRANZ et al. 1986). Analysis of the ability of MPSV/MoMuLV hybrids to function in these cells uncovered determinants responsible for this property both within U3 and in the region of the primer binding site (WEIHER et al. 1987).

5 Human T-Cell Leukemia Viruses

The human T-cell leukemia viruses HTLV-I and HTLV-II, and bovine leukemia virus, BLV, together make up a retrovirus subfamily, each member of which shares with the others unique biological and biochemical properties. Both

HTLV-I and BLV are inefficient leukemogenic agents. Tumor cells are generally clonal and transcriptionally silent for the expression of randomly integrated viral sequences. Culture of these tumor cells frequently results in reactivation of viral gene expression. Molecular genetic analysis has recently provided new insights into the biochemical basis for these properties. These studies were the first to demonstrate a clear role for virally coded genes in the regulation of viral gene expression. This property, coupled with an inability to attribute their weak leukemogenicity to molecular mechanisms associated with other oncogenic retroviruses, make their study a potential source of new insight into the biology of virus-host interactions. Because of the clear demonstration that these novel viral regulatory proteins work through sequences in the LTR, our discussion will focus on these interactions.

5.1 General Structure of the Long Terminal Repeat

Several features of the HTLV-I and -II LTRs distinguish them from those of other retroviruses. (a) An extended R sequence of about 230 bp, generated in part by a polyA addition signal, AATAAA, which lies more than 250 bp upstream from the site of cleavage and polyA addition. (b) A 5' splice donor site which lies within the R sequence. (c) Threefold repeated 21-bp elements within U3 which mediate *trans*-activation by the tax protein. Throughout the LTRs of the two viruses one finds regions of limited sequence homology; in general these sequences are associated with the elements described above.

Early experiments showed that the LTRs of HTLV-I and -II functioned much more efficiently in virus-infected than in uninfected cells (SODROSKI et al. 1984). This phenomenon was termed *trans*-activation. The HTLV-II LTR was essentially inactive in uninfected cells while the HTLV-I LTR was *trans*-activated up to 100-fold by virus infection (SODROSKI et al. 1984). A unique feature of each of these viruses is the presence of a protein-coding region which starts just 3' of the *env* gene and extends into the LTR (SEIKI et al. 1983; SHIMOTOHNO et al. 1984; HASELTINE et al. 1984). Expression of sequences within this region is sufficient for LTR *trans*-activation (SODROSKI et al. 1985). Further analysis (reviewed in YOSHIDA and SEIKI 1987) showed that this region harbors multiple, overlapping reading frames, which for HTLV-I code for a protein of 40K in one reading frame, and for proteins of 27K and 21K in a second reading frame (KIYOKAWA et al. 1985a, b). Similar sequences are found in the equivalent region of the HTLV-II and BLV genomes (SHIMOTOHNO et al. 1984; HASELTINE et al. 1984; RICE et al. 1984; SAGATA et al. 1985). Each of these proteins is expressed from a subgenomic, doubly spliced RNA (SEIKI et al. 1985). The 40K protein is the product of the *tax* gene (previously called *x*, *x-lor*, or *tat*-1) and is responsible for *trans*-activation (SEIKI et al. 1986). The 27K protein, the product of the *rex* gene, acts posttranscriptionally to augment expression of unspliced genomic RNA and singly spliced *env* mRNA (see below). The 21K protein, though expressed in infected cells from the same reading frame as *rex*, has not yet been assigned a function. Both *tax* and *rex* are required for HTLV-II virus replication (CHEN et al. 1985); a similar demonstration has not been possible with HTLV-I. Progress toward understanding the mechanism of *tax* activation has come from defining *tax*-responsive sequence elements within *tax*-regulated promoters.

5.2 Regulation of HTLV-I Expression by *tax*

Dissection of the HTLV-I promoter region and parallel protein binding studies reveal a complex structure, outlined in Fig. 5. A single 21-bp repeat element is relatively unresponsive to *tax* activation; however, it can be made strongly reponsive by oligomerization or weakly responsive by being placed adjacent to the 60-bp fragment (between − 160 and − 117) which normally separates the upstream two repeats from the promoter proximal repeat (BRADY et al. 1987; SHIMOTOHNO et al. 1986; PASKALIS et al. 1986; ROSEN et al. 1985c, 1987). Crude cellular extracts contain multiple proteins which footprint over specific sequences within the HTLV-I and -II LTRs (ALTMAN et al. 1988; NYBORG et al. 1988). Included among these are the following: (a) a factor which covers the sequence AAAAGGTCAG located at about -250 in both LTRs, a region which contributes to basal promoter activity (ROSEN et al. 1985c); (b) a factor(s) which covers each of the 21-bp repeat elements in HTLV-I, and the most upstream of the HTLV-II repeats; (c) a factor which partly covers a CCACC repeat element centered around − 140, within the region which stimulates *tax* responsiveness of a single repeat; (d) a factor which covers the polyadenylation signal AATAAA at − 42. Significantly, similar though not identical patterns of protein binding are seen with extracts from different cell types, including those which express *tax* (ALTMAN et al. 1988; NYBORG et al. 1988). Further analysis has focussed on a better definition of proteins which recognize the *tax*-responsive elements (TREs).

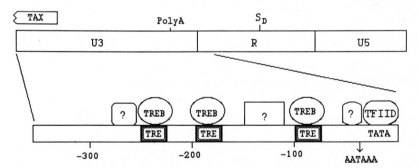

Fig. 5. Schematic structure of the HTLV-I long terminal repeat. U3, R, and U5 are 355, 228, and 176 base pairs long respectively. Noted are the end of the *tax* gene translational reading frame, the polyadenylation signal (*Poly A*) located more than 250 bp upstream from the site of cleavage and polyadenylation, and a splice donor site (S_D) for the processing of subgenomic messenger RNAs. The U3 region is shown in expanded form with the locations of three 21-bp repeat *tax* response elements (*TRE*) and sites of cellular protein binding described in the text

The core of the 21-bp repeat is the sequence TGACGTCT, and mutations within this octamer sequence abolish *tax* responsiveness (JEANG et al. 1988a; TAN et al. 1989). That sequence has been used to isolate and/or characterize cellular proteins which recognize it. UV crosslinking of proteins in crude extracts bound to a labeled oligonucleotide identified a 180K protein whose binding correlated with *tax trans*-activating function and with activation of LTR function in vitro (JEANG et al. 1988a).

A separate biochemical fractionation of HeLa cell nuclear extracts and oligonucleotide affinity chromatography revealed three proteins, termed TREB-1, 2, 3 (for *tax* response element binding protein), which specifically recognize the repeat sequence (TAN et al. 1989). The repeat core sequence, TGACG, is also present in binding sites for the cellular proteins ATF (activating transcription factor) and CREB (the cyclic AMP response element binding factor) (JONES et al. 1988b). Characterization of TREB-1 revealed a 43K protein, which also bound to ATF and CREB recognition sites and which is probably related to ATF and/or CREB (TAN et al. 1989). The nature of the TREB-2 and TREB-3 proteins and their relationship to the 180K protein of JEANG et al. is not known.

5.3 *tax* Activation of Other Promoters

Activation of resting T cells by either antigen or mitogen stimulation results in increased expression of lymphokines and lymphokine receptors and also activates expression from the HIV-1 LTR (see below). Leukemic cells from patients with ATL and human lymphocytes transformed by HTLV-I in vitro also express elevated levels of specific cellular genes known to be involved in T-cell proliferation. Included among these are the gene for subunit α of the IL-2 receptor gene (IL-2Rα) and the genes for IL-2 (in some HTLV-I-transformed cells) and granulocyte/macrophage colony-stimulating factor (GM-CSF) (YOSHIDA and SEIKI 1987). Expression of the Tax protein alone is sufficient to account for this phenomenon as its constitutive presence in a T-cell line leads to elevated expression of these genes (GREENE et al. 1986; WANO et al. 1988). IL-2Rα and GM-CSF are inducible by *tax* alone; IL-2 expression in minimally affected by *tax* but is significantly induced by a combination of *tax* and an additional mitogenic stimulus (WANO et al. 1988). Short-term transfection assays have been used to document the presence of TREs not only within the promoter regions of these inducible genes (SIEKEVITZ et al. 1987a, b; MARUYAMA et al. 1987; CROSS et al. 1987; MIYATAKE et al. 1988a, b; LOWENTHAL et al. 1988; RUBEN et al. 1988; LEUNG and NABEL 1988), but also within the enhancer of the DNA virus, SV40 (MIYATAKE et al. 1988a). A sequence comparison of the *tax*-responsive regions of these promoters with those found within the HTLV-I LTR revealed no common element and motivated efforts to characterize more completely the response elements. The results of these efforts are revealing. The response elements within the HIV LTR, the SV40 enhancer, and the IL-2Rα promoter are binding sites for NF-κB (SIEKEVITZ et al. 1987a, b; MIYATAKE et al. 1988b; LEUNG and NABEL 1988;

RUBEN et al. 1988), a protein first described for its ability to bind to the Igκ light chain enhancer and subsequently implicated in the regulation of several cellular genes (SEN and BALTIMORE 1986; LENARDO et al. 1988). The GM-CSF response is mediated by two closely spaced elements which function independently, and neither of which resembles previously characterized elements (MIYATAKE et al. 1988a). The ability of these elements of confer *tax* responsiveness is mirrored by their ability to permit their associated promoters to respond to T-cell activation signals (MIYATAKE et al. 1988a,b; BOHNLEIN et al. 1988). The close correlation between ability to respond to *tax* and to T-cell activation signals suggests that Tax proteins might function by intervening in the T-cell activation pathway. The relatively strict nuclear localization of Tax proteins (SLAMON et al. 1985; KIYOKAWA et al. 1985a) constrains the point in the pathway at which activation might occur.

5.4 Regulation by *rex*

The Rex protein affects in a qualitative way the pattern of virus-specific mRNA expression. Its presence increases synthesis of viral Gag, Pol, and Env proteins by permitting cytoplasmic accumulation of unspliced and singly spliced viral mRNAs (INOUE et al. 1987; HIDAKA et al. 1988). The mechanism by which this is effected is not yet clear though it appears to involve more than simple inhibition of splicing. The requirements for *rex* action have been mapped within the HTLV-1 genome (SEIKI et al. 1988) and are twofold: a 5' splice donor site which can come either from a 5' HTLV-I LTR or from a heterologous genomic sequence; and an apparently specific sequence within the 3' LTR which lies between 302 and 560 bp from the left end of the LTR, and which must be present on the RNA transcript. If a 3' splice acceptor site is present, *rex* simultaneously suppresses accumulation of spliced RNA in the cytoplasm and stimulates accumulation of unspliced RNA. Accumulation of the latter species appears to be greater than can be accounted for by simple inhibition of splicing. Consistent with this fact is the observation that in the absence of a 3' acceptor site, *rex* still promotes accumulation of full-length RNA in the cytoplasm. In its absence the unspliced nuclear genomic RNA is simply degraded in the nucleus. This result suggests that *rex* provides an efficient pathway for incompletely processed RNAs to exit the nucleus. Although a similar picture has been drawn for BLV (DERSE 1988), the story for HTLV-II is slightly different. There, a signal sufficient for rex_{II} response maps to the 5' LTR (OHTA et al. 1988; ROSENBLATT et al. 1988). Moderate levels of rex_{II} stimulate tax_{II}-activated expression from an LTR fused to a heterologous marked gene, while high levels inhibit expression (ROSENBLATT et al. 1988). The response element maps to a region just 3' to the 5' splice donor site (OHTA et al. 1988). A similar mechanism for the Rev protein of HIV-1 has been proposed and supported by recent experimental data (MALIM et al. 1989). However, the response elements for *rev* fall outside the LTR and will not be discussed further.

6 Human Immunodeficiency Viruses

HIV-1 has been implicated as the causative agent in the acquired immune deficiency disease (AIDS). Viral infection is largely confined to cells which express its receptor, the CD4 (T4) antigen. Included among this population are T helper cells and macrophages. Despite early speculation that the tissue tropism could reflect an inability of the viral LTR to function in non-CD4$^+$ cells, subsequent experiments have shown that it results from a barrier to entry and that the LTR functions in many cell types. The LTR U3, R, and U5 elements are 456, 97, and 82 bp long, respectively. Several properties of the virus and of the isolated LTR point to the LTR as an important target for regulation. These properties include: (a) The ability of a viral gene product, the Tat protein, to *trans*-activate expression of heterologous genes linked to an isolated LTR; (b) the ability of T-cell mitogens to stimulate production of virus from latently infected resting T cells; and (c) the ability of many DNA viruses to stimulate production of HIV-1 particles from co-infected cells. The discussion of the HIV LTR will focus on these three issues and attempt to describe underlying molecular mechanisms.

6.1 Dissection of the Long Terminal Repeat

The HIV-1 LTR was initially subdivided into several functional regions, based upon the ability of various of its fragments to promote synthesis of marker gene sequences or to enhance expression from heterologous promoters in gene transfer experiments. The removal of sequences upstream of − 167 resulted in increased LTR-directed expression, suggesting the presence of a negative regulatory element (NRE) in this region (ROSEN et al. 1985b). The nature of this element has not been explored, nor is its role in the normal process of viral replication understood. An enhancer element, localized to between − 17 and − 137, functioned in cells of varied origin (HeLa, B-cell, cat epithelial) and could be substituted for by heterologous enhancers (from RSV or HTLV-1) (ROSEN et al. 1985b). Finally, sequences which conferred response to the *tat trans*-activator protein were located between − 17 and + 80 and were termed TAR for *trans*-acting response element (ROSEN et al. 1985b). This finding is unusual in that most transcription activator elements are found upstream of TATA elements and suggests that *tat* regulation might be the consequence of a novel control mechanism.

More recent efforts have been directed both towards a more precise localization of sequence elements within these extended regions which contribute to their regulatory function, and toward a more complete description of the cellular or viral proteins which interact with these elements. Studies already completed suggest that the structure of the LTR is complex and harbors binding sites for many proteins. The results of several of these studies are summarized in the diagram shown in Fig. 6. Upstream from the transcription start site are found a TATA element (between − 22 and − 28), three G/C-rich elements (between

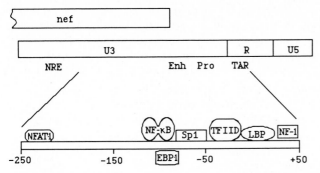

Fig. 6. Schematic structure of the HIV-I long terminal repeat. U3, R, and U5 are 455, 97, and 85 base pairs long, respectively. Noted are the end of the *nef* gene translational reading frame and locations of the negative regulatory element (*NRE*), the 10-base pair repeat enhancer sequences (*Enh*), the promoter (*Pro*), and the tat1 response element (*TAR*). Shown in expanded form are positions of binding sites for cellular proteins discussed in the text

−44 and −75), and two copies of a sequence GGGGACTTTCC which functions as an enhancer element. Purified Sp1 protein binds to the G/C-rich elements and stimulated transcription 10-fold in vitro (JONES et al. 1986). The role of the other elements in HIV expression is discussed below.

6.2 Core Enhancer Element and T-Cell Activation

The 10 base-pair repeat element resembles the core enhancer element of SV40 and mediates the response of the LTR to T-cell activation signals including phytohemagglutinin, the phorbol ester Phorbol myristic acid (PMA), and the *trans*-activator protein (Tax) of HTLV-I (TONG-STARKSEN et al. 1987; NABEL and BALTIMORE 1987; SIEKEVITZ et al. 1987b; KAUFMAN et al. 1987). The element functions in vitro as transcription from the HIV LTR in HeLa cell extracts is six-fold more active if the cells are pretreated with phorbol esters (DINTER et al. 1987). Associated with this activation is the induced binding of cellular proteins (NABEL and BALTIMORE 1987; WU et al. 1988a, b; FRANZA et al. 1987). One of these proteins is NF-κB, a constitutive B-cell transcription factor whose activity and DNA binding is induced in T cells by activation and proliferation signals, and in non-T cells by phorbol esters (SEN and BALTIMORE 1986). This regulated activity probably results from the induced dissociation of an inhibitor protein, IκB (BAEUERLE and BALTIMORE 1988). When bound to the inhibitor, NF-κB is cytoplasmic and inactive. NF-κB purified from a human B-cell tumor line is a protein of 53K which stimulates transcription in vitro from the HIV LTR (KAWAKAMI et al. 1988). A similar activity purified from bovine spleen cells yields a protein of 44K (LENARDO et al. 1988). Binding of this protein to the κB element is greatly stimulated by nucleoside triphosphates. A second factor, HIVEN86A, an 86K protein identified using a microscale DNA affinity purification assay, shows inducible binding both to the HIV 10 bp repeat and to a similar sequence in the promoter region of the IL-2 receptor α gene (BOHNLEIN et al. 1988). The HIV LTR and the IL-2Rα promoter are coordinately regulated by the same T-cell activation signals (LOWENTHAL et al. 1988; MARUYAMA et al. 1987; CROSS et al. 1987; SIEKEVITZ et al. 1987a, b). The relationship between these different factors is not yet established. Further complicating this story is the presence of proteins in nonstimulated cells which recognize the same sequence element (FRANZA et al. 1987; GARCIA et al. 1987; WU et al. 1988, BALDWIN and SHARP 1988; YANO et al. 1987) and the presence further upstream of a binding site for an unrelated protein, NFAT-1, whose binding to the LTR is induced by T-cell activation (SHAW et al. 1988).

6.3 Activation of HIV Expression by Other Agents

The potential role of opportunistic infection by non-HIV pathogens on the activation of latent HIV proviruses has led several investigators to measure the ability of DNA viruses to *trans*-activate the HIV LTR. Viruses implicated in this phenomenon include HTLV-I (SIEKEVITZ et al. 1987b), herpes simplex virus type 1 (HSV-1) (MOSCA et al. 1987; RANDO et al. 1987; GENDELMAN et al. 1986; OSTROVE et al. 1987), human cytomegalovirus (HCMV) (DAVIS et al. 1987b; MOSCA et al. 1987), adenovirus (RICE and MATHEWS 1988), hepatitis B virus (HBV) (SETO et al. 1988; SIDDIQUI et al. 1989), and various papovaviruses (GENDELMAN et al. 1986). Each of these viruses codes for proteins which had previously been shown to activate transcription expression from a wide variety of viral and nonviral promoters. Attempts have been made to identify responsive elements within the HIV LTR for several of these viral proteins. The results of these efforts suggest the presence of multiple activation pathways. The HTLV-I Tax$_1$ protein appears to work through the enhancer/NF-κB sites. The HBV X protein (SIDDIQUI et al. 1989) and the HSV-1 ICPO protein (MOSCA et al. 1987) may work in part through the NF-κB sites, although other elements may also be involved (SETO et al. 1988; NABEL et al. 1988). The adenovirus E1A protein requires no more than a TATA element to *trans*-activate the LTR (NABEL et al. 1988).

Additional regulators of HIV expression include two cytokines, tumor necrosis factor α (TNFα), and IL-1, which activate both the HIV LTR and the promoter of the IL2-Rα gene (LOWENTHAL et al. 1989; OSBORN et al. 1989; OKAMOTO et al. 1989). In all cases activation requires an NF-κB recognition site, and extracts prepared from activated cells have increased amounts of binding factors similar in size to the NF-κB and HIVEN86A proteins described above (LOWENTHAL et al. 1989). However, the mechanisms by which TNFα and phorbol esters alter NF-κB (and/or HIVEN86A) function appear to be different as TNFα will work in cells which are unresponsive to the phorbol ester PMA (OSBORN et al. 1989). The NF-κB site has also been implicated in promoting HIV expression in mature cells of the monocyte lineage (GRIFFIN et al. 1989).

6.4 Negative Regulation by the Nef Protein

Nef (negative factor, previously known as 3′ orf and orfB) is a protein of 25–27K, coded for by sequences which extend from the 3′-end of env to partway through the LTR. Expression of active Nef inhibits virus replication; that is, viral clones with deletions or mutations in nef replicate to higher titers than a wild-type virus, at least in tissue culture (LUCIW et al. 1987; TERWILLIGER et al. 1986). Further studies show that Nef inhibits LTR promoter activity (AHMAD and VENKATESAN 1988; NIEDERMAN et al. 1989) with a target sequence located between − 156 and -338, in the region of the LTR to which the NRE has been mapped (AHMAD and VENKATESAN 1988). The Nef protein is myristoylated at its N-terminus and binds and hydrolyzes GTP in vitro, with sequence similarities to both ras and src (GUY et al. 1987). These properties suggest that Nef is normally located at the inside surface of the plasma membrane, leading to speculation that it functions as a signal transducer analogue which inhibits transcription from the HIV LTR by an indirect mechanism.

6.5 tat Activation, the TAR Element, and Associated Downstream Sequences

The viral tat gene codes for a small, nuclear protein whose activity is required for virus replication (DAYTON et al. 1986; FISHER et al. 1986). The presence of the Tat protein in cells harboring an HIV-1 LTR fused to a linked marker gene leads to significantly increased expression of the marker gene protein. The precise mechanism by which Tat activates expression of viral proteins is not yet known, though activation requires de novo RNA synthesis (GENTZ et al. 1989) and occurs in the absence of new protein synthesis (JEANG et al. 1988b). Different studies have reported that Tat acts strictly at the transcriptional level (PETERLIN et al. 1986; MUESING et al. 1987; RICE and MATHEWS 1988; ARYA and GALLO 1988; JAKOBOVITS et al. 1988), at the transcriptional and post-transcriptional levels (CULLEN 1986; WRIGHT et al. 1986), and predominantly at the post-transcriptional level (ROSEN et al. 1986; FEINBERG et al. 1986). These differences may reflect the complex nature of tat regulation, and their ultimate resolution will require a better understanding of the activation mechanism. The protein itself is short, 86 aa long, and rich in cysteines and basic residues (MUESING et al. 1987; PETERLIN et al. 1986; SEDAIE et al. 1988). Several early observations suggested a novel mechanism for Tat activity. The target of tat activation, the TAR element, was mapped in early deletion studies to sequences downstream of the TATA element, between − 17 and + 44 (ROSEN et al. 1985b; MUESING et al. 1987; HAUBER and CULLEN 1988). The ability of this element to function was both position and orientation dependent (MUESING et al. 1987; PETERLIN et al. 1986), clearly distinguishing it from previously characterized enhancer and promoter elements. A further distinction was the inability of the element to function efficiently when placed at an equivalent position downstream from a heterologous promoter (PETERLIN et al. 1986). Sequences within the transcribed part of this region have the ability to form a stem-loop secondary structure which would be present on all HIV-1 mRNAs (OKAMOTO and WONG-STAAL 1986; MUESING et al. 1987; LE et al. 1988). High resolution nucleotide substitution experiments have recently localized the *tat* response element to the stem-loop structure located between + 19 and + 42 (FENG and HOLLAND 1988; JAKOBOVITS et al. 1988; SELBY et al. 1989; GARCIA et al. 1989). Substitution of any base but the A within the loop sequence CUGGGA significantly decreases *tat* activation (FENG and HOLLAND 1988). Disruption of the adjacent stem structure also decreases *tat* responsiveness; compensating mutations, which restore the ability to form a base-paired stem, also restore responsiveness (FENG and HOLLAND 1988; SELBY et al. 1989; GARCIA et al. 1989). Surprisingly, a mutation in the TATA element prevents *tat* activation (JAKOBOVITS et al. 1988; GARCIA et al. 1989).

Further insight into the significance of these structures comes from a comparative analysis of the related but genetically distinct virus HIV-2. Like HIV-1, HIV-2 expresses a Tat-like protein (ARYA et al. 1987). Tat-1 (from HIV-1) activates both the HIV-1 and HIV-2 LTRs, but Tat-2 (from HIV-2) activates only the HIV-2 LTR (EMERMAN et al. 1987; GUYADER et al. 1987; ARYA 1988). Like HIV-1, the leader sequence of HIV-2 has the capacity to form an extensive secondary structure including three stem loops, located between + 18 and + 52, + 55 and + 84, and + 102 and + 123, each of which has the sequence CUGGG in the loop sequence (ARYA and GALLO 1988; SELBY et al. 1989). Deletion of the most downstream structure has no effect on activation by either Tat protein, but a deletion which extends into the stem of the second structure decreases Tat-2 activation but has no effect on Tat-1 (EMERMAN et al. 1987; ARYA and GALLO 1989). Deletions extending into the promoter proximal structure prevent activation by both Tat proteins. Two recent observations suggest possible points at which *tat* might act.

6.6 Early Termination Products from HIV-1 and HIV-2 LTRs

KAO et al. (1987) showed that in the absence of *tat*, the HIV-LTR promoted synthesis in vivo of transcripts which initiated at the normal site within the LTR but which terminated at + 60. Addition of *tat* to the cells stimulated transcription of sequences downstream from the apparent termination by allowing RNA synthesis to proceed beyond this point. Similar transcripts have recently been detected as products of transcription in vitro from the HIV-1 and HIV-2 LTRs (TOOHEY and JONES 1989). The HIV-1 transcripts were the same length as those seen in vivo; the HIV-2 transcripts were longer, terminating at between + 125 and + 130. In both cases the transcripts terminate at the 3'-end of a stem-loop structure. Whether extension of these products will result from the addition of *tat* to the extract has not yet been determined. Although the localization of the TAR sequence to the stem-loop structure is consistent with an RNA target for *tat* activity, binding sites for several cellular DNA binding proteins are found within the same region (JONES et al. 1988a; GARCIA et al. 1989). The role of these proteins in HIV LTR promoter activity and their potential involvement in regulation by *tat* are currently under investigation (JONES et al. 1988a; GARCIA et al. 1989).

6.7 HIV-1 Leader Sequence Inhibits Translation

It had been noted previously that hybrid mRNAs in which HIV-1 leader sequences were fused to heterologous protein coding sequences were translated inefficiently. PARKIN et al. (1988) recently showed that insertion of the first 11 nucleotides from the 5'-end of the HIV-1 mRNAs significantly inhibits translation of a downstream sequence. Mutations which disrupt predicted secondary structure within the 5' stem-loop structure relieved the inhibition and increased accessibility of the 5' cap structure of the mRNA to translation initiation factors. Compensatory mutations which restored the secondary structure also restored the translation inhibition. Although Tat-1 is probably a nuclear protein (HAUBER et al. 1986), and there was relief of inhibition caused by the addition of *tat* to the experimental systems used, it nonetheless remains possible that one effect of *tat* is to generate mRNAs with a structure that promotes translation.

7 Conclusion

I have attempted in this chapter to illustrate the critical role played by LTR sequences in the molecular biology and pathobiology of retroviruses. For each virus considered, the LTR provides important targets for regulation by cellular or viral proteins. A clear lesson from these studies is that a detailed picture of the molecular mechanisms responsible for phenomena as complex as the oncogenic specificity of Mo-MuLV or the destructiveness of HIV toward the cellular immune system will not come easily. The activity of an LTR in a particular context generally reflects a large number of diverse host-viral interactions. Fortunately, the tools needed to attack these difficult problems from both genetic and biochemical directions are readily available, and progress toward eventual understanding seems inevitable. For the human retroviruses an understanding of these molecular details may lead to improved methods for limiting viral replication and controlling progression of the disease. For both the human and the other viruses, future work on LTR function should produce new insights into fundamental problems in regulation of gene expression.

References

Ahmad N, Venkatesan S (1988) Nef protein of HIV-1 is a transcriptional repressor of HIV-1 LTR. Science 241: 1481–1485

Akroyd J, Fincham VJ, Green AR, Levantis P, Searle S, Wyke JA (1987) Transcription of Rous sarcoma proviruses in rat cells is determined by chromosomal position effects that fluctuate and can operate over long distances. Oncogene 1: 347–354

Altman R, Harrich D, Garcia JA, Gaynor RB (1988) Human T-cell leukemia virus types I and II exhibit different DNase I protection patterns. J Virol 62: 1339–1346

Arrigo S, Yun M, Beemon K (1987) cis-acting regulatory elements within gag genes of avian retroviruses. Mol Cell Biol 7: 388–397

Arya SK (1988) Human and simian immunodeficiency retroviruses: activation and differential transactivation of gene expression. AIDS Res Hum Retroviruses 4: 175–186

Arya SK, Gallo RC (1988) Human immunodeficiency virus type 2 long terminal repeat: analysis of regulatory elements. Proc Natl Acad Sci USA 85: 9753–9757

Arya SK, Beaver B, Jagodzinski L, Ensoli B, Kank PJ, Albert J, Fenyo J, Fenyo EM, Biberfeld G, Zagury JF, Laure F, Essa M, Norrby E, Wong-Staal F, Gallo RC (1987) New human and simian HIV-related retroviruses possess functional transactivator (tat) gene. Nature 328: 548–550

Baldwin AS, Sharp PA (1988) Two transcription factors, NF-κB and H2TFI, interact with a single regulatory sequence in the class I major histocompatibility complex promoter. Proc Natl Acad Sci USA 85: 723–727

Ball JK, McCarter JA (1971) Repeated demonstration of a mouse leukemia virus after treatment with chemical carcinogens. JNCI 46: 751–762

Ball JK, Arthur LO, Dekaban GA (1985) The involvement of a type-B retrovirus in the induction of thymic lymphomas. Virology 140: 159–172

Ball JK, Diggelmann H, Dekaban GA, Grossi GF, Semmler R, Waight PA, Fletcher RF (1988) Alterations in the U3 region of the long terminal repeat of an infectious thymotropic type B retrovirus. J Virol 62: 2985–2993

Barklis E, Mulligan RC, Jaenisch R (1986) Chromosomal position or virus mutation permits retrovirus expression in embryonal carcinoma cells. Cell 47: 391–399

Bauerle PA, Baltimore D (1988) IκB: a specific inhibitor of the NF-κB transcription factor. Science 242: 540–546

Bohnlein E, Lowenthal JW, Siekevitz M, Ballard DW, Franza BR, Greene WC (1988) The same inducible nuclear proteins regulates mitogen activation of both the interleukin-2 receptor-alpha gene and type 1 HIV. Cell 53: 827–836

Boral AL, Okenquist SA, Lenz J (1989) Identification of the SL3-3 virus enhancer core as a T-lymphoma cell-specific element. J Virol 63: 76–84

Bosze A, Thiesen H, Charney P (1986) A transcriptional enhancer with specificity for erythroid cells is located in the long terminal repeat of the Friend murine leukemia virus. EMBO J 5: 1615–1623

Brady J, Jeang K-T, Duvall J, Khoury G (1987) Identification of p 40^{x-} responsive regulatory sequences within the human T-cell leukemia virus type I long terminal repeat. J Virol 61: 2175–2181

Brown DW, Blais BP, Robinson HL (1988) Long terminal repeat (LTR) sequences, env, and a region near the 5' LTR influence the pathogenic potential of recombinants between Rous-associated virus type 0 and 1. J Virol 62: 3431–3437

Buetti E, Kuhnel B (1986) Distinct sequence elements involved in the glucocorticoid regulation of the mouse mammary tumor virus promoter identified by linker scanning mutagenesis. J Mol Biol 190: 379–389

Carlberg K, Ryden TA, Beemon K (1988) Localization and footprinting of an enhancer within the avian sarcoma virus gag gene. J Virol 62: 1617–1624

Cato ACB, Weinmann J (1988) Mineralocorticoid regulation of transcription of transfected mouse mammary tumor virus DNA in cultured kidney cells. J Cell Biol 106: 2119–2125

Cato ACB, Miksicek R, Schutz G, Arnemann J, Beato M (1986) The hormone regulatory element of mouse mammary tumor virus mediates progesterone induction. EMBO J 5: 2237–2240

Cato ACB, Henderson D, Ponta H (1987) The hormone response element of the mouse mammary tumor virus DNA mediates the progestin and androgen induction of transcription in the proviral long terminal repeat region. EMBO J 6: 363–368

Cato ACB, Skroch P, Weinmann J, Butkeraitis P, Ponta H (1988) DNA sequences outside the receptor-binding sites differentially modulate the responsiveness of the mouse mammary tumor virus promoter to various steroid hormones. EMBO J 7: 1403–1410

Celander D, Haseltine WA (1984) Tissue-specific transcription preference as a determinant of cell tropism and leukaemogenic potential of murine retroviruses. Nature 312: 159–162

Celander D, Haseltine WA (1987) Glucocorticoid regulation of murine leukemia virus transcription elements is specified by determinants within the viral enhancer region. J Virol 61: 269–275

Celander D, Hsu BL, Haseltine WA (1988) Regulatory elements within the murine leukemia virus enhancer regions mediate glucocorticoid responsiveness J Virol 62: 1314–1322

Chalepakis G, Arnemann J, Slater E, Bruller H-J, Gross B, Beato (1988) Differential gene activation by glucocorticoids and progestins through the hormone regulatory element of mouse mammary tumor virus. Cell 53: 371–382

Chandler VL, Maler BA, Yamamoto K (1983) DNA sequences bound specifically by glucocorticoid receptor in vitro render a heterologous promoter hormone responsive in vivo. Cell 33: 489–499

Chatis PA, Holland CA, Hartley JW, Rowe WP, Hopkins N (1983) Role for the 3' end of the genome in determining disease specificity of Friend and Moloney murine leukemia virus. Proc Natl Acad Sci USA 80: 4408–4411

Chatis PA, Holland CA, Silver JE, Frederickson TN, Hopkins N, Hartley JW (1984) A 3' end fragment encompassing the transcriptional enhancer of nondefective Friend virus confers erythroleukemogenicity on Moloney leukemia virus. J Virol 52: 248–254

Chattopadhyay SK, Baroudy BM, Holmes KL, Fredrickson TN, Lander MR, Morse III HC, Hartley JW (1989) Biologic and molecular genetic characteristics of a unique MCF virus that is highly leukemogenic in ecotropic virus-negative mice. Virology 168: 90–100

Chen ISY, Slamon DJ, Rosenblatt JD, Shah NP, Quan SG, Wachsman W (1985) The x gene is essential for HTLV replication. Science 229: 54–58

Chodosh LA, Baldwin AS, Carthew RW, Sharp PA (1988) Human CCAAT-binding proteins have heterologous sub-units. Cell 53: 11–24

Choi Y, Henrard D, Lee I, Ross SR (1987) The mouse mammary tumor virus long terminal repeat directs expression in epithelial and lymphoid cells of different tissues in transgenic mice. J Virol 61: 3013–3019

Claude A (1967) An active factor inhibiting body growth in mice: Its origin and mode of action. In: Their H, Rytomaa T (eds) Control of cellular growth in adult organisms. Academic, New York, pp 302–309

Cordingley MG, Hager GL (1988) Binding of multiple factors to the MMTV promoter in crude and fractionated nuclear extracts. Nucleic Acids Res 2: 609–627

Cordingley MG, Riegel AT, Hager GL (1987) Steroid-dependent interaction of transcription factors with the inducible promoter of mouse mammary tumor virus in vivo. Cell 48: 261–270

Cross SL, Feinberg MB, Wolf JB, Holbrook NJ, Wong-Staal F, Leonard WJ (1987) Regulation of the human interleukin-2 receptor α chain promoter: activation of a nonfunctional promoter by the transactivator gene of HTLV-1. Cell 49: 47–56

Cullen BR (1986) Trans-activation of human immunodeficiency virus occurs via a bimodal mechanism. Cell 46: 973–982

Cullen BR, Lomedico PT, Ju G (1984) Transcriptional interference in avian retroviruses-implication for the promoter insertion model of leukemogenesis. Nature 307: 241–245

Cullen BR, Raymond K, Ju G (1985a) Functional analysis of the transcription control region located within the avian retroviral long terminal repeat. Mol Cell Biol 5: 438–447

Cullen BR, Raymond K, Ju G (1985b) Transcriptional activity of avian retroviral long terminal repeats directly correlates with enhancer activity. J. Virol 53: 515–521

Cuypers HT, Selten G, Quint W, Zylstra M, Maandag ER, Boelens W, van Wezenbeek P, Melief C, Berns A (1984) Murine leukemia virus-induced T-cell lymphomagenesis: integration of proviruses in a distinct chromosomal region. Cell 37: 141–150

Darbre P, Page M, DKing RJB (1986) Androgen regulation by the long terminal repeat of mouse mammary tumor virus. Mol Cell Biol 6: 2847–2854

Davis BR, Brightman BK, Chandy KG, Fan H (1987a) Characterization of a preleukemic state induced by Moloney murine leukemia virus: evidence for two infection events during leukemogenesis. Proc Natl Acad Sci USA 84: 4875–4879

Davis MG, Kenney S, Kamine J, Pagano JS, Huang E-S (1987b) Immediate-early gene region of human cytomegalovirus trans-activates the promoter of human immunodeficiency virus. Proc Natl Acad Sci USA 84: 8642–8646

Dayton AI, Sodroski JG, Rosen CA, Goh WC, Haseltine WA (1986) The trans-activator gene of the human T cell lymphotropic virus type III is required for replication. Cell 44: 941–947

DeFranco D, Yamamoto K (1986) The two different factors act separately or together to specify functionally distinct activities at a single transcriptional enhancer. Mol Cell Biol 6: 993–1001

Derse D (1988) Trans-acting regulation of bovine leukemia virus mRNA processing. J Virol 62: 1115–1119

Derse D, Casey JW (1986) Two elements in the bovine leukemia virus long terminal repeat that regulate gene expression. Science 231: 1437–1440

DesGroseillers L, Jolicoeur P (1984) The tandem direct repeats within the long terminal repeat of murine leukemia viruses are the primary determinant of their leukemogenic potential. J Virol 52: 945–952

DesGrosseillers L, Rassert E, Jolicoeur P (1983) Thymotropism of murine leukemia virus is conferred by its long terminal repeat. Proc Natl Acad Sci USA 80: 4203–4207

Dickson C, Smith R, Peters G (1981) In vitro synthesis of polypeptides encoded by the long terminal repeat region of mouse mammary tumor virus DNA. Nature 291: 511–513

Dickson C, Smith R, Brookes S, Peters G (1984) Tumorigenesis by mouse mammary tumor virus: proviral activation of a cellular gene in the common integration region int-2. Cell 37: 529–536

Dinter H, Chiu R, Imagawa M, Karin M, Jones KA (1987) In vitro activation of the HIV-1 enhancer in extracts from cells treated with a phorbol ester tumor promoter. EMBO J 6: 4067–4071

Donehower LA, Fleurdelys B, Hager GL (1983) Further evidence of the protein-coding potential of the mouse mammary tumor virus long terminal repeat: nucleotide sequence of an endogenous proviral long terminal repeat. J Virol 45: 941–949

Dyson PJ, Cook PR, Searle S, Wyke JA (1985) The chromatin structure of Rous sarcoma proviruses is changed by factors that act in trans in cell hybrids. EMBO J 4: 413–420

Emerman M, Temin HM (1984) Genes with promoters in retrovirus vectors can be independently suppressed by an epigenetic mechanism. Cell 39: 459–467

Emerman M, Guyander M, Montagnier L, Baltimore D, Muesing MA (1987) The specificity of the human immunodeficiency virus type 2 transactivator is different from that of human immunodeficiency virus type 1. EMBO J 6: 3755–3760

Evans RM (1988) The steroid and thyroid hormone receptor superfamily. Science 240: 889–895

Fan H, Mittal S, Chute H, Chao E, Pattengale PK (1986) Rearrangements and insertions in the Moloney murine leukemia virus long terminal repeat alter biological properties in vivo and in vitro. J Virol 60: 204–214

Fan H, Chute H, Chao E, Pattengale PK (1988) Leukemogenicity of Moloney murine leukemia viruses carrying polyoma enhancer sequences in the long terminal repeat is dependent on the nature of the inserted polyoma sequences. Virology 166: 58–65

Fasel N, Pearson K, Buetti E, Diggelmann H (1982) The region of mouse mammary tumor virus DNA containing the long terminal repeat includes a long coding sequence and signals for hormonally regulated transcripts. EMBO J 1: 3–7

Feinberg MB, Jarrett RF, Aldovini A, Gallo RC, Wong-Staal F (1986) HTLV-III expression and production involve complex regulation at the levels of splicing and translation of viral RNA. Cell 46: 807–817

Feinberg MBV, Holbrook N, Wong-Staal F, Greene WC (1987) Activation of interleukin 2 and interleukin 2 receptor (Tac) promoter expression by the trans-activator (tat) gene product of human T-cell leukemia virus, type I. Proc Natl Acad Sci USA 84: 5389–5393

Feng S, Holland EC (1988) HIV-1 *tat* trans-activation requires the loop sequence within *tar*. Nature 334: 165–167

Fisher AG, Feinberg MB, Josephs SF, Harper ME, Marselle LV, Reyes G, Gonda MA, Aldovini A, Debouk C, Gallo RC, Wong-Staal F (1986) The trans-activator gene of HTLV-III is essential for virus replication. Nature 320: 367–371

Flamant F, Gurin CC, Sorge JA (1987) An embryonic DNA-binding protein specific for the promoter of the retrovirus long terminal repeat. Mol Cell Biol 7: 3548–3553

Flanagan JR, Krieg AM, Max EE, Khan AS (1989) Negative control region at the 5′ end of murine leukemia virus long terminal repeats. Mol Cell Biol 9: 739–746

Folks TM, Clouse DA, Justement J, Rabson A, Duh E, Kehrl JH, Fauci AS (1989) Tumor necrosis factor α induces expression of human immunodeficiency virus in a chronically infected T-cell clone. Proc Natl Acad Sci USA 86: 2365–2368

Franz T, Hilberg F, Seliger B, Stocking C, Ostertag W (1986) Retroviral mutants efficiently expressed in embryonal carcinoma cells. Proc Natl Acad Sci USA 83: 3292–3296

Franza BR, Josephs SF, Gilman MZ, Ryan W, Clarkson B (1987) Characterization of cellular proteins recognizing the HIV enhancer using a microscale DNA-affinity precipitation assay. Nature 330: 391–395

Fujisawa J-I, Seiki M, Sato M, Yoshida M (1986) A transcriptional enhancer sequence of HTLV-I is responsible for trans-activation mediated by p40^x of HTLV-I. EMBO J 5: 713–718

Garcia JA, Wu FK, Mitsuyasu R, Gaynor RB (1987) Interactions of cellular proteins involved in the transcriptional regulation of the human immunodeficiency virus. EMBO J 6: 3761–3770

Garcia JA, Harrich D, Soultanakis E, Wu F, Mitsuyasu R, Gaynor RB (1989) Human immunodeficiency virus type 1 LTR TATA and TAR region sequences required for transcriptional regulation. EMBO J 8: 765–778

Gendelman HE, Phelps W, Feigenbaum L, Ostrove JM, Adachi A, Howley PM, Khoury G, Ginsberg HS, Martin MA (1986) Trans-activation of the human immunodeficiency virus long terminal repeat sequence by DNA viruses. Proc Natl Acad Sci USA 83: 9759–9763

Gentz R, Chen C-H, Rosen CA (1989) Bioassay for trans-activation using purified human immunodeficiency virus tat-encoded protein: trans-activation requires mRNA synthesis. Proc Natl Acad Sci USA 86: 821–824

Gimble JM, Duh E, Ostrove JM, Gendelman HE, Max EE, Rabson AB (1988) Activation of the human immunodeficiency virus long terminal repeat by herpes simplex virus type 1 is associated with induction of a nuclear factor that binds to the NF-kB/core enhancer sequence. J Virol 62: 4104–4112

Golemis E, Li Y, Fredrickson TN, Hartley JW, Hopkins N (1989) Distinct segments within the enhancer region collaborate to specify the type of leukemia induced by nondefective Friend and Moloney viruses. J Virol 63: 328–337

Goodenow MM, Hayward WS (1987) 5' long terminal repeats of myc-associated proviruses appear structurally intact but are functionally impaired in tumors induced by avian leukosis viruses. J Virol 61: 2489–2498

Goodwin GH (1988) Identification of three sequence-specific DNA binding proteins which interact with the Rous sarcoma virus enhancer and upstream promoter elements. J Virol 62: 2186–2190

Gorman CM, Merlino GT, Willingham MC, Pastan I, Howard BH (1982) The Rous sarcoma virus long terminal repeat is a strong promoter when introduced into a variety of eukaryotic cells by DNA-mediated transfection. Proc Natl Acad Sci USA 79: 6777–6781

Gorman CM, Rigby PWJ, Lane DP (1985) Negative regulation of viral enhancers in undifferentiated embryonic stem cells. Cell 42: 519–526

Gowda S, Rao AS, Kim YW, Guntaka RV (1988) Identification of sequences in the long terminal repeat of avian sarcoma virus required for efficient transcription. Virology 162: 243–247

Graham DE, Medina D, Smith GH (1984) Increased concentration of an indigenous proviral mouse mammary tumor virus long terminal repeat-containing transcript is associated with neoplastic transformation of mammary epithelium in C3H/Sm mice. J Virol 49: 819–827

Graham M, Adams JM, Corey S (1985) Murine T lymphomas with retroviral inserts in the chromosome 14 locus for plasmacytoma variant translocations. Nature 314: 740–745

Graves BJ, Eisenberg SP, Coen DM, McKnight SL (1985a) Alternate utilization of two regulatory domains within the Moloney murine sarcoma virus long terminal repeat. Mol Cell Biol 5: 1959–1968

Graves BJ, Eisenman RN, McKnight SL (1985b) Delineation of transcriptional control signals within the Moloney murine sarcoma virus long terminal repeat. Mol Cell Biol 5: 1948–1958

Green, AR, Wyke JA (1988) Integrated proviruses as probes for chromosomal position effects in mammalian cells and their hybrids. Cancer Surv 7: 335–349

Green AR, Searle S, Gillespie DAF, Bissell M, Wyke JA (1986) Expression of integrated Rous sarcoma viruses: DNA rearrangements 5' to the provirus are common in transformed rat cells but not seen in infected but untransformed cells. EMBO J 5: 707–711

Griffin GE, Leung K, Folks TM, Kunkel S, Nabel GJ (1989) Activation of HIV gene expression during monocyte differentiation by induction of Nf-κB. Nature 339: 70–73

Guilhot S, Hampe A, d'Auriol L, Galibert F (1987) Nucleotide sequence analysis of the LTRs and env genes of SM-FeSv and GA-FeSV. Virology 161: 252–258

Gustafson TA, Miwa T, Boxer LM, Kedes L (1988) Interaction of nuclear proteins with muscle-specific regulatory sequences of the human cardiac α-actin promoter. Mol Cell Biol 8: 4110–4119

Guy B, Kieny MP, Riviere U, Le Peuch C, Dott K, Girard M, Montagnier L, Lecocq J-P (1987) HIV F/3' orf encodes a phosphorylated GTP-binding protein resembling an oncogene product. Nature 330: 265–269

Guyader M, Emerman M, Sonigo P, Clavel F, Montagnier L, Alizon M (1987) Genome organization and transactivation of the human immunodeficiency virus type 2. Nature 326: 662–669

Hallberg B, Grundstrom T (1988) Tissue specific sequence motifs in the enhancer of the leukaemogenic mouse retrovirus SL-3. Nucleic Acids Res 16: 5927–5944

Ham J, Thomson A, Needham M, Webb P, Parker M (1988) Characterization of response elements for androgens, glucocorticoids, and progestins in mouse mammary tumor virus. Nucleic Acids Res 16: 5263–5276

Hanecak R, Mittal S, Davis BR, Fan H (1986) Generation of infectious Moloney murine leukemia viruses with deletions in the U3 portion of the long terminal repeat. Mol Cell Biol 6: 4634–4640

Hanecak R, Pattengale PK, Fan H (1988) Addition or substitution of simian virus 40 enhancer sequences into the Moloney murine leukemia virus (M-MuLV) long terminal repeat yields infectious M-MuLV with altered biological properties. J Virol 62: 2427–2436

Haseltine WA, Sodroski J, Patarca R, Briggs D, Perkins D, Wong-Staal F (1984) Structure of 3' terminal region of type II human T lymphotropic virus: evidence for new coding region. Science 225: 419–421

Hauber J, Cullen BR (1988) Mutational analysis of the trans activation-responsive region of the human immunodeficiency virus type I long terminal repeat. J Virol 62: 673–679

Hauber J, Perkins A, Heimer EP, Cullen BR (1986) Trans-activation of human immunodeficiency virus gene expression is mediated by nuclear events. Proc Natl Acad Sci USA: 6364–6368

Hayward WS, Neel BG, Astrin SM (1981) Activation of a cellular onc gene by promoter insertion in ALV-induced lymphoid leukosis. Nature 290: 465–480

Herman SA, Coffin JM (1986) Differential transcription from the long terminal repeats of integrated avian leukosis virus DNA. J Virol 60: 497–505

Hidaka M, Inoue J, Yoshida M, Seiki M (1988) Post-transcriptional regulator (rex) of HTLV-1 initiates expression of viral structural proteins but suppresses expression of regulatory proteins. EMBO J: 519–523

Hilberg F, Stocking C, Ostertag W, Grez M (1987) Functional analysis of a retroviral host-range mutant: altered long terminal repeat sequences allow expression in embryonal carcinoma cells. Proc Natl Acad Sci USA 84: 5232–5236

Hodgson CP, Arora P, Fisk RZ (1987) Nucleotide sequence of the long terminal repeat of the avian retrovirus RAV-1: evolution of avian retroviruses. Nucleic Acids Res 15: 2393

Holland CA, Wozney J, Chatis PA, Hopkins N, Hartley JW (1985) Construction of recombinants between molecular clones of murine retrovirus MCF 247 and Akv: determinant of an in vitro host range property that maps in the long terminal repeat. J Virol 53: 152–157

Holland CA, Thomas CY, Chattopadhyay SK, Koehne C, O'Donnell PV (1989) Influence of enhancer sequences on thymotropism and leukemogenicity of mink cell focus-forming viruses. J Virol 63: 1284–1292

Hsu C-LL, Fabritius C, Dudley J (1988) Mouse mammary tumor virus proviruses in T-cell lymphomas lack a negative regulatory element in the long terminal repeat. J Virol 62: 4644–4652

Huang AL, Ostrowski MC, Berard D, Hager GL (1981) Glucocorticoid regulation of the Ha-MuSV p21 gene conferred by sequences from mouse mammary tumor virus. Cell 27: 245–255

Huang C-C, Hammond C, Bishop JM (1984) Nucleotide sequence of v-fps in the PRCII strain of avian sarcoma virus. J Virol 50: 125–131

Hynes N, van Ooyen AJJ, Kennedy N, Herrlich P, Ponta H, Groner B (1983) Subfragments of the large terminal repeat cause glucocorticoid-responsive expression of mouse mammary tumor virus and of an adjacent gene. Proc Natl Acad Sci USA 80: 3637–3641

Inoue J-I, Seiki M, Taniguchi T, Tsuru S, Yoshida M (1986) Induction of interleukin 2 receptor gene expression by p40^x encoded by human T-cell leukemia virus type I. EMBO J 5: 2883–2888

Inoue J-I, Yoshida M, Seiki M (1987) Transcriptional (p40^x) and post-transcriptional (p27^{x-III}) regulators are required for the expression and replication of human T-cell leukemia virus type I genes. Proc Natl Acad Sci USA 84: 3653–3657

Ishimoto A, Takimoto M, Adachi A, Kakuyama M, Kato S, Kakimi K, Fukuoka K, Ogiu T, Matsuyama M (1987) Sequences responsible for erythroid and lymphoid leukemia in the long terminal repeats of Friend-mink cell focus-forming and Moloney murine leukemia viruses. J Virol 61: 1861–1866

Jahner D, Haase K, Mulligan R, Jaenisch R (1982) De novo methylation and expression of retroviral genomes during mouse embryogenesis. Nature 298: 623–628

Jakobovits A, Smith DH, Jakobovits EB, Capon DJ (1988) A discrete element 3' of human immunodeficiency virus 1 (HIV-1) and HIV-2 mRNA initiation sites mediates transcriptional activation by an HIV trans activator. Mol Cell Biol 3: 2555–2561

Jeang K-T, Boros I, Brady J, Radonovich M, Khoury G (1988a) Characterization of cellular factors that interact with the human T-cell leukemia virus type I p40^x-responsive 21-base-pair sequence. J Virol 62: 4499–4509

Jeang K-T, Shank PR, Kumar A (1988b) Transcriptional activation of homologous viral long terminal repeats by the human immunodeficiency virus type 1 or the human T-cell leukemia virus type I tat proteins occurs in the absence of de novo protein synthesis. Proc Natl Acad Sci USA 85: 8291–8295

Jones KA, Kadonaga JT, Luciw PA, Tjian R (1986) Activation of the AIDS retrovirus promoter by the cellular transcription factor, Sp1. Science 231: 755–759

Jones KA, Luciw PA, Duchange N (1988a) Structural arrangements of transcriptional control domains within the 5'-untranslated leader regions of the HIV-1 and HIV-2 promoters. Genes Dev 2: 1101–1114

Jones NC, Rigby PWJ, Ziff EB (1988b) Trans-acting protein factors and the regulation of eukaryotic transcription: lessons from studies on DNA tumor viruses. Genes Dev 2: 267–281

Ju G, Cullen BR (1985) The role of avian retroviral LTRs in the regulation of gene expression and viral replication. Adv Virus Res 30: 179–223

Kan NC, Flordellis CS, Mark GE, Duesberg PH, Papa TS (1984) Nucleotide sequence of avian carcinoma virus MH2: two potential onc genes, one related to avian virus MC29 and the other related to murine sarcoma virus 3611. Proc Natl Acad Sci USA 81: 3000–3004

Kao SY, Calman AF, Luciw PA, Peterlin BM (1987) Anti-termination of transcription within the long terminal repeat of HIV-1 by tat gene product. Nature 330: 489–493

Karnitz L, Poon D, Weil PA, Chalkley R (1989) Purification and properties of the Rous sarcoma virus internal enhancer binding factor. Mol Cell Biol 9: 1929–1939

Kaufman JD, Valandra G, Roderiquez G, Bushar G, Giri C Norcross MA (1987) Phorbol ester enhances human immunodeficiency virus-promoted gene expression and acts on a repeated 10-base-pair functional enhancer element. Mol Cell Biol 7: 3759–3766

Kawakami K, Scheidereit C, Roeder RG (1988) Identification and purification of a human immunoglobulin-enhancer-binding protein (NF-κB) that activates transcription from a human immunodeficiency virus type 1 promoter in vitro. Proc Natl Acad Sci USA 85: 4700–4704

Kelly M, Holland CA, Lung ML, Chattopadhyay SK, Lowy DR, Hopkins N (1983) Nucleotide sequence of the 3' end of MCF 247 murine leukemia virus. Jr Virol 45: 291–298

Khan AS, Martin MA (1983) Endogenous murine leukemia proviral long terminal repeats contain a unique 190-base-pair insert. Proc Natl Acad Sci USA 80: 2699–2703

Kitamura N, Kitamura A, Toyoshima K, Hirayama Y, Yoshida M (1982) Avian sarcoma virus Y73 genome sequence and structural similarity of its transforming gene product to that of Rous sarcoma virus. Nature 297: 205–208

Kiyokawa T, Kawaguchi T, Seiki M, Yoshida M (1985a) Association with nucleus of pX gene product of human T-cell leukemia virus type I. Virology 147: 462–465

Kiyokawa T, Seiki M, Iwashita S, Imagawa K, Shimizu F, Yoshida M (1985b) p27^{x-III} and p21^{x-III}, proteins encoded by the pX sequence of human T-cell leukemia virus type I. Proc Natl Acad Sci USA 82: 8359–8363

Klock G, Strahle U, Schutz G (1987) Oestrogen and glucocorticoid responsive elements are closely related but distinct. Nature 329: 734–736

Kuhnel B, Buetti E, Diggelmann H (1986) Functional analysis of the glucocorticoid regulatory elements present in the mouse mammary tumor virus long terminal repeat: a synthetic distal binding site can replace the proximal binding domain. J Mol Biol 190: 367–378

Kuo W-L, Vilander LR, Huang M, Peterson DO (1988) A transcriptionally defective long terminal repeat within an endogenous copy of mouse mammary tumor virus proviral DNA. J Virol 62: 2394–2402

Kwon BS, Weissman SM (1984) Mouse mammary tumor virus-related sequences in mouse lymphocytes are inducible by 12-O-tetradecanoyl phorbol 13-acetate. J Virol 52: 1000–1004

Laimins LA, Gruss P, Pozatti R, Khoury G (1984a) Characterization of enhancer elements in the long terminal repeat of a Moloney murine sarcoma virus. J Virol 49: 183–189

Laimins LA, Tsichlis P, Khoury G (1984b) Multiple enhancer domains in the 3' terminus of the Prague strain of Rous sarcoma virus. Nucleic Acids Res 12: 6427–6442

Landshulz WH, Johnson PF, Adashi EY, Graves BJ, McKnight SL (1988) Isolation of a recombinant copy of the gene encoding C/EBP. Genes Dev 2: 786–800

Langer SJ, Ostrowski MC (1988) Negative regulation of transcription in vitro by a glucocorticoid response element is mediated by a trans-acting factor. Mol Cell Biol 8: 3872–3881

Le S-Y, Chen J-H, Braun MJ, Gonda MA, Maizel JV (1988) Stability of RNA stem-loop structure and distribution of non-random structure in the human immunodeficiency virus (HIV-1). Nucleic Acids Res 15: 5153–5168

Lee F, Mulligan R, Berg P, Ringold G (1981) Glucocorticoids regulate expression of dihydrofolate reductase cDNA in mouse mammary tumor virus chimaeric plasmids. Nature 294: 228–232

Lee WT-L, Prakash O, Klein D, Sarkar NH (1987) Structural alterations in the long terminal repeat of an acquired mouse mammary tumor virus provirus in a T-cell leukemia of DBA/2 mice. Virology 159: 39–48

Lenardo MJ, Kuang A, Gifford A, Baltimore D (1988) NF-κB protein purification from bovine spleen: nucleotide stimulation and binding site specificity. Proc Natl Acad Sci USA 85: 8825–8829

Lenz J, Celander D, Crowther RL, Patarca R, Perkins DW, Haseltine WA (1984) Determination of the leukemogenicity of a murine retrovirus by sequences within the long terminal repeat. Nature 308: 467–470

Leung K, Nabel GJ (1988) HTLV-I transactivator induces interleukin-2 receptor expression through an NF-kB like factor. Nature 333: 776–778

Levy DE, McKinnon RD, Brolaski MN, Gautsch JW, Wilson MC (1987) The 3′ long terminal repeat of a transcribed yet defective endogenous retroviral sequence is a competent promoter of transcription. J Virol 61: 1261–1265

Li Y, Holland CA, Hartley JW, Hopkins N (1984) Viral integration near c-myc in 10–20% of MCF 247-induced AKR lymphomas. Proc Natl Acad Sci USA 81: 6808–6811

Li Y, Golemis E, Hartley JW, and Hopkins N (1987) Disease specificity of non-defective Friend and Moloney murine leukemia viruses is controlled by a small number of nucleotides. J Virol 61: 693–700

Liegler TJ, Blair PB (1986) Direct detection of exogenous mouse mammary tumor virus sequences in lymphoid cell of BALB/cfC3H female mice. J Virol 59: 159–162

Linial M, Gunderson N, Groudine M (1985) Enhanced transcription of c-myc in bursal lymphoma cells requires continuous protein synthesis. Science 230: 1126–1132

Linney E, Davis B, Overhauser J, Chao E, Fan H (1984) Non-function of a Moloney murine leukemia virus regulatory sequence in F9 embryonal carcinoma cells. Nature 308: 470–472

Loh TP, Sievert LL, Scott RW (1987) Proviral sequences that restrict retroviral expression in mouse embryonal carcinoma cells. Mol Cell Biol 10: 3775–3784

Loh TP, Sievert LL, Scott RW (1988) Negative regulation of retrovirus expression in embryonal carcinoma cells mediated by an intragenic domain. J Virol 62: 4086–4095

Lowenthal JW, Ballard DW, Bohnlein E, Greene WC (1989) Tumor necrosis factor α induces proteins that bind specifically to κB-like enhancer elements and regulate interleukin 2 receptor α-chain gene expression in primary human T lymphocytes. Proc Natl Acad Sci USA 86: 2331–2335

Lowenthal JW, Böhnlein E, Ballard DW, Greene WC (1988) Regulation of interleukin 2 receptor α subunit (Tac or CD25 antigen) gene expression; Binding of inducible nuclear proteins to discrete promoter sequences correlates with transcriptional activation. Proc Natl Acad Sci USA 85: 4468–4472

Luciw PA, Bishop JM, Varmus HE, Capecchi MR (1983) Location and function of retroviral and SV40 sequences that enhance biochemical transformation after microinjection of DNA. Cell 33: 705–716

Luciw PA, Chen-Mayer C, Levy JA (1987) Mutational analysis of the human immunodeficiencyvirus (HIV): the orf-B region down regulates virus replication. Proc Natl Acad Sci USA 84: 1434–1438

Maekawa T, Itoh F, Okamoto T, Kurimoto M, Imamoto F, Ishii S (1989) Identification and purification of the enhancer-binding factor of human immunodeficiency virus-1: multiple proteins and binding to other enhancers. J Biol Chem 264: 2826–2831

Maity SN, Golumbek PT, Karsenty G, de Crombrugghe B (1988) Selective activation of transcription by a novel CCAAT binding factor. Science 241: 582–585

Malim MH, Hauber J, Le SY, Maizel JV, Cullen BR (1989) The HIV rev trans-activator acts through a structured target sequence to activate nuclear transport of unspliced viral messenger RNA. Nature 338: 254–257

Majors JE, Varmus HE (1983a) A small region of the mouse mammary tumor virus long terminal repeat confers glucocorticoid hormone regulation on a linked heterologous gene. Proc Natl Acad Sci USA 80: L 5866–5870

Majors JE, Varmus HE (1983b) Nucleotide sequence of an apparent proviral copy of env mRNA defines determinant of expression of the mouse mammary tumor virus env gene. J Virol 47: 495–504

Maruyama M, Shibuya H, Harada H, Tatakeyama M, Seiki M, Fumjita T, Inoue J-I, Yoshida M, Taniguchi T (1987) Evidence for aberrant activation of the interleukin-2 autocrine loop by HTLV-I-encoded p40^x and T3/Ti complex triggering. Cell 48: 342–350

Mayer BJ, Hamaguchi M, Hanafusa H (1988) A novel viral oncogene with structural similarity tophospholipase C. Nature 332: 272–275

Michalides R, Wagenaar E (1986) Site-specific rearrangements in the long terminal repeat of extra mouse mammary tumor proviruses in murine T-cell leukemias. Virology 154: 76–84

Michalides R, Wagenaar E, Weijers P (1985) Rearrangement in the long terminal repeat of extra mouse mammary tumor proviruses in T-cell leukemias of mouse strain GR result in a novel enhancer-like structure. Mol Cell Biol 5: 823–830

Miksicek R, Heber A, Schmid W, Dnaesch U, Posseckert G, Beato M, Schutz G (1986) Glucocorticoid responsiveness of the transcriptional enhancer of Moloney murine sarcoma virus. Cell 467: 283–290

Miksicek R, Borgmeyer W, Nowock J (1987) Interaction of the TGGCA-binding protein with upstream sequences is required for efficient transcription of mouse mammary tumor virus. EMBO J 6: 1355–1360

Miyatake S, Seiki M, Malefijt D, Heike T, Fujisawa J-I, Takebe Y, Nishida J, Shlomai J, Tokata T, Arai K-I, Arai N (1988a) Activation of T cell-derived lymphokine genes in T cells and fibroblasts: effects of human T cell leukemia virus type I p40ˣ protein and bovine papilloma virus encoded E2 protein. Nucleic Acids Res 16: 5581–5587

Miyatake S, Seiki M, Yoshida M, Arai K-I (1988b) T-cell activation signals and human T-cell leukemia virus type I-encoded p40ˣ protein activate the mouse granulocyte-macrophage colony-stimulating factor gene through a common DNA element. Mol Cell Biol 8: 5581–5587

Morley KL, Toohey MG, Peterson DO (1987) Transcriptional repression of a hormone-responsive promoter. Nucleic Acids Res 15: 6973–6989

Morris DW, Bradshaw HD, Billy HT, Munn RJ, Cardiff RD (1989) Isolation of a pathogenic clone of mouse mammary tumor virus. J Virol 63: 148–158

Mosca JD, Bednarik DP, Raj NBK, Rosen CA, Sodroski JG, Haseltine WA, Hayward GS, Pitha PM (1987) Activation of human immunodeficiency virus by herpesvirus infection: Identification of a region within the long terminal repeat that responds to a trans-acting factor encoded by herpes simplex virus 1. Proc Natl Acad Sci USA 84: 7408–7412

Muesing MA, Smith DH, Capon DJ (1987) Regulation of mRNA accumulation by a human immunodeficiency virus trans-activator protein. Cell 48: 691–701

Nabel G, Baltimore D (1987) An inducible transcription factor activates the expression of human immunodeficiency virus in T lymphocytes. Nature 326: 711–713

Nabel GJ, Rice SA, Knipe DM, Baltimore D (1988) Alternative mechanisms for activation of human immunodeficiency virus enhancer in T cells. Science 239: 1299–1302

Neckameyer WS, Wang L-H (1985) Nucleotide sequence of avian sarcoma virus UR2 and comparison of its transforming gene with other members of the tyrosine protein kinase oncogene family. J Virol 53: 879–884

Niederman TMJ, Thielan BJ, Ratner L (1989) Human immunodeficiency virus type 1 negative factor is a transcriptional silencer. Proc Natl Acad Sci USA 86: 1128–1132

Norton PA, Coffin JM (1987) Characterization of Rous sarcoma virus sequences essential for viral gene expression. J Virol 61: 1171–1179

Nunn M, Weiher H, Bullock P, Duesberg P (1984) Avian erythroblastosis virus E26: nucleotide sequence of the tripartitite onc gene and of the LTR, and analysis of the cellular prototype of the viral ets sequence. Virology 139: 330–339

Nusse R, van Ooyen A, Cos D, Fung YK, Varmus HE (1984) Mode of proviral activation of a putative mammary oncogene (int-1) on mouse chromosome 15. Nature 307: 131–136

Nyborg JK, Dynan WS, Chen IS-Y, Wachsman W (1988) Binding of host-cell factors to DNA sequences in the long terminal repeat of human T-cell leukemia virus type I: implications for viral gene expression. Proc Natl Acad Sci USA 85: 1457–1461

O'Donnell PV, Fleissner E, Lonial H, Koehne C, Reicin A (1985) Early clonality and high-frequency proviral integration into the c-myc locus in AKR leukemias. J Virol 55: 500–503

Ohta M, Nyunoya N, Tanaka H, Okamoto T, Akagi T, Shimotohno K (1988) Identification of a cis-regulatory element involved in accumulation of human T-cell leukemia virus type II genomic mRNA. J Virol 62: 4445–4451

Ohtani K, Nakamura M, Saito S, Noda T, Ito Y, Sugamura K, Hinuma Y (1987) Identification of two distinct elements in the long terminal repeat of HTLV-I responsible for maximum gene expression. EMBO J 6: 389–395

Okamoto T, Matsuyama T, Mori S, Hamamoto Y, Kobayashi N, Yamamoto N, Josephs SF, Wong-Staal F, Shimotohno K (1989) Augmentation of human immunodeficiency virus type 1 gene expression by tumor necrosis factor α. AIDS Res Hum Retrov 5: 131–138

Okamoto T, Wong-Staal F (1986) Demonstration of virus-specific transcriptional activator(s) in cells infected with HTLV-III by an in vitro cell-free system. Cell 47: 29–35

Osborn L, Kunkel S, Nabel GJ (1989) Tumor necrosis factor and interleukin 1 stimulate the human immunodeficiency virus enhancer by activation of the nuclear factor kB. Proc Natl Acad Sci USA 86: 2336–2340

Ostrove JM, Leonard J, Weck KE, Rabson AB, Gendelman HE (1987) Activation of the human immunodeficiency virus by herpes simplex virus type 1. J Virol 61: 3726–3732

Overbeek PA, Lai S-P, Van Quill KR, Westphal H (1986) Tissue-specific expression in transgenic mice of a fused gene containing RSV terminal sequences. Science 231: 1574–1577

Overhauser J, Fan H (1985) Generation of glucocorticoid responsive Moloney murine leukemia virus by insertion of regulatory sequences from murine mammary tumor virus into the long terminal repeat. J Virol 54: 133–141

Parkin NT, Cohen EA, Darveau A, Rosen C, Haseltine W, Sonenberg N (1988) Mutational analysis of the 5′ non-coding region of human immunodeficiency virus type 1: effects of secondary structure on translation. EMBO J 7: 2831–2837

Paskalis H, Felber BK, Pavlakis GN (1986) Cis-acting sequences responsible for the transcriptional activation of human T-cell leukemia virus type I constitute a conditional enhancer. Proc Natl Acad Sci USA 83: 6558–6562

Payne GS, Courtneidge SA, Crittenden LB, Fackley AM, Bishop JN, Varmus HE (1981) Analyses of avian leukosis viral DNA and RNA in bursal tumors suggest a novel mechanism for retroviral oncogenesis. Cell 25: 311–322

Payvar FD, DeFranco D, Firestone GL, Edgar B, Wrange O, Okret S, Gustafsson JA, Yamamoto KR (1983) Sequence-specific binding of glucocorticoid receptor to MTV DNA at sites within and upstream of the transcribed region. Cell 35: 381–392

Perlmann T, Wrange O (1988) Specific glucocorticoid receptor binding to DNA reconstituted in a nucleosome. EMBO J 7: 3073–3079

Peterlin BM, Luciw PA, Barr PJ, Walker WD (1986) Elevated levels of mRNA can account for the trans-activation of human immunodeficiency virus. Proc Natl Acad Sci USA 83: 9734–9738

Peterson DO (1985) Alterations in chromatin structure associated with glucocorticoid-induced expression of endogenous mouse mammary tumor virus genes. Mol Cell Biol 5: 1104–1110

Ponta H, Kennedy N, Sckroch R, Hynes NE, Groner B (1985) The hormonal response region in the mouse mammary tumor virus long terminal repeat can be dissociated from the proviral promoter and has enhancer properties. Proc Natl Acad Sci USA 82: 1020–1024

Prywes R, Roeder RG (1987) Purification of the c-fos enhancer-binding protein. Mol Cell Biol 7: 3482–3489

Quint W, Boelens W, van Wezenbeed P, Cuypers T, Robanus-Maandag E, Selten G, Berns A (1984) Generation of AKR mink cell focus-forming viruses: a conserved single-copy xenotrope-like provirus provides recombinant long terminal repeat sequences. J Virol 50: 432–438

Raceviskis J, Prakash O (1984) Proteins encoded by the long terminal repeat region of mouse mammary tumor virus: identification by hybrid-selected translation. J Virol 51: 604–610

Rando RF, Pellett PE, Luciw PA, Bohan CA, Srinivasan A (1987) Transactivation of human immunodeficiency virus by herpesviruses. Oncogene 1: 13–18

Reddy EP, Reynolds RK, Watson DK, Schultz RA, Lautenberger J, Papas TS (1983) Nucleotide sequence analysis of the proviral genome of avian myelocytomatosis virus (MC29). Proc Natl Acad Sci USA 80: 2500–2504

Redmond SMS, Dickson C (1983) Sequence and expression of the mouse mammary tumor virus env gene. EMBO J 2: 125–131

Rice AP, Mathews MB (1988) Transcriptional but not translational regulation of HIV-1 by the tat gene product. Nature 332: 551–553

Rice NR, Stephens RM, Couez D, Deschamp J, Kettmann R, Burny A, Gilden R (1984) The nucleotide sequence of the env and post-env region of bovine leukemia virus. Virology 138: 82–93

Richard-Foy H, Hager GL (1987) Sequence-specific positioning of nucleosomes over the steroid inducible MMTV promoter. EMBO J 6: 2321–2328

Ringold GM (1985) Steroid hormone regulation of gene expression. Annu Rev Pharmacol Toxicol 25: 529–566

Robinson H, Jensen L, Coffin JM (1985) Sequences outside of the long terminal repeat determine the lymphomogenic potential of Rous-associated virus type 1. J Virol 55: 752–759

Robinson HL, Blais BM, Tsichlis PN, Coffin JM (1982) At least two regions of the viral genome determine the oncogenic potential of avian leukosis viruses. Proc Natl Acad Sci USA 79: 1225–1229

Rosen CA, Haseltine WA, Lenz J, Ruprecht R, Cloyd MW (1985a) Tissue selectivity of murine leukemia virus infection is determined by long terminal repeat sequences. J Virol 55: 862–866

Rosen CA, Sodroski JG, Haseltine W (1985b) The location of cis-acting regulatory sequences in the human T cell lymphotropic virus type III (HTLV-III/LAV) long terminal repeat. Cell 41: 813–823

Rosen CA, Sodroski JG, Haseltine WA (1985c) Location of cis-acting regulatory sequences in the human T-cell leukemia virus type I long terminal repeat. Proc Natl Acad Sci USA 82: 6502–6506

Rosen CA, Sodroski JG, Goh WC, Dayton AI, Lippke J, Haseltine WA (1986) Post-transcriptional regulation accounts for the trans-activation of the human T-lymphotropic virus type III. Nature 319: 555–559

Rosen CA, Park R, Sodroski JG, Haseltine WA (1987) Multiple sequence elements are required for regulation of human T-cell leukemia virus gene expression. Proc Natl Acad Sci USA 84: 4919–4923

Rosen CA, Sodroski JG, Kettman R, Haseltine WA (1988) Activation of enhancer sequences in type II human T-cell leukemia virus and bovine leukemia virus long terminal repeats by virus-associated trans-acting regulatory factors. J Virol 57: 738–744

Rosenblatt JD, Cann AJ, Slamon DJ, Smalberg IS, Shah NP, Fujii J, Wachsman W, Chen IS-Y (1988) HTLV-II transactivation is regulated by the overlapping tax-rex nonstructural genes. Science 240: 916–919

Ross SR, Solter D (1985) Glucocorticoid regulation of mouse mammary tumor virus sequences in transgenic mice. Proc Natl Acad Sci USA 82: 5880–5884

Ruben S, Poteat H, Tan T-H, Kawakami K, Roeder R, Haseltine W, Rosen CA (1988) Cellular transcription factors and regulation of IL-2 receptor gene expression by HTLV-I tax gene product. Science 241: 89–92

Ruddell A, Linial M, Schubach W, Groudine M (1988) Lability of leukosis virus enhancer-binding protein in avian hematopoeitic cells. J Virol 62: 2728–2735

Ryden TA, Beemon K (1989) Avian retroviral long terminal repeats bind CCAAT/enhancer-binding protein. Mol Cell Biol 9: 1155–1164

Sagata N, Yasunaga T, Tsuzuku-Kawamura J, Ohishi K, Ogawa Y, Ikawa Y (1985) Complete nucleotide sequence of the genome of bovine leukemia virus: its evolutionary relationship to other retroviruses. Proc Natl Acad Sci USA 823: 677–681

Saito S, Nakamura M, Ohtani K, Ichijo M, Sugamura K, Hinmuma Y (1988) Trans-activation of the simian virus 40 enhancer pX product of human T-cell leukemia virus type I. J Virol 62: 644–648

Salmons B, Groner B, Calberg-Bacq CM, Ponta H (1985) Production of mouse mammary tumor virus upon transfection of a recombinant proviral DNA into cultured cells. Virology 144: 101–114

Scheidereit C, Geisse S, Westphal HM, Beato M (1983) The glucocorticoid receptor binds to defined nucleotide sequences near the promoter of mouse mammary tumor virus. Nature 304: 749–752

Schwartz DE, Tizard R, Gilbert W (1983) Nucleotide sequence of Rous sarcoma virus. Cell 32: 853–869

Sealey L, Chalkley R (1987) At least two nuclear proteins bind specifically to the Rous sarcoma virus long terminal repeat enhancer. Mol Cell Biol 7: 787–798

Sedaie MR, Benter T, Wong-Staal F (1988) Site-directed mutagenesis of two trans-regulatory genes (tat-III, trs) of HIV-I. Science 239: 910–913

Seiki M, Hattori S, Hirayama Y, Yoshida M (1983) Human adult T cell leukemia virus: complete nucleotide sequence of the provirus genome integrated in leukemia cell DNA. Proc Natl Acad Sci USA 80: 3618–3622

Seiki M, Hikikoshi A, Taniguchi T, Yoshida M (1985) Expression of the pX gene of HTLV-1: general splicing mechanism in the HTLV family. Science 228: 1532–1534

Seiki M, Inoue J-I, Hidaka M, Yoshida M (1988) Two cis-acting elements responsible for posttranscriptional trans-regulation of gene expression of human T-cell leukemia virus type I. Proc Natl Acad Sci USA 85: 7124–7128

Selby MJ, Bain ES, Luciw PA, Peterlin BM (1989) Structure, sequence, and position of the stem-loop in tar determine transcriptional elongation by tat through the HIV-1 long terminal repeat. Genes Dev 3: 547–558

Selten G, Cuypers HT, Zijlstra M, Melieft C, Berns A (1984) Involvement of c-myc in M-MuLV-inducer T-cell lymphomas of mice: frequency and mechanisms of activation. EMBO J 3: 3215–3222

Sen R, Baltimore D (1986) Inducibility of κ immunoglobulin enhancer-binding protein NF-κB by a posttranslational mechanism. Cell 47: 921–928

Seto E, Yen TSB, Peterlin BM, Ou J-H (1988) Trans-activation of the human immunodeficiency virus long terminal repeat by the hepatitis B virus X protein. Proc Natl Acad Sci USA 85: 8286–8290

Shackleford G, Varmus HE (1988) Construction of a clonable, infectious, and tumorigenic mouse mammary tumor virus provirus and a derivative genetic vector. Proc Natl Acad Sci USA 85: 9655–9659

Shah NP, Wachsman W, Cann AJ, Souza L, Slamon DJ, Chen IS-Y (1986) Comparison of the trans-activation capabilities of the human T-cell leukemia virus type I and II X proteins. Mol Cell Biol 6: 3626–3631

Shaw J-P, Utx PJ, Durand DB, Toole JJ, Emmel EA, Crabtree GR (1988) Identification of a putative regulator of early T cell activation genes. Science 241: 202–205

Shimotohno K, Wachsman W, Takahashi Y, Golde DW, Miwa M, Sugimura T, Chen IS-Y (1984) Nucleotide sequence of the 3' region of an infectious human T-cell Leukemia virus type II genome. Proc Natl Acad Sci USA 81: 6657–6661

Shimotohno K, Takano M, Teruuchi T, Miwa M (1986) Requirement of multiple copies of a 21-nucleotide sequence in the U3 regions of human T-cell leukemia virus type I and II long terminal repeats for trans-acting activation of transcription. Proc Natl Acad Sci USA 83: 8112–8116

Shinnick T, Lerner R, Sutcliffe JG (1981) Nucleotide sequence of Moloney murine leukemia virus. Nature 293: 543–548

Short MK, Okenquist SA, Lenz J (1987) Correlation of leukemogenic potential of murine retroviruses with transcriptional tissue preference of the viral long terminal repeats. J Virol 61: 1067–1072

Siddiqui A, Gaynor R, Srinivasan A, Mapoles J, Farr RW (1989) Trans-activation of viral enhancers including long terminal repeat of the human immunodeficiency virus by the hepatitis B virus X protein. Virology 169: 479–484

Siekevitz M, Feinberg MB, Holbrook N, Wong-Staal F, Greene WC (1987a) Activation of interleukin 2 and interleukin 2 receptor (Tac) promoter expression by the trans-activator (tat) gene product of human T-cell leukemia virus, type I. Proc Natl Acad Sci USA 84: 5389–5393

Siekevitz M, Josephs SF, Dukovich M, Peffer N, Wong-Staal F, Greene WC (1987b) Activation of the HIV-1 LTR by T cell mitogens and the trans-activator protein of HTLV-I. Science 238: 1575–1578

Sinn E, Muller W, Pattengale P, Tepler I, Wallace R, Leder P (1987) Coexpression of MMTV/v-Ha-ras and MMTV/c-myc genes in transgenic mice: synergistic action of oncogenes in vivo. Cell 49: 465–475

Slamon DJ, Prsee MF, Souza LM, Murdock DC, Cline MJ, Golde DW, Gasson JC, Chen IS-Y (1985) Studies of the putative transforming protein of the type I human T-cell leukemia virus. Science 228: 1427–1430

Smith DR, Vennstrom B, Hayman MJ, Enrietto PJ (1985) Nucleotide sequence of HBI, a novel recombinant MC29 derivative with altered pathogenic properties. J Virol 56: 969–977

Smith GH, Young LJT, Benjamini E, Medina D, Cardiff RD (1987) Proteins antigenically related to peptides encoded by the mouse mammary tumor virus long terminal repeat sequence are associated with intracytoplasmic A particles. J Gen   68: 473–486

Sodroski JG, Rosen CA, Haseltine WA (1984) Trans-acting transcriptional activation of the long terminal repeat of human T lymphotropic viruses in infected cells. Science 225: 381–385

Sodroski J, Rosen C, Goh WC, Haseltine W (1985a) A transcriptional activator protein encoded by the x-lor region of the human T-cell leukemia virus. Science 228: 1430–1434

Sodroski JG, Goh WC, Rosen CA, Salahuddin SZ, Aldovini A, Franchini G, Wong-Staal F, Gallo RC, Sugamura K, Hinuma Y, Haseltine WA (1985b) Trans-activation of the human T-cell leukemia virus long terminal repeat correlates with expression of the x-lor protein. J Virol 55: 831–855

Sonnenberg A, van Balen P, Hilgers J, Schuuring E, Nusse R (1987) Oncogene expression during progression of mouse mammary tumor cells; activity of a proviral enhancer and the resulting expression of int-2 is influenced by the state of differentiation. EMBO J 6: 121–125

Speck NA, Baltimore D (1987) Six distinct nuclear factors interact with the 75-base-pair repeat of the Moloney murine leukemia virus enhancer. Mol Cell Biol 7: 1101–1110

Steffen D (1984) Proviruses are adjacent to c-myc in some murine leukemia virus-induced lymphomas. Proc Natl Acad Sci USA 81: 2097–2101

Stewart CL, Stuhlmann H, Jahner D, Jaenisch R (1982) De novo methylation, expression and infectivity of retroviral genomes introduced into embryonal carcinoma cells. Proc Natl Acad Sci USA 79: 4098–4102

Stewart TA, Pattengale PK, Leder P (1984) Spontaneous mammary adenocarcinomas in transgenic mice that carry and express MTV/myc fusion genes. Cell 38: 627–637

Stewart TA, Hollingshead PG, Pitts SL (1988) Multiple regulatory domains in the mouse mammary tumor virus long terminal repeat revealed by analysis of fusion genes in transgenic mice. Mol Cell Biol 8: 473–479

Stoltzfus CM, Chang L-J, Cripe TP, Turek LP (1987) Efficient transformation by Prague A Rous sarcoma virus plasmid DNA requires the presence of cis-acting regions within the gag gene. J Virol 61: 3401–3409

Swanstrom R, DeLorbe WJ, Bishop JM, Varmus HE (1981) Nucleotide sequence of cloned unintegrated avian virus DNA: viral DNA contains direct and inverted repeats similar to those in transposable elements. Proc Natl Acad Sci USA 78: 124–128

Taketo M, Tanaka M (1987) A cellular enhancer of retrovirus gene expression in embryonal carcinoma cells. Proc Natl Acad Sci USA 84: 3748–3752

Tan T-H, Horikoshi M, Roeder RG (1989) Purification and characterization of multiple nuclear factors that bind to the TAX-inducible enhancer within the human T-cell leukemia virus I long terminal repeat. Mol Cell Biol 9: 1733–1745

Terwilliger E, Sodroski JG, Rosen CA, Haseltine WA (1986) Effects of mutations within the 3′ orf open reading frame region of human T-cell lymphotropic virus type III (HTLV-III/LAV) on replication and cytopathogenicity. J Virol 60: 754–760

Thiesen H-J, Bosze Z, Henry L, Charnay P (1988) A DNA element responsible for the different tissue specificities of Friend and Moloney retroviral enhancers. J Virol 62: 614–618

Thornell A, Hallberg B, Grundstrom T (1988) Differential protein biding in lymphocytes to a sequence in the enhancer of the mouse retrovirus SL3-3. Mol Cell Biol 8: 1625–1637

Tong-Starksen SE, Luciw PA, Peterlin BM (1987) Human immunodeficiency virus long terminal repeat responds to T-cell activation signals. Proc Natl Acad Sci USA 84: 6845–6849

Toohey MG, Jones KA (1989) In vitro formation of short RNA polymerase II transcripts that terminate within the HIV-1 and HIV-2 promoter-proximal downstream regions. Genes Dev 3: 265–282

Treisman R (1987) Identification of a polypeptide that binds to the c-fos serum response element. EMBO J 6: 2711–2717

Tsubara Y, Imai S, Morimoto J, Tsubura A (1986) Histological distribution of MTV antigen in mice detected by immuno-peroxidase staining. Acta Pathol Jpn 36: 481–486

Van Beveren C, Rands C, Chattopadhyay K, Lowy DR, Verma IM (1982) Long terminal repeat of murine retroviral DNAs: sequence analysis, host-proviral junctions, and preintegration site. J Virol 41: 542–556

van Ooyen AJJ, Michalides R, Nusse R (1984) Structural analysis of a 1.7kb mouse mammary tumor virus-specific RNA. J Virol 45: 362–370

Varmus HE (1987) Cellular and viral oncogenes. In: Stamatoyannopoulos G, Nienhuis AW, Leder P, Majerus PW (eds) Molecular basis of blood diseases. Saunders, Philadelphia pp 271–346

Viglianti GA, Mullins JI (1988) Functional comparison of transactivation by simian immunodeficiency virus from rhesus macaques and human immunodeficiency virus type 1. J Virol 62: 4523–4532

Villemur R, Rassart E, DesGroseillers L, Jolicoeur (1983) Molecular cloning of viral DNA from leukemogenic Gross passage A murine leukemia virus and nucleotide sequence of its long terminal repeat. J Virol 45: 539–546

Von der Ahe D, Janich S, Scheidereit C, Renkavitz R, Schütz G, Beato M (1985) Glucocorticoid and progesterone receptors bind to the same sites in two hormonally regulated promoters. Natur 313: 706–709

Walsh K (1989) Cross-binding of factors to functionally different promoter elements in c-fos and skeletal actin genes. Mol Cell Biol 9: 2191–2201

Wano Y, Feinberg M, Hosking JB, Bogerd H, Greene WC (1988) Stable expression of the tax gene of type I human T-cell leukemia virus in human T cells activates specific cellular genes involved in growth. Proc Natl Acad Sci USA 85: 9733–9737

Weiher H, Barklis E, Ostertag W, Jaenisch R (1987) Two distinct sequence elements mediate retroviral gene expression in embryonal carcinoma cells. J Virol 61: 2742–2746

Wellinger RJ, Garcia M, Vessaz A, Diggelmann H (1986) Exogenous mouse mammary tumor virus proviral DNA isolated from a kidney adenocarcinoma cell line contains alterations in the U3 region of the long terminal repeat. J Virol 60: 1–11

Westaway D, Payne G, Varmus HE (1984) Proviral deletions and oncogene base-substitutions in insertionally mutagenized c-myc alleles may contribute to the progression of avian bursal tumors. Proc Natl Acad Sci USA 81: 843–847

Wheeler DA, Butel JS, Medina D, Cardiff RD, Hager GL (1983) Transcription of mouse mammary tumor virus: identification of a candidate mRNA for the long terminal repeat gene product. J Virol 46: 42–49

Wright CM, Felber BK, Pasklis H, Pautakis GN (1986) Expression and characterisation of the *trans*-activator of HTLV-III/LAV virus. Science 234: 988–992

Wu F, Garcia J, Mitsuyasu R, Gaynor R (1988a) Alterations in binding characteristics of the human immunodeficiency virus enhancer factor. J Virol 62: 218–225

Wu FK, Garcia JA, Harrich D, Gaynor RB (1988b) Purification of the human immunodeficiency virus type 1 enhancer and TAR binding proteins EBP-1 and UBP-1, EMBO J 7: 2117–2129

Yamamoto KR (1985) Steroid receptor regulated transcription of specific genes and gene networks. Annu Rev Genet 19: 209–252

Yano O, Kanellopoulos J, Kieran M, Le Bail O, Israel A, Kourilsky P (1987) Purification of KBF1, a common factor binding to both H-2 and α-microglobulin enhancers. EMBO J 6: 3317–3324

Yoshida M, Seiki M (1987) Recent advances in the molecular biology of HTLV-I: trans-activation of viral and cellular genes. Annu Rev Immunol 5: 541–559

Yoshimura FH, Davison B, Chafflin K (1985) Murine leukemia virus long terminal repeat sequences can enhance gene activity in a cell type-specific manner. Mol Cell Biol 5: 2832–2835

Zaret KS, Yamamoto (1984) Reversible and persistent changes in chromatin structure accompany activation of a glucocorticoid-dependent enhancer. Cell 38: 29–38

Translational Suppression in Gene Expression in Retroviruses and Retrotransposons*

T. JACKS

1 Introduction

The past 5 years have brought an exciting and very unexpected solution to a long-standing question in retrovirology: the mechanism of expression of the *pol* gene. Since the earliest studies of retroviral gene expression, the mechanism by which *pol*, the gene that encodes the critical enzymes reverse transcriptase, integrase, and sometimes protease, acts had remained an enigma. Experiments carried out recently seem to have finally settled this issue, as the *pol* genes of several retroviruses and one retrotransposon have been shown to be expressed by one or another form of translational suppression. This solution to the problem of *pol* gene expression is as unexpected as it is unusual. Even 5 year ago there was general agreement in this field that mRNA splicing would ultimately be found to be responsible for expression of the *pol* functions.

Whitehead Institute, Nine Cambridge Center, Cambridge, MA 02142, USA
*This work is supported by a Merck Postdoctoral Fellowship from the Helen Hay Whitney Foundation

By way of introduction to these current findings, I have chosen to review the history of this one-time enigma. This historical treatment is worthwhile both because it provides a backdrop for recent discoveries and illustrates how our preconceptions about the way things work can sometimes lead us astray.

pol is the central of the three replication genes carried by all replication-competent retroviruses (WEISS et al. 1984). It is preceded by the *gag* gene (encoding the structural genes of the virus core) and followed by the *env* gene (encoding the glycoproteins of the viral membrane) (WEISS et al. 1984). Examination of the mRNAs encoded by retroviral proviruses in the mid-1970s immediately suggested how *gag* and *env* were expressed. Two major messages were found in infected cells: one (the genome-length message) carried *gag* at its 5′-terminus, and another (the spliced subgenomic mRNA) with *env* in the 5′ proximal position (HAYWARD 1977; WEISS et al. 1977). Following the general rule in eukaryotic cells that limits translation to the 5′-most open reading frame in a given mRNA (KOZAK 1978), these two messages should (and do) encode the Gag and Env proteins (VON DER HELM and DUESBERG 1975; PAWSON et al. 1976; PURCHIO et al. 1977; KERR et al. 1976; MURPHY et al. 1979; STACEY et al. 1977). What then is the mRNA for the *pol* gene?

The solution to what might have been called the "*pol* problem" came from the analysis of *pol*-encoded proteins in virus-infected cells. Using an antiserum specific for the *pol* product reverse transcriptase and another directed against a Gag antigen, OPPERMAN et al. (1977) showed that the primary translation product of the *pol* gene of RSV was, in fact, a Gag-Pol fusion protein. Pulse-chase experiments showed that this fusion protein was not the precursor to the Gag protein, which was present in infected cells approximately 20-fold more abundantly than the Gag-Pol protein (OPPERMANN et al. 1977). Moreover, tryptic peptide analysis of the Gag-Pol fusion proteins of RSV and MLVs indicated that they contained most, if not all, of the sequences present in the respective Gag proteins (OPPERMAN et al. 1977; JAMJOON et al. 1977; RETTENMEIR et al. 1979). Thus, the *pol* problem was transformed into the perhaps more interesting *gag-pol* problem: how could an apparently single species of mRNA (the genome-length mRNA) give rise to both the Gag and Gag-Pol proteins?

At the time the *gag-pol* problem was defined, two hypotheses were advanced as potential solutions. According to the suppression hypothesis (Fig. 1), the genome-length mRNA is translated to yield both the Gag and Gag-Pol proteins, with the latter arising upon occasional suppression of the signal(s) that normally terminates translation at the end of the *gag* gene. The splicing hypothesis, on the other hand, calls for the inefficient processing of the genome-length message to generate a rare species of "*gag-pol*" mRNA in which the two genes are joined in one long open reading frame (Fig. 1).

The first attempt to discern the actual mechanism of *pol* gene expression came in 1978 when PHILIPSON and coworkers (1978) translated MLV virion RNA (vRNA) in an in vitro translation system supplemented with yeast suppressor tRNAs. Several groups had previously shown that cell-free translation of MLV or RSV vRNA (or purified genome-length mRNA) yielded gag and gag-pol proteins

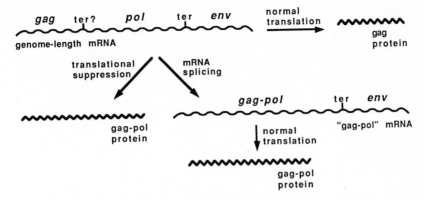

Fig. 1. Models for *pol* gene expression. Normal translation of the retroviral genome-length mRNA is shown to give rise to Gag protein. Generation of the Gag-Pol protein from this mRNA could be accomplished by either translational suppression of the signal(s) that normally terminates translation at the end of *gag* and prevents translation into *pol* or production of a specific "*gag-pol*" mRNA (in which the coding domains of *gag* and *pol* are fused into one long open reading frame) through mRNA splicing

in ratios similar to those observed in infected cells (VON DER HELM and DUESBERG 1975; PAWSON et al. 1976; PURCHIO et al. 1977; KERR et al. 1976; MURPHY et al. 1979).[1] PHILIPSON et al. (1978) noted that addition of yeast amber suppressor tRNA to an MLV-vRNA-programmed rabbit reticulocyte lysate translation reaction enhanced production of the Gag-Pol protein at the expense of the Gag protein. This observation strongly suggested that the MLV *gag* and *pol* genes were in the same translational reading frame and separated by a single amber termination codon, a configuration that was at least consistent with the suppression hypothesis. This presumed *gag-pol* configuration was later confirmed by DNA sequencing of an MLV provirus (SHINNICK et al. 1981), but neither the sequence nor the in vitro suppression of the *gag* terminator guranteed that translational suppression was the actual mechanism of MLV *gag-pol* expression in vivo.

In fact, shortly after the report that the MLV Gag-Pol protein could be synthesized in vitro by the addition of nonsense suppressor tRNAs, a similar experiment performed with RSV vRNA produced a contrary result. As had been found with MLV, WEISS et al. (1978) observed that in vitro translation of RSV vRNA in the presence of yeast amber suppressor tRNA reduced the yield of Gag protein. However, rather than producing a corresponding increase in the level of the Gag-Pol protein, this treatment resulted in appearance of a novel, extended Gag protein and no additional Gag-Pol protein. The conclusion from this experiment was that the RSV *gag* gene is terminated by an amber stop codon, but

---

[1] Note that the fact that vRNA can be translated to yield both Gag and Gag-Pol proteins does not by itself distinguish between the suppression and splicing hypotheses since virions could contain both the genome-length mRNA and the potentially very similar, spliced *gag-pol* mRNA

unlike the situation with MLV this terminator is not immediately followed by an inframe *pol* gene. At least one more terminator or a difference in reading frame WEISS and co-authors reasoned stands between the RSV *gag* and *pol* genes. Since they doubted that multiple stop codon or frameshift suppression would be adequately efficient to yield the observed ratio of Gag to Gag-Pol proteins, these authors argued that the most likely mode of *gag-pol* expression of RSV was via the production of a spliced *gag-pol* mRNA (see Fig. 1).

The nucleotide sequence of RSV reported by SCHWARTZ et al. (1983) clarified the genetic structure of the RSV *gag-pol* region. The conclusions drawn from this sequence, however, might have further delayed the ultimate solution to the *gag-pol* problem. Consistent with the in vitro translation data, SCHWARTZ et al. (1983) found that the RSV *gag* gene terminates with the amber stop codon and that this stop codon is followed by a second one in the *gag* reading frame some 111 nucleotides downstream. The *pol* open reading frame (identified by its position relative to *gag* and the presence of a coding region whose predicted amino acid sequence matched the known N-terminal acid sequence of RSV reserse transcriptase) is in a different translational reading frame than *gag*. The 5′-end of the *pol* open reading frame overlaps the 3′-end of *gag* by 58 nucleotides in the − 1 direction. As defined by SCHWARTZ et al. (1983) however, the 5′-end of the *pol* "gene" begins with the portion known to encode reverse transcriptase, located 20 nucleotides downstream of the *gag* terminator. While acknowledging the possibility that ribosomes could shift reading frame during translation of the 58 nucleotide *gag-pol* overlap, these workers firmly concluded that the only reasonable way to synthesize the RSV Gag-Pol protein would be form an RNA derived from the genome-length mRNA by splicing that carried the *gag* and *pol* genes fused in-frame.

The view, first formed with respect to RSV, soon dominated the field of retrovirology generally. This bias is indicated most obviously in the treatment of the subject in the comprehensive review, *RNA Tumor Viruses* (WEISS et al. 1984). Largely based on the evidence presented above, the authors of several chapters allude to the near necessity for an RSV *gag-pol* mRNA. At one point it is claimed that such a species "must" exist (p. 581). Since the replication strategies of the different retroviruses are similar, it was also generally believed that MLV, for which stop codon suppression was at least a structural possibility, and other retroviruses also expressed the Gag-Pol protein from a separate, spliced mRNA.

The splicing hypothesis gained more credibility with the first nucleotide sequence of human T-cell leukemia virus type I (HTLV-I) SEIKI et al. 1983). This sequence included a 300 nucleotide "intergenic" region between *gag* and *pol* that was closed in all three reading frames by multiple termination codons. As such, translation from *gag* into *pol* along the genome-length mRNA would require multiple suppression events. Although physical evidence for a spliced *gag-pol* mRNA was lacking for this or any other virus, this presumed *gag-pol* "intron" seemed to leave no alternative.

In the year 1983, then, the *gag-pol* problem seemed ostensibly solved, awaiting only the isolation and characterization of the elusive *gag-pol* mRNA. In the intervening 6 years, however, the consensus opinion has taken an about-face: the weight of the available evidence favors the view that translational suppression accounts for Gag-Pol synthesis in all retroviruses and many retrotransposons. In the body of this review, I will discuss the experiments that led to the transformation of opinion away from the splicing hypothesis and toward translational suppression. But first, I will conclude this introduction by briefly considering how the incorrect solution became so popular.

The general acceptance of the splicing hypothesis occurred primarily on account of the interpretation of the data concerning RSV (WEISS et al. 1977; SCHWARTZ et al. 1983) and the seemingly irrefutable evidence from HTLV-1 (SEIKI et al. 1983). These papers are, in fact, often cited as evidence for splicing in retroviral *pol* gene expression. With hindsight one can now suggest that both WEISS et al. (1977) and SCHWARTZ et al. (1983) should have been more even-handed with regard to the possible mechanisams of *pol* gene expression. However, they cannot be faulted for favoring a mechanism that was fast becoming the norm in eukaryotic gene expression (mRNA splicing) over one that had no physiological precedent (frameshift suppression). And while these publications strongly influenced the field's perception of the *gag-pol* problem, they actually only solidified an existent bias found generally in favor of mRNA splicing.

More importantly, the conclusions drawn from the RSV data set the stage for what seemed at the time to be overwhelming evidence for splicing in HTLV-1 (SEIKI et al. 1983). In this case there appeared to be no need for interpretation. And, indeed, even now, if faced with a genetic wasteland between the *gag* and *pol* genes of a given virus, one would have to conclude that splicing would be required to generate a joint Gag-Pol protein for that virus. But, in fact, no such retrovirus is known to exist. The originally sequenced clone of HTLV-1 is almost certainly noninfectious. Based on the sequences of two additional HTLV-1 clones (HIRAMATSU et al. 1987; NAM and HATANAKA 1986), it is now clear that the region between HTLV-1 *gag* and *pol* is a coding domain. The region comprises an open reading frame whose predicted product is homologous to known retroviral proteases. Furthermore, the so-called *pro* gene overlaps the 3'-end of *gag* and the 5'-end of *pol*. This overlapping, three gene structure has been observed in several other retroviruses as well (Fig. 2).

Thus, the death knell for the suppression hypothesis was sounded on account of the sequence of a noninfectious clone. This sequence and the interpretations of it, both by the authors and the retrovirological community at large, clearly illustrate the danger of preconceptions. While SEIKI et al. (1983) acknowledge that their clone was not known to be infectious, they nonetheless drew conclusions about HTLV-1 replication based on it. Given that splicing was the accepted mechanism of RSV *gag-pol* expression, the discovery of a putative intron between HTLV-1 *gag* and *pol* did not signal that something might be amiss. It should be noted that a second group later "confirmed" the presence of an intergenic region between *gag* and *pol* of HTLV-1 by sequencing a second, noninfectious HTLV-1 provirus (RATNER et al. 1985b). These are not example of making the data fit the

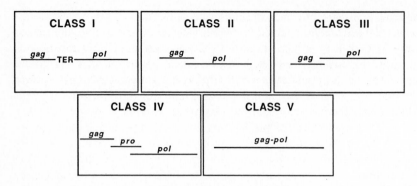

Fig. 2. The genetic structure of the *gag-pol* domains of retroviruses and retrotransposons. *Class I*: *gag* and *pol* in the same translational reading frame separated by a single termination codon (*TER*) MLV (SHINNICK et al. 1981), FeLV (YOSHINAKA et al. 1985b), and baboon endogenous virus (TAMURA et al. 1983) exhibit this arrangement. Class II: *pol* directly overlapping *gag* in the -1 reading frame. Examples of this type include: RSV (SCHWARTZ et al. 1983), HIV-1 (WAIN-HOBSON et al. 1985; RATNER et al. 1985a, SANCHEZ-PESCADOR et al. 1985), HIV-2 (GUYADER et al. 1987), simian immunodeficiency virus (CHAKRABARTI et al. 1987), Visna virus (SONIGO et al. 1985), equine infectious anemia virus (STEPHENS et al. 1986), mouse intracisternal A particle (MEITZ et al. 1987), 17.6 (SAIGO et al. 1985), and gypsy (MARLOR et al. 1987). Class III: *pol* directly overlapping *gag* in the +1 direction. The yeast transposable elements Tyl (CLARE and FARABAUGH 1985; MELLOR et al. 1985) and Ty2 (WILSON et al. 1986) and the murine element L1Md (LOEB et al. 1986) are in this class. Class IV: *gag* and *pol* separated by a third gene (*pro* encoding the viral protease) that overlaps them both. The *pro* and *pol* genes lie in the −1 frame relative to the genes that precede them (*gag* and *pro*). Retroviruses in the class IV category include: MMTV (JACKS et al. 1987; MOORE et al. 1987), simian retrovirus type 1 (POWER et al. 1986), Mason-Pfizer monkey virus (SONIGO et al. 1986), bovine leukemia viurs (SAGATA et al. 1985; RICE et al. 1985), HTLV-1 (NAM and HATANAKA 1986; HIRAMATSU et al. 1987), and HTLV-2 (SHIMOTOHNO et al. 1985). Class V: *gag* and *pol* domains contained in one long open reading frame. Three retrotransposons, *copia* (MOUNT and RUBIN 1985), *Tal* (VAYTAS and AUSUBEL 1988), and *Tnt1* (GRANDBASTIEN et al. 1989), belong to this class

theory; the sequencing data are presumably accurate. Yet the overinterpretation of the data, in light of the uncertainty about the clones, was clearly fitted to the prevailing theory and, as is discussed from here on, an incorrect theory at that.

2 Retrovirus and Retrotransposon Nucleotide Sequences and *gag-pol* Structures

The past 6 years have brought an explosion of nucleotide sequence 5 of retroviruses and retrotransposons from species ranging from yeast to humans. The genetic structures in the *gag-pol* regions of these elements fall into five classes. As shown in Fig. 2, the first class of elements carry *gag* and *pol* in the same translational reading frame separated by a single amber termination codon (Class I). In Class II elements, the 5′-end of the *pol* open reading frame overlaps, the 3′-end of *gag*, with the *pol* frame offset by one nucleotide in the 5′ direction (−1) with respect to the *gag* frame. Class III elements also display directly overlapping *gag* and *pol* genes, but for these the *pol* frame is + 1 relative to the *gag* frame. Six known retroviruses carry an additional open reading frame between *gag* and *pol* that overlaps them both (Class IV). This open reading frame encodes the viral protease and is termed variously "*prt*" and "*pro*"; *pro* is in the − 1 frame relative to *gag* and in the + 1 frame relative to *pol*. Finally, three retrotransposons appear to include both the *gag* and *pol* coding domains in one continuous open reading frame (Class V). For those elements that have overlapping genes, the size of the overlap (defined as the sequence shared by the two open reading frames) ranges from 14 to 205 nucleotides.

3 Discovery of Translational Suppression
During *gag-pol* Synthesis

Members of each of the first four classes of viruses and transposons shown in Fig. 2 are currently known or believed to utilize translational suppression in the synthesis of their Gag fusion proteins. The experiments that led to these conclusions will be described in turn below. As for the retrotransposons designated Class V, in which *gag* and *pol* coding domains share the same long open reading frame, translational suppression is not required for *gag-pol* expression. The mechanism of *gag* expression in these elements is discussed in Sect. 6.

3.1 Class I: Termination Suppression

The first compelling evidence in favor of translational suppression during Gag-Pol synthesis for any retrovirus or retrotransposon came from amino acid sequence analysis of the protease protein of MLV in 1985 (YOSHINAKA et al. 1985a). This protein is initially expressed as part of the MLV Gag-Pol protein; it is responsible for cleaving itself and other mature viral proteins from their precursors. Crude mapping and sequence comparisons had suggested that the MLV protease was encoded upstream of the reverse transcriptase domain, near the 5′-end of *pol* (LEVIN et al. 1984). The N-terminal sequence of the purified protease produced by YOSHINAKA et al. (1985a) revealed that in fact the protein is encoded across the *gag-pol* junction. The first four amino acids of the protease are encoded by the last four codons of *gag*; the fifth amino acid is a glutamine; and the remainder of the protein is encoded by *pol*, beginning with the codon that immediately follows the *gag* terminator. From this amino acid sequence, it was simple to deduce the mechanism of MLV *gag-pol* expression: suppression of the *gag* amber termination codon by a glutamine-charged tRNA. Since all of the nucleotides at the *gag-pol* junction were required to encode the protease, a spliced *gag-pol* mRNA was definitively excluded.

YOSHINAKA et al. (1985b) subsequently sequenced the protease protein of FeLV, another member of the Class I elements shown in Fig. 2. The amino acid sequence once again revealed that the FeLV Gag-Pol protein is expressed via insertion of a glutamine residue in response to the *gag* amber terminator.

Termination suppression at the end of the MLV *gag* gene is not restricted to a UAG terminator. FENG et al. (1989b) have recently reported efficient suppression of the two other termination codons, UAA and UGA, when placed at the end of MLV *gag*. Proviruses harboring either UAA or UGA terminators yielded wild-type levels of virus and *pol* gene products after transfection into tissue culture cells, and in vitro translation of mRNAs transcribed from these mutants produced the normal ratio (1:20) of Gag-Pol to Gag proteins. The fact that all three termination codons are efficiently suppressed at this site suggests that features of the surrounding sequence influence the suppression event (see Sect. 4.2). It is not known which amino acids are inserted in response to the UAA and UGA codons in this setting.

3.2 Class II: − 1 Ribosomal Frameshifting

Once termination suppression had been demonstrated for MLV Gag-Pol synthesis, attention quickly turned to retroviruses and retrotransposons whose *gag* and *pol* genes overlapped. If the basic replication strategies of different retroviruses are similar, these viruses should utilize another form of translational suppression, frameshift suppression, in the synthesis of their Gag fusion proteins. JACKS and VARMUS (1985) tested this possibility for RSV by cloning a DNA fragment derived from the *gag-pol* domain downstream of the *Salmonella* phage 6 (SP6) promoter. In vitro transcription of this clone by SP6 RNA polymerase yielded a homogeneous population of mRNA that mimicked, at least in the *gag-pol* region, the RSV genome-length mRNA. Translation of this synthetic mRNA in a rabbit reticulocyte lysate translation reaction would be expected to generate the Gag polyprotein. However, if some fraction of the ribosomes were able to shift into the -1 reading frame during translation of the 58 nucleotide *gag-pol* overlap, the Gag-Pol protein would also be produced. The result was clear-cut: Both Gag and Gag-Pol proteins were observed, and their ratio (approximately 20:1) closely matched that observed in RSV-infected cells (OPPERMAN et al. 1977). After excluding transcriptional frameshifting and in vitro splicing of the SP6-produced mRNA, these authors concluded that the RSV Gag-Pol protein could be synthesized in vitro from the genome-length mRNA via ribosomal frameshifting. Moreover, the efficiency of frameshifting observed in vitro (∼ 5%) was sufficient to suggest that frameshifting was the mechanism of RSV *gag-pol* expression in vivo as well.

The same experimental strategy was later used to ascertain whether ribosomal frameshifting was responsible for *gag-pol* expression of human immunodefiency virus type 1 (HIV-1) (JACKS et al. 1988a), another of the Class II elements (Fig. 2). Just as with RSV, in vitro translation of a synthetic mRNA

Table 1. Heptanucleotide frameshift sites. Common 7-nucleotide sequence motifs are present in all retroviral and retrotransposon overlaps known or presumed to contain sites of frameshifting. The heptanucleotides are shown (*upper case*) along with their neighboring sequences and their distance (in nucleotides) upstream of the 0-frame termination codon. *Triplets* denote codons in the 0-frame. References for nucleotide sequences are found in the legend to Fig. 2. Table is adapted from JACKS et al. 1988b)

Retrovirus or retrotransposon	Overlap	Sequence	Distance upstream of 0-frame terminator
RSV	gag/pol	ACA AAU UUA UAG	0
HIV–1	gag/pol	AAU UUU UUA GGG	198
HIV–2	gag/pol	GGU UUU UUA GGA	267
SIV	gag/pol	GGU UUU UUA GGC	213
Gypsy	gag/pol	AAU UUU UUA GGG	51
MMTV	pro/pol	CAG GAU UUA UGA	0
SRV–1	pro/pol	GGA AAU UUU UAA	0
MPMV	pro/pol	GGA AAU UUU UAA	0
17.6	gag/pol	GAA AAU UUU CAG	30
Mouse IAP	gag/pol	CUG GGU UUU CCU	3
MMTV	gag/pro	UCA AAA AAC UUG	3
BLV	gag/pro	UCA AAA AAC UAA	0
HTLV–1	gag/pro	CCA AAA AAC UCC	18
HTLV–2	gag/pro	GGA AAA AAC UCC	18
EIAV	gag/pol	CCA AAA AAC GGG	195
BLV	pro/pol	CCU UUA AAC UAG	0
HTLV–1	pro/pol	CCU UUA AAC CAG	156
HTLV–2	pro/pol	CCU UUA AAC CUG	18
SRV–I	gag/pro	CAG GGA AAC GAC	147
MPMV	gag/pro	CAG GGA AAC GGG	147
Visna	gag/pol	CAG GGA AAC AAC	45

carrying the HIV-1 *gag* and *pol* genes in their genomic, out-of-frame configuration yielded both Gag and Gag-Pol proteins. The Gag to Gag-Pol protein ratio observed in vitro for HIV-1 was approximately 10:1, suggesting that frameshifting is more efficient on the HIV-1 mRNA than on the RSV message. It is not known whether this higher efficiency also occurs in vivo, since there are not yet accurate estimates of the ratio of Gag to Gag-Pol proteins in HIV-1-infected cells.

While the other retroviruses belonging to this class have not been directly tested, they are likely to utilize ribosomal frameshifting also. Putative frameshift signals are present in the *gag-pol* overlaps of each of them (see Table 1).

3.3 Class III: + 1 Ribosomal Frameshifting

In two known retrotransposons, the *pol* reading frame is offset by one nucleotide in the 3′ direction relative to *gag*. Thus, translation from *gag* into *pol* would require + 1 ribosomal frameshifting for these elements. The *gag-pol* expression in one member of this class, TY of *Saccharomyces cerevisiae*, has been examined by the laboratories of Farabough and Kingsman and Kingsman. Both groups have monitored expression of the *pol*-like gene (*tyb*) by inserting a reporter gene (lacZ or α-interferon) just downstream of the *tya*(*gag*)-*tyb* overlap. Despite the absence of an initiator methionine codon in the *pol* frame upstream of the reporter genes, a high level of expression of these genes was observed (CLARE and FARABOUGH 1985; MELLOR et al. 1985). Furthermore, Western blot analysis detected the reporter proteins at a molecular weight consistent with them being fused to the product of the upstream *tya* gene. Synthesis of this fusion protein did not appear to require mRNA splicing, as Northern blot and S1 nuclease analysis failed to detect a spliced mRNA species. As had been true in the earlier studies characterizing retroviral mRNAs, this type of analysis cannot exclude a very small splice in the *gag-pol* overlap. However, it is suggestive that Ty-1 utilizes ribosomal frameshifting in the expression of its Gag-Pol protein.

This claim has been strengthened by further experiments performed by the same two groups. WILSON et al. (1986) reported that the more sensitive S1 analysis, capable of detecting a splice as small as five nucleotides, still failed to detect a spliced *tya-tyb* mRNA in yeast cells. CLARE et al. (1988) used direct mRNA sequencing to rule out both splicing and mRNA editing of the *tya-tyb* mRNA. Thus, production of the Tya-Tyb fusion protein is a posttranscriptional event, almost certainly + 1 ribosomal frameshifting. CLARE et al. (1988) also noted that the β-galactosidase activity in a yeast strain containing a frameshift-requiring lacZ fusion was only fivefold below that obtained with an "in-frame" control, indicating a frameshifting efficiency of approximately 20%.

3.4 Class IV: Double Ribosomal Frameshifting

The retroviruses in this class represent the greatest challenge to the suppression hypothesis. In order to continue translation from *gag* to *pol* on the genome-length mRNAs of these viruses, ribosomes would have to change reading frames twice, first during translation of the *gag-pro* overlap and then again in the *pro-pol* overlap (Fig. 2). (Both of these frameshifts would be in the − 1 direction.) Ribosomes that only shifted frame in the *gag-pro* overlap would be expected to generate a Gag-Pro fusion protein. Such a fusion has been observed in cells infected by MMTV (DICKSON and ATTERWILL 1979). Furthermore, if the ratio of the Gag to Gag-Pro-Pol proteins of viruses in this class is similar to the Gag to Gag-Pol protein ratios seen in RSV- and MLV-infected cells (and this appears to be true for, at least, MMTV), the efficiency of frameshifting in at least one of the two overlaps would need to be higher than the 5%–10% previously observed for RSV (JACKS·and VARMUS 1985) and HIV-1 (JACKS et al. 1988a). (Two successive frameshift events of 10% efficiency would result in a Gag to Gag-Pro-Pol protein ratio of 100 to 1.)

Ribosomal frameshifting on MMTV mRNA has been examined in two ways. MOORE et al. (1987) and JACKS et al. (1987) used the same in vitro assay for frameshifting as discussed above. They synthesized artificial mRNAs in vitro containing the *gag-pro-pol* portion of the MMTV genome. In addition to yielding the Gag protein, in vitro translation of these messages produced a Gag-Pro fusion protein and to a lesser extent a Gag-Pro-Pol fusion, the two expected products of frameshifting. The identities of the products were confirmed by immunoprecipitation and by truncation of the DNA templates at numerous positions prior to transcription. The comparative yield of the Gag-specific protein and the two Gag fusions indicated frameshifting efficiencies in the *gag-pro* and *pro-pol* overlaps of approximately 25% and 10%, respectively. Thus, one in four translating ribosomes changes frame in the *gag-pro* overlap, and of those, one in ten shifts into the *pol* frame in the *pro-pol* overlap. The ratio of the presumed Gag, Gag-Pro, and Gag-Pro-Pol proteins seen in MMTV-infected cells is approximately 30:10:1 (DICKSON and ATTERWILL 1979). Once again, the frameshifting efficiencies derived in vitro are consistent with this being the mechanism of expression in vivo as well.

Oroszlan's group has addressed the problem of suppression in MMTV as was done for MLV: protein purification and amino acid sequencing. HIZI et al. (1987) purified from MMTV virions a protein termed p30, suspected to be the C-terminal cleavage product of the *gag-pro* fusion, p110$^{gag-pro}$. Indeed, upon determining the entire amino acid sequence of p30, these workers could demonstrate that the protein was encoded by both the *gag* and *pro* genes and identify the position on the mRNA at which the reading frame switched. At one of two adjacent codons within the *gag-pro* overlap, the amino acid sequence indicated, ribosomes shifted by one nucleotide in the 5' direction, moving from the *gag* frame into the *pro* frame. The nature of this frameshift site will be discussed in more detail below.

4 Mechanistic Considerations

The experiments discussed in the previous section have at once solved the *gag-pol* problem and introduced another set of problems altogether. What features of retroviral or retrotransposon mRNA allow or encourage such high-level suppression? The spontaneous rate of frameshifting (at least in *E. coli*) is approximately 3×10^5 per codon (KURLAND 1978), and yet at certain codons in MMTV and TY mRNA frameshifting occurs at the staggering frequency of one in four or five. Termination suppression occurs at the end of the MLV and FeLV *gag* genes at least one hundred times more often then at typical stop codons (CAPONE et al. 1986). What *trans*-acting factors, cellular or viral, are involved in these processes? While our understanding of these issues is far from complete, there has been some progress recently. Where appropriate, I will compare these fledgling models for suppression in retroviral genes with those emerging in other systems, particularly in *E. coli*.

4.1 *cis*-Acting Sequences

Identification of Suppression Sites. By deducing the site of a suppression event, one can potentially learn a great deal about the event itself. This does not apply to termination suppression, of course; by definition suppression occurs at the terminator. In contrast, productive frameshifting can occur at any point along the mRNA where the involved genes overlap. In some cases the overlaps between retroviral genes are greater than 200 nucleotides in length (see Table 1).

The only definitive method of localizing a frameshift site is to sequence the relevant portion of the "trans-frame" protein (defined as a protein encoded by at least two overlapping open reading frames via ribosomal frameshifting). As discussed above, Hizi et al. (1987) used this approach to localize the point of transition from the *gag* to *pro* frames of MMTV to either an AAC-asparagine or a UUG-leucine codon in the *gag* frame within the *gag-pro* overlap. (The prsence of an overlapping leucine codon in the *pro* frame leads to this ambiguity.) Three other -1 frameshift sites have been deduced by amino acid sequencing, all from trans-frame proteins synthesized in vitro in a rabbit reticulocyte system. Jacks and coworkers (1988a,b) have cloned portions of the *gag-pol* overlaps of RSV and HIV-1 downstream of an initiator methionine and a short leader sequence. Translation of mRNA transcribed in vitro from these templates would be expected to produce trans-frame proteins whose N-termini would be within 15 amino acids of the sites of frameshifting. The mRNAs were translated in the presence of several different radioactive amino acids, and the amino acid sequence of the purified proteins deduced from the radioactivity profile of the products of progressive Edman degradation. These analyses identified the same type of codon, a UUA-leucine, as the frameshift site in both the RSV and HIV-1 *gag-pol* overlaps. Amino acid sequencing of the product of a functional point mutant in the RSV frameshift site demonstrated that frameshifting will also occur at a UUU-phenylalanine codon in this context (Jacks et al. 1988b).

Amino acid sequence information is not yet available for the TY transframe protein. However, deletion analysis has implicated a short sequence within the *tya-tyb* overlap. This 11-nucleotide sequence is conserved between the otherwise fairly divergent types of TY elements, TY-1 and TY-2 (Wilson et al. 1986). Furthermore, a 14-nucleotide sequence containing these 11 nucleotides is sufficient to direct + 1 frameshifting when placed in an unrelated mRNA (Clare et al. 1988). Thus, this sequence appears to be necessary and sufficient for + 1 frameshifting in yeast cells. Precisely where or by what mechanism the frameshift event occurs must await amino acid sequencing and more detailed mutational analysis.

Heptanucleotide Consensus Sequences for − 1 Frameshift Sites. The study of the − 1 frameshift events has benefitted from the numerous documented or suspected examples (see Fig. 2). Even before they were confirmed by amino acid sequencing, the AAC-asparagine codon in the MMTV *gag-pro* overlap and the UUA-leucine codons in the RSV and HIV-1 *gag-pol* overlaps were suspected to be involved in frameshifting, simply because these same codons are found in the overlaps of several other retroviruses and some retrotransposons. In fact, as shown in Table 1, the overlaps of all of the elements in Classes II and IV of Fig. 2 contain one of the three following sequences: U UUA, U UUU, or A AAC, where the triplet is a codon in the upstream open reading frame. [While the U UUU sequence has not been shown to be the site of frameshifting in any of its native contexts, this sequence will substitute for the natural RSV site (JACKS et al. 1988b; see above).]

The similarity between the overlap sequences actually extends upstream of these putative frameshift sites. In every case save one, these sites are preceded by runs of three A, U, or G residues (Table 1). (The U UUA sequence in the MMTV *pro-pol* overlap, the one exception, is preceded by the sequence GGA.) These similarities suggest that the − 1 frameshift signals encompass seven nucleotides: two adjacent codons and the nucleotide that precedes them.

A Model for − 1 Frameshifting: Simultaneous Slippage. The conserved structure of the documented or suspected − 1 frameshift sites suggests how they might function (JACKS et al. 1988b). This model is shown for the RSV sequence A AAU UUA in Fig. 3. Normal translation delivers the ribosome to the conformation depicted in step I: the AAU codon resident in the P site complexed with tRNA^{Asn} carrying the nascent peptide and the adjacent UUA codon decoded by tRNA^{Leu} in the A site. Slippage by both tRNAs by one nucleotide in the 5′ direction leads to the conformation shown in step II with both tRNAs paired to the overlapping *pol* frame codons, AAA and UUU. Assuming conventional Watson-Crick base-pairs between the tRNA anticodons and their *gag*-frame codons, this *pol*-frame pairing

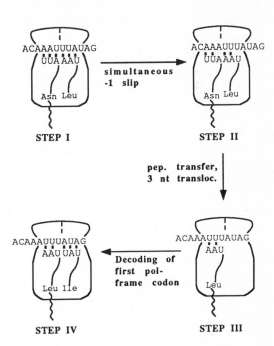

Fig. 3. Simultaneous slippage model for frameshifting. *Step I:* Peptidyl-tRNA^{Asn} and aminoacyl-tRNA^{Leu} are bound to the *gag*-frame codons AAU and UUA. *Step II:* Slippage by both tRNAs by one nucleotide in the 5′ direction results in mispairing to the *pol*-frame codons AAA and UUU. *Step III:* Peptidyl transfer and 3-nucleotide translocation brings the first decoded *pol*-frame codon, AUA, into the ribosomal A site. *Step IV:* Entry of the aminoacyl-tRNA^{Ile} into the A begins translation in *pol*. This model is illustrated for the RSV *gag-pol* frameshift site, but all of the other heptanucleotide sequences shown in Table 1 could substitute for it. Adapted from JACKS et al. (1988b)

would involve only the first two anticodon positions of each tRNA. Peptidyl transfer and three-nucleotide translocation then brings the tRNA^{Leu} (and the nascent peptide) to the P site, delivering the *pol*-frame codon AUA-isoleucine to the A site (step III). Normal translation in the *pol* frame begins with the decoding of the AUA codon by tRNA^{Ile} (step IV). The other heptanucleotide sequences shown in Table 1 could substitute for the RSV sequence in Fig. 3. Although in some cases different tRNAs species would be required, the basic mechanism of single nucleotide slippage by adjacent tRNAs is maintained.

Evidence in Favor of the Simultaneous Slippage Model. Support for the simultaneous slippage model has come not only from the amino acid sequences discussed above but also from mutational analysis of several frameshift sites. The − 1 slippage at the so-called A-site codon (for example, the RSV UUA codon; Fig. 3) is consistent with the amino acid sequences of the trans-frame proteins of MMTV, RSV, and HIV-1 (HIZI et al. 1987; JACKS et al. 1988a,b). These sequences implicate the predicted *gag*-frame codons and show that the first *pol*-frame codon decoded is that which directly overlaps the A-site codon. Certain alternative mechanisms for frameshifting at this site would predict different amino acid sequences. For example, if the tRNA reading the A-site codon were to translocate five nucleotides instead of the normal three or slip by two nucleotides in the 3′ direction, the overlapping *pol*-frame codon would be bypassed, and the first decoded *pol*-frame codon would be the next one in line. However, the amino acid sequence analysis alone cannot confirm the -1 slippage model. A mechanism such as 2-nucleotide translocation by the A-site tRNA would also predict the observed amino acid sequences.

The simultaneous − 1 slippage model of frameshifting in retroviral overlaps (Fig. 3) is more strongly supported by the effects of point mutations in the frameshift sites in the RSV and HIV-1 *gag-pol* overlaps. For both of these viruses, frameshifting occurs at UUA codons preceded by another U residue. The proposed model predicts that all three of the U residues in the sequence U UUA are necessary for frame shifting as part of the O- or -1-frame codons bound by the tRNA^{Leu} before and after slippage (Fig. 3). Indeed, mutation of any of the U residues in this sequence in the RSV frameshift site to any other nucleotide eliminates production of the *gag-pol* protein in vitro (JACKS et al. 1988b). Frameshifting in the HIV-1 overlap is also abolished if either of the first two U residues of the U UUA sequence are changed to C or the final U to any nucleotide (JACKS et al. 1988a; WILSON et al. 1988).[2]

The evidence cited above quite convincingly established simple tRNA slippage as the mechanism by which ribosomes are redirected into the -1 frame

---

[2] Interestingly, mutations of the A position in the U UUA sequences of RSV and HIV-1 are not inhibitory, and, in fact, changing the A to U causes an approximately twofold increase in activity in both cases (JACKS et al. 1988b; WILSON et al. 1988). These results suggest that in addition to tRNA^{Leu}, tRNA^{Phe} can also mediate frameshifting along a run of U residues in these contexts. Indeed, amino acid sequencing of a trans-frame protein produced by the RSV A-to-U mutant has shown a phenylalanine residue at the transition from the *gag* to *pol* frames. The sequence U UUU is also thought to be the naturally occurring frameshift site in several retroviral genes (see Table 1)

during frameshifting in retroviral overlaps. The claims that the responsible tRNAs are in the ribosomal A site when the slip occurs and that this slip is coupled with a similar one by the adjacent P-site tRNA (Fig. 3) are less well grounded. As predicted by the model, mutations in the run of three A residues that precede the RSV U UUA sequence do inhibit frameshifting in vitro (by approximately 80%), and a mutation affecting nucleotides directly preceding these A residues has no obvious effect on frameshifting (JACKS et al. 1988b). Furthermore, mutations in the *gag* termination codon, which directly follows the UUA codon, also do not inhibit frameshifting in vitro. These mutations might have been expected to influence frameshifting if the tRNA^{Leu} were to slip into the P site rather than in the A site. Also, mutations in the central position of the HIV-1 P-site codon UUU strongly inhibit frameshifting. Finally, the mere conservation of the heptameric sequence motif in all Class II and Class IV overlaps is very suggestive that two adjacent codons are involved in the process. Nevertheless, disruption of the run of A residues upstream of the RSV U UUA sequence does not abolish frameshifting (these mutants function at approximately 20% the wild-type activity), suggesting that slippage by the P-site tRNA may not be obligatory during the process of frameshifting but might merely facilitate slippage by the A-site tRNA.

Other Examples of tRNA Slippage in Frameshifting. tRNA slippage along homopolymeric sequences has been proposed to account for frameshifting in a number of systems. Stretches of U residues have been suggested as the sites of frameshifting in gene 10 of bacteriophage T7 (DUNN and STUDIER 1983) and in leaky + 1 and − 1 frameshift-mutant alleles of the yeast mitochondrial gene *oxi*1 (Fox and WEISS-BRUMMER 1980). Frameshifting in the release factor II (RFII) gene of *E. coli* has been shown to involve mispairing of the tRNA reading the last 0-frame codon with the overlapping + 1-frame codon (WEISS et al. 1988). WEISS and co-workers (1987) have also demonstrated tRNA slippage by one or more nucleotides in both the 5′ and 3′ directions along numerous synthetic homopolymeric sequences in *E. coli*.

Unlike the simultaneous slippage model for frameshifting in retroviral overlaps, none of these examples is thought to involve slippage by tRNAs at both ribosomal sites. In fact, both for the RFII gene and the synthetic homopolymeric sequences in *E. coli*, the positioning of stop codons adjacent to the frameshift sites greatly increases the frameshifting efficiency (WEISS et al. 1987). This finding suggests that tRNA slippage occurs in the ribosomal P site, while the terminator is in the A site. The positive effect of the stop codons on frameshifting in these settings could result from their extending the time that the frameshift-mediating tRNAs are in the P site (due to slower decoding of the terminator), thereby increasing the probability of P-site tRNA slippage. A different mechanism for achieving this end during frameshifting in retroviral genes is discussed below.

Presumed + 1 Frameshift Sites. In the yeast transposable elements TY-1 and TY-2 the frameshift sites have been grossly defined by the observation that these two elements shared a common 11-nucleotide sequence in their *tya-tyb* overlaps

(WILSON et al. 1986) and, more persuasively, by the demonstration that a 14-nucleotide sequence containing this 11-mer allows frameshifting when placed in a heterologous genetic context (CLARE et al. 1988). The conserved sequence, 5'U CUU AGG CCA C3' (where triplets denote codons in the *tya* frame), is clearly not related to the heptanucleotide frameshift sites described above. Despite the difference in the polarity of the frameshift events, one might have expected that Ty elements possess a similar motif, with the nucleotide sequence arranged to allow tandem tRNAs to shift into the +1 frame. However, this sequence is not indicative of slippage by even one tRNA, nor, in fact, of any alternative mechanism.

Experiments performed in *E. coli* might shed some light on the mechanism of frameshifting with TY RNA. Recently, SPANJAARD and VAN DUIN (1988) observed high-level +1 frameshifting during translation of introduced, adjacent AGG-arginine codons in an otherwise normal mRNA in *E. coli* cells. They postulate that the low abundance of the *E. coli* tRNA isoacceptor that reads AGG results in failure to decode this AGG-AGG doublet properly. Similarly, WEISS and GALLANT (1983) and ATKINS et al. (1979) have reported frameshifting in *E. coli* cells or in vitro translation extracts upon alterations in the concentrations of various charged tRNA species. Frameshifting in these contexts could be a result of improper pairing of a noncognate tRNA in the vacant ribosomal A site (ATKINS et al. 1979) or pairing by a cognate tRNA to an out-of-frame codon (WEISS and GALLANT 1983). In all cases, increasing the concentration of the tRNA corresponding to the "hungry codon" inhibits or eliminates frameshifting. The putative frameshift site in TY may function analogously, since both the CUU and AGG codons (found within the implicated 11-nucleotide sequence) are rarely used in yeast cells and, therefore, probably have correspondingly rare tRNAs (BENNETZEN and HALL 1982).

Although the LINE element L1Md is listed in Fig. 2 as a second example of an element with a directly +1 overlapping *pol* gene, there is as yet no direct evidence that this element utilizes frameshifting to produce a fusion protein. Given the sequence of the 14-nucleotide overlap region in L1Md (LOEB et al. 1986), it is not evident where or how frameshifting would occur there. None of the five codons in the upstream (*gag*-like) frame are conspicuously rare, nor is there a long homopolymeric run of nucleotides. Development of an in vitro assay would greatly facilitate study of frameshifting for this element.

4.2 Additional *cis*-Acting Signals: A Role for RNA Secondary Structure in Suppression

Given that random errors in translation, such as read-through of a termination codon or shift in reading frame, are infequent, the high-level suppression events that occur in retroviral and retrotransposon genes would seem to require specialized signals in the mRNA in order to amplify the frequency of ribosomal miscues. In part these signals must involve the sequence at the point of suppression, along with its neighboring nucleotide context. I have already discussed the documented and presumed frameshift sites of several retrovirus and retrotransposon genes, and these do encompass sequences several nucleotides in length. While the nucleotide requirements around the *gag* terminators of MLV and FeLV are not known, we presume that the context of the stop codon is equally important here. Indeed, the efficient suppression of UAA and UGA stop codons at the end of MLV *gag* (FENG et al. 1989b) strongly suggests a role for "context" in this case as well. Also, termination suppression in *E. coli* is strongly influenced by the identity of the nucleotide that immediately follows the stop codon (BOSSI 1983; MILLER and ALBERTINI 1983).

There is growing evidence, however, that attention to only the sequence that immediately flank the suppression site might be too narrowly focussed. At least in the case of heptanucleotide − 1 frameshift signals (see above), these very sequences appear in the correct reading frame in numerous cellular genes for which there is no evidence (or suspicion) of frameshifting (JACKS et al. 1988b; WILSON et al. 1988). In addition, the heptanucleotide sequences found in the MMTV *gag-pro* and *pro-pol* overlaps (as well as the other nucleotides of the overlaps) are insufficient to direct frameshifting in a novel genetic context (JACKS et al. 1987).

Stem-loop Structures and − 1 Frameshifting. The failure of the MMTV *gag-pro* and *pro-pol* overlaps to act in isolation (JACKS et al. 1987) demonstrates that frameshifting efficiency can be affected by sequences outside of the frameshift site. In this case, the negative effect could result from inhibition by surrounding sequences in the nonfunctional mRNAs or the absence of a necessary positive element normally present either upstream or downstream of the frameshift sites in MMTV mRNA. In favor of the latter possibility, JACKS et al. (1987) noted potential stem-loop structures downstream of the two MMTV overlaps. RICE et al. (1985) and SAGATA et al. (1985) had previously called attention to the potential for stem-loop structures downstream of the *gag-pro* overlaps of BLV. In fact, the sequences downstream of all of the putative frameshift sites listed in Table 1 can be folded into stem-loop structures of reasonable stability. A representative set of these is shown in Fig. 4. The structures vary somewhat in the length of the stems and loops, considerably in their base composition, and slightly in the distance between the base of the stem and the frameshift site, but for every retrovirus and retrotransposon known (or suspected) to utilize − 1 frameshifting a stem-loop structure can be drawn within 9 nucleotides of the last base of the putative frameshift site.

Direct support for the involvement of RNA secondary structure during ribosomal frameshifting in retroviral genes has come from mutational analysis of the sequences downstream of the RSV frameshift site (JACKS et al. 1988b). Deletion mutations that remove *pol* sequences beginning 23 nucleotides downstream of the base of the stem-loop do not affect frameshifting efficiency in vitro, whereas mutations that remove any or all of the stem structure severely inhibit frameshifting. Interestingly, one mutation that deletes sequences just up to the

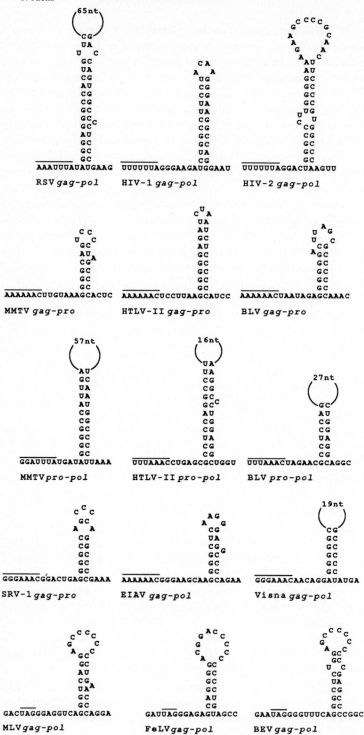

RSV *gag-pol*   HIV-1 *gag-pol*   HIV-2 *gag-pol*

MMTV *gag-pro*   HTLV-II *gag-pro*   BLV *gag-pro*

MMTV *pro-pol*   HTLV-II *pro-pol*   BLV *pro-pol*

SRV-1 *gag-pro*   EIAV *gag-pol*   Visna *gag-pol*

MLV *gag-pol*   FeLV *gag-pol*   BEV *gag-pol*

base of the RSV stem also inhibits frameshifting, suggesting a possible necessary interaction between sequences in the loop and those downstream of the stem (a so-called pseudo-knot structure; see below). In addition, these deletion mutations were used to demonstrate that a 147-nucleotide sequence from RSV, containing the frameshift site and stem-loop, are sufficient to direct frameshifting in a heterologous genetic context (JACKS et al. 1988b).

To confirm that the RSV stem-loop structure per se is necessary for efficient frameshifting (rather some portion of its primary sequence), JACKS et al. (1988b) constructed site-directed mutations in the stem. Translation of mRNAs containing either of two complementary mutations in the 5′ and 3′ arms of the stem failed to produce any observable Gag-Pol protein. However, when these two mutations were combined in the same mRNA, returning the potential for base-pairing, frameshifting was restored to approximately 50% of the wild-type level.

Given the demonstrated need for mRNA secondary structure during frameshifting in the RSV *gag-pol* region, a similar requirement in other relevant retroviral and retrotransposon genes would seem likely. At least for the −1 frameshift events, the similarity between the putative frameshift sites (Table 1) suggests a conservation of mechanism, and, as discussed above, all of these frameshift sites are followed by sequences that could assume a secondary structure (see Fig. 4). However, experiments performed on HIV-1 show that high-level frameshifting can occur in at least some of these frameshift sites in the absence of obvious downstream secondary structure. MADHANI et al. (1988) constructed a large series of mutations in the region downstream of the HIV-1 frameshift site. For all but one of these mutations, the in vitro frameshifting activity was indistinguishable from wild type. It is not clear why the single mutation had an inhibitory effect. Similarly, WILSON et al. 1988 reported high-level frameshifting in vitro and in yeast cells on a short HIV-1 sequence that does not include the nucleotides involved in the potential stem-loop structure. Thus, at least for HIV-1, a stem-loop structure is not required for efficient frameshifting in vitro or in vivo.

One possible explanation for the differing requirements for different retroviruses has recently arisen from the work of BRIERLEY et al. (1989) concerning a different type of virus altogether. These workers, who had previously provided evidence that the coronavirus avian infectious bronchitis virus (IBV) utilizes frameshifting (BRIERLEY et al. 1988; see also Sect. 6), have now carefully defined the sequences necessary for efficient frameshifting in vitro. In addition to the nucleotides of the presumed frameshift site, UUUAAAC (a site also seen in several retroviral overlaps; Table 1), approximately eighty nucleotides immediately downstream are also required. From the previous work on retroviruses described above, one would assume that these downstream sequences would form a stem-loop structure. However, by constructing numerous mutations and

◄ ────────────────────────────────────

Fig. 4. Potential stem-loop structures located downstream of retroviral frameshift and termination suppression sites. Predicted stem-loop structures are shown relative to known or suspected sites of suppression (*overlined*). References for nucleotide sequences are found in the legend to Fig. 2

compensatory mutations, BRIERLEY et al. (1989) have shown quite convincingly that the notion of a simple stem-loop is incorrect. Rather, this downstream region must fold into a more complex three-dimensional structure, most likely a pseudo-knot, for efficient frameshifting to proceed.

This finding may help explain two remaining questions about retroviral frameshifting. First, for RSV, where the potential exists for base-pairing between loop nucleotides and sequences downstream of the stem, a requirement for pseudo-knot formation would explain the inhibitory effects of a deletion mutation that leaves the basic stem-loop structure intact (JACKS et al. 1988b; see above). BRIERLEY et al. (1989) have also noted that while many other proposed retroviral stem-loop structures could also form pseudo-knot structures, the proposed HIV-1 structure cannot. Perhaps the HIV-1 frameshift sequence has evolved to the point where a contribution from the downstream structure is not required, and the potential stem-loop structure present there is either unrelated to frameshifting or is a vestigial remnant of a former pseudo-knot. It is also possible that the less energetically stable simple stem-loop structure subtly enhances frameshifting efficiency from what is already a particularly "leaky" frameshift site.

Status of Secondary Structure in +1 Frameshifting and Termination Suppression. Given that retroviruses and retrotransposons do utilize similar strategies to express their *gag*-related gene products, and since they all presumably evolved from some primordial "retro-element", we might expect that the various types of translational suppression would be mechanistically related. However, as already discussed above, this does not seem to hold when comparing the structure of the putative −1 and +1 frameshift sites. Also, there is no evidence that mRNA secondary structure is required for frameshifting in the TY-1 overlap (CLARE et al. 1988).

On the other hand, recent experiments addressing the sequence requirements for suppression of the MLV *gag* terminator have suggested that this event may also be dependent on some type of mRNA structure in the neighboring *pol* sequence. FELSENSTEIN and GOFF (1989), assaying MLV termination suppression in vivo, found inhibitory effects by mutations in several nucleotide positions downstream of the *gag* terminator. Although not yet conclusive, these results suggest that the necessary *pol* sequences assume a required secondary (or tertiary) structure. As shown in Fig. 4, potential stem-loop structures exist downstream of the *gag* terminator in the three viruses known or believed to use termination suppression.

Possible Functions for Stem-loop Structures. The presence of an adjacent stem-loop structure could enhance suppression efficiency in several ways. For frameshift suppression, the downstream structure might actually force a fraction of ribosomes at the frameshift site into the −1 frame. The structure (either the stem or loop) might be the binding site for a ribosomal protein, soluble translation factor, or ribosomal RNA. This interaction could destabilize the codon-anticodon interaction which would promote tRNA slippage or mispairing of a tRNA to a termination codon. Arguing against any sequence-specific interaction, though, is the lack of primary sequence similarity between the various stem-loops (Fig. 4).

A downstream stem-loop structure could also function by simply slowing translation through the suppression site, allowing increased time for the suppression event to occur. In the case of RSV *gag-pol* suppression, the presence of the stem-loop does cause a subset of ribosomes to pause at or near the frameshift site (JACKS et al. 1988b). Translational time-course experiments performed on various RSV mRNA have shown a distinct but transient protein species that comigrates with the expected product of pausing at the frameshift site. The abundance of this "pause product" is greatly reduced when the time-course is performed on an mRNA in which the stem structure has been perturbed. The effect of pausing could be to broaden the time window during which tRNA slippage could occur, thereby increasing the likelihood that a frameshift would have taken place prior to the ensuing tRNA translocation. Pausing at a stem-loop structure could increase the efficiency of termination suppression if the position of the paused ribosome precluded entry by the release factor but not the suppressor tRNA.

The concept of increased "error" with decreased translation rate runs counter to the generally accepted notion that accuracy is sacrificed for increased speed of translation (YARUS and THOMPSON 1983). Several lines of evidence suggest that the need for rapid protein synthesis prevents ribosomes from exercising their full potential to discriminate between cognate and noncognate tRNAs. Reducing the rate of translation by drugs or ribosomal mutations can decrease the frequency of missense errors (THOMPSON and KARIM 1982; THOMPSON 1988). However, YARUS and THOMPSON (1983) have pointed out that errors requiring kinetically slow reactions might be enhanced if translation itself were slowed. Thus, frame maintenance and proper termination may be normally achieved, at least in part, by limiting the time that ribosome-bound tRNAs have to sample the alternative reading frames or for potential suppressor tRNAs to access a termination codon. This hypothesis could be tested directly by examining the effects on translational suppression by agents that artificially slow translation.

4.3 *trans*-Acting Factors

In addition to the *cis*-acting sequences at the suppression sites and possible nearby structures, translational suppression in retroviral and retrotransposon genes must be dependent on certain *trans*-acting factors. At the very least, the tRNA species that carry out the suppression events are necessary conspirators. Specialized factors, viral or cellular, ribosomal proteins, and ribosomal RNAs could also potentially be involved.

Suppressor tRNAs. To date the only implicated *trans*-acting factor for any of these suppression events is a rare glutamine tRNA species able to suppress amber stop codons. This tRNA was isolated by KUCHINO et al. (1987) by virtue of its ability to suppress efficiently the amber terminator at the end of the coat gene of tobacco mosaic virus. Interestingly, the level of this tRNA species is significantly higher in mouse NIH 3T3 cells that are infected with MLV compared with uninfected 3T3 cells, suggesting that MLV infection might specifically induce expression of the gene for this tRNA. This is an intriguing result since it implies that the virus actively promotes translational suppression rather than simply providing the necessary *cis*-acting sequences and relying on the host for the rest.

The result is also surprising for several reasons. First, it has been known for some time that in vitro translation of MLV vRNA results in a Gag to Gag-Pol ratio that approximates the ratio observed in infected cells (KERR et al. 1976; MURPHY and ARLINGHAUS 1978). FENG et al. (1989a) have recently used a similar in vitro assay to compare the amount of suppressor tRNA activity in normal and MLV-infected cells, and they find no difference between the two cell types. PANGANIBAN (1988) has constructed a vector for assaying termination suppression in vivo containing approximately 300 nucleotides surrounding the *gag* terminator of AKV (a mouse retrovirus derived from an endogenous retrovirus harbored by AKR mouse strains and closely related to MLV). Introduction of this vector into several cell types resulted in approximately 10% suppression of the amber terminator. Significantly, NIH 3T3 cells infected with an amphotropic murine retrovirus did not show an increased level of suppression. Finally, high-level suppression also occurs at both UAA and UGA stop codons placed at the end of MLV *gag* (FENG et al. 1988b). While the glutamine tRNA proposed to be induced by MLV infection might also act on a UAA terminator, it is unlikely to account for UGA suppression (FENG et al. 1989b). Thus, if MLV infection does induce expression of the relevant glutamine tRNA species, this induction appears superfluous, at least in the systems in which it has been studied to date. Perhaps increased production of the suppressor tRNA is only necessary during infection of certain cell types or in the context of the whole animal where host antiviral factors might otherwise limit suppression frequency.

None of the frameshift-mediating tRNAs has been isolated to date. The fact that retroviral Gag-fusion proteins have been detected in several cell types and in vitro translation systems suggests that the tRNAs involved in -1 frameshift are widely distributed. It is interesting that all of the putative -1 frameshift sites include one of three A-site codons: UUU, UUA, or AAC (Table 1). Perhaps the tRNAs that decode these codons are particularly suited for slippage.

Frameshift-suppressor tRNAs have been detected following genetic selection in bacteria and yeast (RIDDLE and ROTH 1970; ROTH and CARBON 1973; ROTH 1974; KOHNO and ROTH 1978; BOSSI and ROTH 1981; GABER and CULBERTSON 1984; BOSSI and SMITH 1984). The most common of these suppressors have an extra nucleotide in the anticodon loop and seem to function by occupying four message nucleotides instead of the normal three, forcing the ribosome into the $+1$ reading frame. This type of RNA could function to suppress the $+1$ frameshift in TY-1, although they have not been observed in wild-type yeast strains. One -1 frameshift suppressor tRNA has been characterized from *Salmonella* (D. J. O'MAHONEY et al. 1988, unpublished observations). It lacks one of the normal anticodon loop nucleotides and is thought to cause -1 frameshifting by translocating, or otherwise occupying, just two message nucleotides. This suppressor is probably not a good model for tRNAs that cause -1 frameshifting by slippage, however.

Non-tRNA Factors. In order to understand suppression mechanisms at the molecular level, one must first identify all of the players. In addition to the relevant codons and tRNAs that read them and the other *cis*-acting mRNA sequences, suppression certainly involves other factors. Ribosomal proteins, for example, are known to affect the fidelity of translation (STRINGINI and GORINI 1970; ROSSET and GORINI 1969). Mutant elongation factors may also enhance the frequency of termination suppression (CULBERTSON et al. 1982). Frameshifting in the RFII gene of *E. coli* requires an interaction between 16S ribosomal RNA (the sequence that normally recognizes the Shine-Dalgarno sequence during translational initiation) and the mRNA sequence just upstream of the frameshift site (WEISS et al. 1988). Defining the additional factors involved in suppression in retroviral and retrotransposon genes may require establishing a genetic selection in which, for example, cell viability is dependent on a translational suppression event. Such a selection might best be carried out in a genetically tractable system like bacteria or yeast, assuming that the suppression event of interest occurs in that system.

With the possible exception of virus infection raising the level of suppressor tRNA (KUCHINO et al. 1987; see above), viral proteins do not seem to be required for termination suppression or frameshifting. The efficiencies of suppression observed on mRNAs in vitro (including mRNAs from which no viral products could be produced) appear to rival the in vivo levels. Also, termination suppression on a short sequence from AKV occurs equally well in virus-infected and uninfected cells (PANGANIBAN 1988).

5 Physiological Effects

In this section I have included those subjects that relate more to the consequences of translational suppression rather than its mechanism.

Efficiency of Suppression. Through the analysis of various normal and mutant suppression sites, it has become clear that a wide range of suppression efficiencies are possible. For example, frameshifting occurs in the MMTV *gag-pro* overlap at approximately 25% efficiency (JACKS et al. 1987; MOORE et al. 1987), while a point mutation in the RSV frameshift site reduces the efficiency there to about 1% (JACKS et al. 1988b). Thus, depending on the exact nature of the *cis*-acting sequences at the suppression site, the relative amount of the product of suppression could be anywhere from 1 part in 4 to 1 in 100. Why then did the different sequences (and their corresponding efficiencies) evolve in the different viruses?[3] In some instances, one can make a reasonable guess. For those viruses that require two successive frameshift events to access their *pol* genes [the Class IV viruses with *pro* genes intervening between *gag* and *pol* (Fig. 2)], it is expected that at least the first of them should be quite efficient or else very little of the Gag-Pro-Pol protein would be produced. But why, for example, the frameshifting efficiencies in the RSV and HIV-1 *gag-pol* overlaps should be 5% and 10%, respectively, and not 25% is not known.

The issue of suppression efficiency is particularly interesting because the available evidence suggests that the ratio of Gag to its fusion proteins may strongly influence virus replication. FELSENSTEIN and GOFF (1988) have shown that a nonfunctional mutant of MLV in which the *gag* terminator has been converted to a glutamine codon is only weakly rescued by the expression of an exogenous *gag* gene. The implication of this result is that the normal 20:1 Gag to Gag-Pol ratio is necessary for maximal MLV virion production. For RSV, P. PRYCIAK et al. (1988, unpublished observations) found inhibition of virus production by mutations previously shown to affect in vitro frameshifting efficiency. RSV production is impaired not only by mutations that eliminate frameshifting in vitro, but also by only partially inhibitory and one partially stimulatory mutation. Thus, even subtle alterations in the ratio of Gag to Gag-Pol can have significant effects. Perhaps due to the geometry of the viral capsid, a proper ratio of Gag to its fusion proteins is necessary during virus assembly. The different suppression efficiencies observed for different viruses may reflect subtle differences in the ways in which their core subunits are assembled.

Affecting Suppression Efficiency as a Means of Virus Inhibition. If virus replication is sensitive to subtle changes in the ratio of Gag to its fusion proteins, it might be possible to block virus production with agents that either inhibit or stimulate suppression frequency. KUCHINO et al. (1988) have recently reported that Avarol, a substance isolated from the sponge *Dysidea avara*, inhibits the MLV-infection-induced expression of the glutamine tRNA species thought to suppress the *gag* terminator. Thus, the observed inhibition of virus production by Avarol may be mediated, albeit indirectly, by an inhibition of termination suppression. Other, more direct inhibitors or stimulators of suppression frequency could be imagined, but none has as yet been described. Such an agent would be potentially valuable as an inhibitor of HIV-1, especially if the cellular side effects were limited. It is not currently known whether any eukaryotic cellular

---

[3] A separate, but equally interesting question is how do these different *cis*-acting sequences deliver different frameshifting efficiencies? With the exception of certain cases involving frameshift site mutations (where mutations may disrupt potential base pairing between a tRNA and an alternate-frame codon), the answer is unknown. Efficiency probably results from a combination of the nature of the site structure, and relative abundance of the suppressor tRNAs, and, where applicable, the stability and positioning of the stem-loop structure. Evidence for the first point comes from comparing the frameshifting efficiency of the wild-type RSV *gag* gene with that of a mutant that substitutes the MMTV *gag-pro* frameshift site for the natural one (JACKS et al. 1988b). While this mutant site functions more efficiently than the wild-type one (10% versus 5%), the efficiency is not as high as is obtained on this sequence in its native setting

genes require frameshifting or termination suppression for their expression (see below). However, even if such genes do exist and their expression is necessary for cellular viability, conditions probably exists that affect suppression levels sufficiently to disrupt virus production without causing cellular toxicity.

Significance of the Sites of Suppression. For those elements that utilize termination suppression for *gag-pol* expression or whose frameshift sites correspond to the last codons of the 0-frame (see Table 1), the resulting fusion proteins carry the complete protein sequence encoded by the upstream gene. For example, the Gag moieties of the Gag-Pol proteins of MLV and RSV (whose frameshift site covers the last two *gag* codons) exactly match Gag proteins themselves. However, several putative frameshift sites are not positioned at the end of the upstream genes (Table 1). In these cases, the trans-frame proteins have substituted sequences encoded in the -1 frame of the overlap for the sequences normally present at the C-terminus of the uni-frame protein. Again, by way of example, the HIV-1 frameshift site is located very near the 5′-end of the 205-nucleotide *gag-pol* overlap (JACKS et al. 1988a). As such, the final 65 aa of the Gag protein are not present in the Gag-Pol fusion; rather the amino acids encoded by the last 65 *pol*-frame codons of the overlap are in their place. Whether this amino acid sequence difference is functionally significant, though, is unclear. Indeed, LOEB et al. (1989) have argued that most of the *gag-pol* sequence encoded by the *pol*-frame codons of the overlap are functionally unimportant, since there is little sequence similarity in this region between the two isolates of HIV, HIV-1 and HIV-2. These workers have suggested that the *pol*-encoded sequences may merely serve as a spacer between the Gag and protease domains in the Gag-Pol protein. (The N-terminus of the protease is encoded near the 3′-end of the *gag-pol* overlap.) Another intriguing suggestion is that these sequences (and, by extension, others similarly located) may be maintained because they serve a necessary function in the suppression event itself, such as forming a portion of a stem-loop structure (LOEB et al. 1989; see Fig. 2 and Sect. 4.2).

6 Additional Examples, Counter-Examples, and Future Examples

In the introduction to this review, I discussed the history of the *gag-pol* problem, particularly the emergence of an consensus solution that was based in large part on preconceptions about how eukaryotes controlled their genes. The recent discovery of translational suppression as the actual solution to the *gag-pol* problem in, at least, several cases has increased our appreciation of the variety of available genetic control mechanisms. This broadened view has and will continue to aid in the discovery of additional examples of translational suppression in the control of eukaryotic gene expression. Ironically, though, the knowledge that some retroviruses and retrotransposons utilize translational suppression mechanisms might also have fostered the belief that all *gag-pol*-like genes will be controlled in a similar fashion. This preconception, radically different from the one that slowed progress in the understanding of the *gag-pol* problem only a few years ago, is probably incorrect as well.

Counter-examples. There are classes of "retro-elements" that seem to express their *pol* genes without the use of termination suppression or ribosomal frameshifting. For the retrotransposons *copia* of *Drosophila*, *Ta1* of *Arabidopsis*, and *Tnt1* of tobacco, synthesis of a Gag-Pol protein requires only standard translation (MOUNT and RUBIN 1985, VOYTAS and AUSUBEL 1988; GRANDBASTIEN et al. 1989). As shown in Fig. 2, these transposons carry both the *gag* and *pol* coding domains in one continuous open reading frame and, thus, present an interesting twist on the problem: How to express the Gag protein alone. Possibilities include ribosomal frameshifting near the end of the *gag* domain or cleavage of some fraction of the Gag-Pol protein prior to core assembly. It is also possible that the Gag-Pol protein is sufficient for core assembly. However, the most likely explanation is that these elements produce a separate, *gag*-specific message. An mRNA species seemingly containing only the *gag* portion of the *copia gag-pol* gene has been observed in *Drosophila* cells (FLAVELL et al. 1981). Such an mRNA could be synthesized either by premature transcriptional termination or mRNA splicing.

HBV and CaMV, generally considered DNA viruses, require reverse transcription in their life cycles. The *pol* genes of these viruses all lie downstream of and overlap (in the + 1 direction) the genes encoding the viral core proteins. Due to the conservation of this overlapping structure and the use of ribosomal frameshifting by the related retro-elements, one might expect that these DNA viruses would express a core-Pol fusion protein via + 1 ribosomal frameshifting. However, in vitro translation of mRNAs containing the CaMV (GORDON et al. 1988) and HBV (CHANG et al. 1989) core-*pol* overlaps fail to produce the relevant fusion proteins. In addition, recent genetic evidence strongly suggests that CaMV (PENSWICK et al. 1988) and, at least, duck HBV (SCHLICHT et al. 1989; CHANG et al. 1989) express their *pol* genes by internal translational initiation within the *pol* gene, producing a separate Pol protein. Perhaps the differences between the replication strategies of these viruses and RNA viruses obviates the need for a core-Pol protein. Why the core and *pol* genes should overlap, then, is unclear.

Additional Examples of Translational Suppression. Control of expression by translational suppression in eukaryotic cells is not limited to the genes of retroviruses and retrotransposons. Indeed, termination suppression was described by PELHAM (1978) for the coat gene of TMV in 1978. Rattle snake mosaic virus (PELHAM 1979) and two alphaviruses, sindbis virus (STRAUSS et al. 1983) and Semliki forest virus (STRAUSS et al. 1984), are also believed to utilize termination suppression.

Ribosomal frameshifting has been proposed by BRIERLY et al. (1987) to account for expression of a long open reading frame (F2) of the avian coronavirus infectious bronchitis virus (IBV). F2 partially overlaps the upstream open reading frame, F1, in the −1 direction. Although an F1-F2 fusion protein has not been observed in IBV-infected cells, in vitro translation of mRNAs containing the F1-F2 overlap yields proteins consistent with ribosomal frameshifting. In addition, the IBV overlap includes the sequence U UUA AAC [believed to be the frameshift site for several retroviruses (Table 1)], and this sequence is followed closely by a potential stem-loop structure (BRIERLY et al. 1987; see above). Recent mutational analysis has confirmed the requirement for this heptanucleotide sequence and a complex downstream structure in frameshifting in vitro (BRIERLY et al. 1989; see above). Thus, frameshifting in the IBV F1-F2 overlap is almost certainly mechanistically related to frameshifting in retroviral genes.

A computer-assisted search of nucleotide sequence data bases for the putative heptanucleotide frameshift sites listed in Table 1 has uncovered another group of viral genes that may utilize frameshifting (JACKS et al. 1988b). These include genes of tobacco etch virus (ALLISON et al. 1986) and three alphaviruses: sindbis virus (RICE and STRAUSS 1981), semliki forest virus (GAROFF et al. 1980), and Ross river virus (DALGARNO et al. 1983). As yet, there is no independent evidence that frameshifting occurs in any of these genes, however.

Translational Suppression in Cellular Genes. Generally, viral mechanisms, including mechanisms of gene expression, mimic those of the host cell. Thus, with the discovery of translational suppression in certain retroviral and retro-transposon genes came the expectation that cellular examples would quickly follow. At present, however, there is but one example of a frameshift-controlled cellular gene [the RFII gene of *E. coli* (CRAIGEN et al. 1985; see above)] and no known examples of cellular genes that require termination suppression. One explanation for the dearth of cellular counterparts is the relatively small fraction of cellular genes that have been examined at the DNA sequence level. Also, the fact that termination suppression and ribosomal frameshifting have only recently achieved recognition as viable control mechanisms might have led to potential examples being previously overlooked. Two groups have used computer-assisted nucleotide sequence data base searches to find possible eukaryotic frameshift-controlled cellular genes (JACKS et al. 1988b; WILSON et al. 1988). Although several genes were found to contain putative heptanucleotide frameshift sites (see Table 1), none had additional features (downstream secondary structures, extended alternative open readings frames) that would indicate that frameshifting might actually occur there.

One could argue that without the constraints of maintaining a small genome size and with available mechanisms such as alternative mRNA splicing and mRNA editing, the eukaryotic cell has outmoded or never evolved genes that would require this type of translational control. Until the first eukaryotic cellular example is discovered, this position is impossible to refute. Armed with the information gleaned from retroviruses and retrotransposons, however, if such cellular example exist, their discovery should not be far off.

Acknowledgements. I thank Judy Levin, Alan Rein, and Kevin Felsenstein for communicating results prior to publication.

120   T. Jacks

References

Allison R, Johnston R, Dougherty WG (1986) The nucleotide sequence of the coding region of tobacco etch virus genomic RNA: evidence for synthesis of a single polypeptide. Virology 154: 9–20

Atkins JF, Gesteland RF, Ried BR, Anderson CW (1979) Normal tRNAs promote ribosomal frameshifting. Cell 18: 1119–1131

Bennetzen JL, Hall BD (1982) Codon selection in yeast. J Biol Chem 257: 3026–3031

Bossi L (1983) Context effects: Translation of AUG codon by suppressor tRNA is affected by the sequence following UAG in the message. J Mol Biol 164: 73–87

Bossi L, Roth JR (1981) Four-base codons ACCA, ACCU and ACCC are recognized by frameshift suppressor sufJ. Cell 25: 489–496

Bossi L, Smith (1984) Suppressor sufJ: a novel type of tRNA mutant that induces translational frameshifting. Proc Natl Acad Sci USA 81: 6105–6109

Brierly I, Boursnell M, Birns M, Bilmoria B, Block V, Brown T, Inglis S (1987) An efficient ribosomal frameshifting signal in the polymerase-encoding region of the coronavirus IBV. EMBO J 6: 3779–3785

Brierly I, Digard P, Inglis SC (1989) Characterization of an efficient ribosomal frameshifting signal: requirement for an RNA pseudoknot. Cell 57: 537–547

Capone JP, Sedivy JM, Sharp PA, Rajbhandary VC (1986) Introduction of UAG, UAA, and UGA nonsense mutations at a specific site in Escherichia coli chloramphenicol acetyltransferase gene: use in measurement of amber, ochre, and opal suppression in mammalian cells. Mol Cell Biol 6: 3059–3067

Chakrabarti L, Guyader M, Alizon M, Daniel MD, Desrosiers RC, Tiollais P, Sonigo P (1987) Sequence of simian immunodeficiency virus from macaque and its relationship to other human and simian retroviruses. Nature 328: 543–547

Chang L-J, Pryciak P, Ganem D, Varmus HE (1989) Biosynthesis of the reverse transcriptase of hepatitis B virus involves de novo translational initiation not ribosomal frameshifting. Nature 337: 364–368

Clare J, Farabaugh P (1985) Nucleotide sequence of a yeast Ty element: evidence for an unusual mechanism of gene expression. Proc Natl Acad Sci USA 82: 2829–2833

Clare JJ, Belcourt M, Farabough PJ (1988) Efficient translational frameshifting occurs within a conserved sequence of the overlap between the two genes of a yeast Ty1 transposon. Proc Natl Acad Sci USA 85: 6816–6820

Craigen WJ, Cook RG, Tate WP, Caskey CT (1985) Bacterial peptide chain release factors: conserved primary structure and possible frameshift regulation of release factor 2. Proc Natl Acad Sci USA 82: 3616–3620

Culbertson MR, Gaber RF, Cummins CM (1982) Frameshift suppression in Saccharomyces cerevisiae V. Isolation and genetic characterization of nongroup-specific suppressors. Genetics 102: 361–378

Cummins CM, Culbertson MR, Knapp G (1985) Frameshift suppressor mutations outside the anti-codon in yeast proline rRNAs containing an intervening sequence. Mol Cell Biol 5: 1760–1771

Dalgarno L, Rice CM, Strauss JH (1983) Ross River virus 26S RNA: complete nucleotide sequence and deduced sequence of encoded structural proteins. Virology 129: 170–187

Dickson C, Atterwill M (1979) Composition, arrangement and cleavage of the mouse mammary tumor virus polyprotein precursor Pr77gag and p110gag. Cell 17: 1003–1012

Dunn JJ, Studier FW (1983) Complete nucleotide sequence of bacteriophage T7 DNA and the locations of T7 genetic elements. J Mol Biol 166: 477–535

Felsenstein KM, Goff SP (1988) Expression of the gag-pol fusion protein of Moloney murine leukemia virus without gag protein does not induce virion formation or proteolytic processing. J Virol 62: 2179–2182

Felsenstein KM, Goff SP (1989) (manuscript in preparation)

Feng Y–X, Hatfield DL, Rein A, Levin JG (1989a) Translational read through of the murine leukemia virus gag gene amber codon does not require virus-induced alteration of tRNA. J Virol 63: 2405–2410

Feng Y–X, Levin JG, Hatfield DL, Schaefer TS, Gorelick RJ, Rein A (1989b) Suppression of UAA and UGA termination codons in mutant murine leukemia viruses. J Virol 63: 2870–2873

Flavell AJ, Levis R, Simon MA, Rubin GM (1981) The 5′ termini of RNAs encoded by the transposable element copia. Nucleic Acids Res 9: 6279–6291

Fox TD, Weiss-Brummer B (1980) Leaky + 1 and − 1 frameshift mutations at the same site in a yeast mitochondrial gene. Nature 288: 60–63

Garoff H, Frischauf AM, Simons K, Leharch H, Delius H (1980) Nucleotide sequence of cDNA coding for Semliki Forest virus membrane glycoproteins. Nature 288: 236–241

Gordon K, Pfeiffer P, Futterer J, Hohn T (1988) In vitro expression of cauliflower mosaic virus genes. EMBO J 7: 309–317

Grandbastien M–A, Spielmann A, Caboche M (1989) Tnt1, a mobile retroviral-like transposable element of tobacco isolated by plant cell genetics. Nature 337: 376–380

Guyader M, Emerman M, Sonigo P, Claver F, Montagnier L, Alizon M (1987) Genome organization and transcription of the human immunodeficiency virus type 2. Nature 326: 662–669

Hayward WS (1977) Size and genetic content of viral RNAs in avian oncovirus-infected cells. J Virol 24: 47–63

Hiramatsu K, Nishida J, Naito A, Yoshikura H (1987) Molecular cloning of the closed circular provirus of human T cell leukemia virus type I: a new open reading frame in the gag-pol region. J Gen Virol 68: 213–218

Hizi A, Henderson LE, Copeland TD, Sowden RC, Hixson CV, Oroszlan S (1987) Characterization of mouse mammary tumor virus gag-pol gene products and the ribosomal frameshift by protein sequencing. Proc Natl Acad Sci USA 84: 7041–7046

Jacks T, Varmus HE (1985) Expression of the Rous sarcoma virus pol gene by ribosomal frameshifting. Science 230: 1237–1242

Jacks T, Townsley K, Varmus HE, Majors J (1987) Two efficient ribosomal frameshift events are required for synthesis of mouse mammary tumor virus gag-related polypeptides. Proc Natl Acad Sci USA 84: 4298–4302

Jacks T, Power MD, Masiarz FR, Luciw PA, Barr PJ, Varmus HE (1988a) Characterization of ribosomal mutations in HIV-1 gag-pol expression. Nature 331: 280–283

Jacks T, Madhani HD, Masiarz FR, Varmus HE (1988b) Signals for ribosomal frameshifting in the Rous sarcoma virus gag-pol region. Cell 55: 447–458

Jamjoon GA, Naso RB, Arlinghaus RB (1977) Further characterization of intracellular precursor polypeptides of Rauscher leukemia virus. Virology 78: 11–34

Kerr IM, Olshevsky U, Lodish HF, Baltimore D (1976) Translation of murine leukemia virus RNA in a cell-free system from animal cells. J Virol 18: 627–635

Kohno T and Roth JR (1978) A Salmonella frameshift suppressor that acts at runs of A residues in the messenger RNA. J Mol Biol 126: 37–52

Kozak M (1978) How do eucaryotic ribosomes select initiation regions in messenger RNA? Cell 15: 1109–1123

Kuchino Y, Beker H, Akita N, Nishimura S (1987) Natural UAG suppressor tRNA is elevated in mouse cell infected with Moloney murine leukemia virus. Proc Natl Acad Sci USA 84: 2668–2672

Kuchini Y, Nishimura S, Schroder HC, Rottmann M, Muller WEG (1988) Selective inhibition of formation of suppressor glutamine tRNA in Moloney murine leukemia virus-infected NIH3T3 cells by Avarol. Virology 165: 518–526

Kurland CG (1978) Reading frame errors on ribosomes. In: Celis JE, Smith JD (eds) Nonsense mutations and tRNA suppressors. Academic, London pp 98–108

Levin JG, Hu SC, Rein A, Messer LI, Gerwin B (1984) Murine leukemia virus mutant with a frameshift in the reverse transcriptase coding region: implications for pol gene structure. J Virol 51: 470–478

Loeb DD, Padgett RW, Hardies SC, Shehee WR, Comer MB, Edgell MH, Hutchison CA (1986) The sequence of a large L1Md element reveals a tandemly repeated end and several features found in retrotransposons. Mol Cell Biol 6: 168–182

Loeb DD, Hutchison CA, Edgell MH, Farmerie WG, Swanstrom R (1989) Mutational analysis of the HIV-1 protease suggests functional homology with aspartic proteinases. J Virol 63: 111–121

Madhani HD, Jacks T, Varmus HE (1988) Signals for the expression of the HIV pol gene by ribosomal frameshifting. In: Franza R, Cullen B, Wong-Stall F (eds) Control of HIV Gene Expression. Cold Spring Harbor Laboratory, Cold Spring Harbor pp 119–125

Marlor RL, Parkhurst SM, Corces VG (1986) The Drosophila melanogaster gypsy transposable element encodes putative gene products homologous to retroviral proteins. Mol Cell Biol 6: 1129–1134

Meitz JA, Grossman Z, Lueders KK, Kuff EL (1987) Nucleotide sequence of a complete mouse intracisternal A-particle genome: no relationship to known aspects of particle assembly and function. J Virol 61: 3020–3029

Mellor J, Fulton SM, Dobson MJ, Wilson W, Kingsman SM, Kingsman AJ (1985) A retrovirus-like strategy for expression of a fusion protein encoded by the yeast transposon Tyl. Nature 313: 243–246

Miller JH, Albertini AM (1983) Effects of surrounding sequence on the suppression of nonsense codons. J Mol Biol 164: 59–71

Moore R, Dixon M, Smith R, Peters G, Dickson C (1987) Complete nucleotide sequence of a milk-transmitted mouse mammary tumor virus: two frameshift suppression events are required for translation of gag and pol. J Virol 61: 480–490

Mount SM, Rubin GM (1985) Complete nucleotide sequence of the Drosophila transposable element copia: homology between copia and retroviral proteins. Mol Cell Biol 5: 1630–1638

Murphy EC, Arlinghaus RB (1978) Cell-free synthesis of Rauscher murine leukemia virus "gag" and "gag-pol" precursor polypeptides from virion 35S RNA in a mRNA-dependent translation system derived from mouse tissue culture cells. Virology 86: 329–343

Murphy EC, Campos D, Arlinghaus RB (1979) Cell-free synthesis of Raucher murine leukemia virus "gag" and "env" gene products from separate cellular mRNA species. Virology 93: 293–302

Nam SH, Hatanaka M (1986) Identification of a protease gene of human T-cell leukemia virus type I (HTLV-I) and its structural comparison. Biochem Biophys Res Commun 139:129

Oppermann L, Bishop JM, Varmus HE, Levintow L (1977) A joint product of the genes gag and pol of avian sarcoma virus: a possible precursor of reverse transcriptase. Cell 12: 993–1005

Panganiban AT (1988) Retroviral gag gene amber codon suppression is caused by an intrinsic cis-acting component of the viral mRNA. J Virol 62: 3574–3580

Pawson TP, Martin GS, Smith AE (1976) Cell-free translation of virion RNA from non-defective and transformation-defective Rous Sarcoma viruses. J Virol 19: 950–967

Pelham HRB (1978) Leaky UAG termination codon in tobacco mosaic virus RNA. Nature 272: 469–471

Pelham HRB (1979) Translation of tobacco rattle snake virus RNAs in vitro: four proteins from three RNAs. Virology 97: 256–265

Penswick T, Hubler R, Hohn T (1988) A viable mutation in cauliflower mosaic virus, a retroviruslike plant virus, separates its capsid protein and polymerase genes. J Virol 62: 1460–1463

Philipson L, Andersson P, Olshevsky U, Weinberg R, Blatimore D, Gesteland R (1978) Translation of MuLV and MSV RNAs in nuclease-treated reticulocye extracts: Enhancement of the gag-pol polypeptide with yeast suppressor tRNA. Cell 13: 189–199

Power MD, Marx PA, Bryant ML, Gardner MD, Barr PJ, Luciw PA (1986) Nucleotide sequence of SRV-1, a type D simian acquired immune deficiency syndrome retrovirus. Science 231: 1567–1572

Purchio AF, Erikson E, Erikson RL (1977) Translation of 35S and of subgenomic regions of avian sarcoma virus RNA. Proc Natl Acad Sci USA 74: 4661–4665

Ratner L, Hazeltine W, Patarca R, Livak KJ, Starcich B, Josephs SF, Doran ER, Rafalski JA, Whitehorn EA, Baumeister K, Ivanoff L, Petteway SR, Pearson ML, Lautenberger JA, Papas TS, Ghrayeb J, Chang NT, Gallo RC, Wong-Staal F (1985a) Complete nucleotide sequence of the AIDS virus, HTLV-III. Nature 313: 277–284

Ratner L, Josephs SF, Starcich B, Hahn B, Shaw GM, Gallo RC, Wong-Staal F (1985b) Nucleotide sequence analysis of a varient human T-cell leukemia virus (HTLV-Ib) provirus with a deletion in Px-1. J Virol 54: 781–790

Rettenmier W, Karess RE, Anderson SM, Hanafusa H (1979) Tryptic peptide analysis of avian oncovirus gag and pol gene products. J Virol 32: 102–113

Rice CM, Strauss JH (1981) Nucleotide sequence of the 26S mRNA of Sindbis virus and deduced sequence of the encoded virus structural proteins. Proc Natl Acad Sci USA 78: 1062–2066

Rice NR, Stephens RM, Burny A, Gilden RV (1985) The gag and pol genes of bovine leukemia virus: nucleotide sequence and analysis. Virology 142: 357–377

Riddle D, Carbon J (1973) A nucleotide addition in the anticodon of a glycine tRNA. Nature 242: 230–234

Riddle DL, Roth JR (1970) Suppressors of frameshift mutations in Salmonella typhimurium. J Mol Biol 54: 131–144

Rosset R, Gorini L (1969) A ribosomal ambiguity mutation. J Mol Biol 39: 95–112

Roth JR (1974) Frameshift mutations. Annu. Rev Genet 8: 319–346

Sagata N, Yasunaga T, Tsuzuku-Kawamura J, Ohishi K, Ogawa Y, Ikawa Y (1985) Complete nucleotide sequence of the genome of bovine leukemia virus: its evolutionary relationship to other retroviruses. Proc Natl Acad Sci USA 82: 677–681

Saigo K, Kugimiya W, Matsu Y, Inouye S, Yoshioka K, Yuki S (1984) Identification of the coding sequence for a reverse transcriptase-like enzyme in a transposable genetic element in Drosophila melanogaster. Nature 312: 659–661

Sanchez-Pescador R, Power MD, Barr PJ, Steimer KS, Stempier MM, Brown-Shimer SL, Gee WW, Renard A, Randolf A, Levy JA, Dina D, Luciw PA (1985) Nucleotide sequence and expression of an AIDS-associated retrovirus (ARV-2) Science 227: 484–492

Schlicht H–J, Radziwill G, Schaller H (1989) Synthesis and encapsidation of duck hepatitis B virus reverse transcriptase do not require formation of core polymerase fusion proteins. Cell 56: 85–92

Schwartz DE, Tizard R, Gilbert W (1983) Nucleotide sequence of Rous sarcoma virus. Cell 32: 853–869

Seiki M, Hattori Y, Hirayama Y, Yoshida M (1983) Human adult T-cell leukemia virus: complete nucleotide sequence of the provirus genome integrated in leukemia cell DNA. Proc Natl Acad Sci USA 80: 3618–3622

Shimotohno K, Takahashi Y, Shimizu N, Gojobori T, Golde DW, Chen ISY, Miwa M, Sugimura T (1985) Complete nucleotide sequence of an infectious clone of human T-cell leukemia virus type II: an open reading frame for the protease gene. Proc Natl Acad Sci USA 82: 3101–3105

Shinnick TM, Lerner RA, Sutcliffe JG (1981) Nucleotide sequence of Moloney murine leukemia virus. Nature 293: 543–548

Sonigo P, Alizon M, Staskus K, Klatzmann D, Cole S, Danos O, Retzel E, Tiollais P, Haase A, Wain-Hobson S (1985) Nucleotide sequence of the visna lentivirus: relationship with the AIDS virus. Cell 42: 369–382

Sonigo P, Barker C, Hunter E, Wain-Hobson S (1986) Nucleotide sequence of Mason-Pfizer monkey virus: an immunosuppressive D-type retrovirus. Cell 45: 375–385

Spanjaard RA, van Duin J (1988) Translation of the sequence AGG-AGG yields 50% ribosomal frameshifting. Proc Natl Acad Sci USA 85: 7967–7971

Stacey DW, Allfrey VG, Hanafusa H (1977) Microinjection analysis of envelope-glycoprotein messenger activities of avian leukosis virus RNAs. Proc Natl Acad SCi USA 74: 1614–1618

Stephens RM, Casey JW, Rice NR (1986) Equine infectious anemia virus gag and pol genes: relatedness to visna and AIDS virus. Science 231: 589–594

Strauss EG, Rice CM, Strauss JH (1983) Sequence coding for the alphavirus nonstructural protein is interrupted by an opal terminator codon. Proc Natl Acad Sci USA 80: 5271–5275

Strauss EG, Rice CM, Strauss JH (1984) Complete nucleotide sequence of the genomic RNA of sindbis virus. Virology 133: 92–110

Stringini P, Gorini L (1970) Ribosomal mutations affecting efficiency of amber suppression. J Mol Biol 47: 517–530

Tamura TA (1983) Provirus of M7 baboon endogenous virus, nucleotide sequence of the gag-pol region. J Virol 47: 137–145

Thompson RC (1988) Ef-Tu provides an internal kinetic standard for translational accuracy. Trends Biochem Sci 13: 91–93

Thompson RC, Karim AM (1982) The accuracy of protein biosynthesis is limited by its speed: high fidelity selection by ribosomes of aminoacyl-tRNA ternary complexes containing GTP[γS]. Proc Natl Acad Sci USA 79: 4922–4926

Vaytas DF, Ausubel FM (1988) A copia-like transposable element family in Arabidopsis thalina. Nature 336: 242–244

Von der Helm K, Duesberg PH (1975) Translation of Rous sarcoma virus RNAs in cell-free systems from ascites Kerbs II cells. Proc Natl Acad Sci USA 72: 614–618

Wain-Hobsen S, Sonigo P, Danos O, Cole S, Alizon M (1985) Nucleotide sequence of the AIDS virus, LAV. Cell 40: 9–17

Weiss R, Gallant J (1983) Mechanism of ribosome frameshift during translation of the genetic code. Nature 302: 389–393

Weiss R, Teich N, Varmus H, Coffin J (eds) (1984) RNA tumor viruses. Cold Spring Harbor Laboratory, Cold Spring Harbor, New York

Weiss RB, Dunn DM, Atkins JF, Gesteland RF (1987) Slippery runs, shifty stops, backward steps and forward hops: -2, -1, $+5$, and $+6$ ribosomal frameshifting. Cold Spring Harbor Symp Quant Biol 52: 687–693

Weiss RB, Dunn DM, Dahlberg AE, Atkins JF, Gesteland RF (1988) Reading frame switch caused by base-pair formation between the 3' end of 16S rRNA and the mRNA during elongation of protein synthesis in Escherichia coli. EMBO J 7: 1503–1507

Weiss SR, Varmus HE, Bishop JM (1977) The size and genetic composition of virus-specific RNAs in the cytoplasm of cells producing avian sarcoma-leukemia viruses. Cell 12: 983–992

Weiss SR, Hackett PB, Oppermann H, Ullrich A, Levintow L, Bishop JM (1978) Cell-free translation of avian sarcoma virus RNA: suppression of the gag termination codon does not augment synthesis of the joint gag/pol product. Cell 15: 607–614

Wilson W, Braddock M, Adams SE, Rathjen PD, Kingsman SM, Kingsman AJ (1988) HIV expression strategies: ribosomal frameshifting is directed by a short sequence in both mammalian and yeast systems. Cell 55: 1159–1169

Wilson W, Malim MH, Mellor J, Kingsman AJ, Kingsman SM (1986) Expression strategies of the yeast retrotransposon Ty: a short sequence directs ribosomal frameshifting. Nucleic Acids Res 14: 7001–7016

Yarus M, Thompson RC (1983) Precision of protein biosynthesis. In: Beckwith JR, Davies JE, Gallant JA (eds) Gene function in prokaryotes. Cold Spring Harbor Laboratory, Cold Spring Harbor

Yoshinaka Y, Katoh I, Copeland TD, Orozslan SJ (1985a) Murine Leukemia virus protease is encoded by the gag-pol gene and is synthesized through suppression of an amber termination codon. Proc Natl Acad Sci USA 82: 1618–1622

Yoshinaka Y, Katoh I, Copeland TD, Oroszlan SJ (1985b) Translational readthrough of an amber termination codon during synthesis of feline leukemia virus protease. J Virol 55: 870–873

Retroviral RNA Packaging:
Sequence Requirements and Implications

M. L. LINIAL and A. D. MILLER

1 Introduction

Unlike many animal viruses, infection by retroviruses generally does not lead to cessation of host RNA synthesis. Despite the high levels of host RNA in infected cells, the vast majority of retroviral particles contain a precise genomic complex consisting of two molecules of genomic RNA, rather than cellular or subgenomic viral mRNAs. Thus, the retroviral genome must be selected for encapsidation against a high background of cellular RNAs. It is therefore surprising that the retroviral genome is structurally similar to that of cellular mRNA. For instance, both molecules contain a $5'$ m^7G cap and several hundred A residues at the $3'$ terminus (reviewed in COFFIN 1984a, 1985). Viral subgenomic mRNAs are even

Division of Basic Sciences, Fred Hutchinson Cancer Research Center, 1124 Columbia Street, Seattle, WA 98104, USA more similar to genomic RNA. The ability of the retroviral particle to choose correctly genomic RNA from the vast excess of heterologous molecules implies that specific sequences are present within the genome which direct the efficient encapsidation of the correct RNAs. Analysis of spontaneous and engineered mutants of both avian and murine retroviruses has in fact revealed that *cis*-acting sequences are involved and are present in the retroviral genome.

The localization of such packaging sequences has had important implications for gene transfer technology. Deletion of packaging sequences has allowed the construction of retroviral packaging cell lines which produce particles deficient in genomic RNA. Inclusion of packaging sequences in retroviral vectors or in nonretroviral transcription units results in efficient packaging of RNAs transcribed from these constructs in packaging cells. However, much still remains to be learned about the structure and specificity of the *cis*-acting packaging sequences. Even less is known about viral gene products which might specifically interact in *trans* with the packaging sequences to ensure encapsidation of the proper RNAs capable of infectious virion production. Genetic analysis suggests that RNA packaging requires functional *gag* gene products, but the nature of the RNA:protein interaction is unknown.

A unique feature of the retroviral life cycle is the conversion of genomic viral RNA into proviral DNA which ultimately becomes integrated into the host cell's genome. Retroviral particles contain the virally encoded RNA-dependent DNA polymerase (reverse transcriptase) which carries out a complex set of reactions necessary for complete proviral synthesis (reviewed in VARMUS and SWANSTROM 1984). Reverse transcriptase is encapsidated into particles independently of genomic RNA (GERWIN and LEVIN 1977). Thus, any imprecision in the selection of RNA for encapsidation could have an effect on the host cell's genetic organization. On rare occasions, retroviral subgenomic mRNA molecules or nonretroviral RNA molecules might be encapsidated, reverse transcribed, and integrated into the infected cell genome. Nonretroviral RNA which is encapsidated might also be incorporated into the retroviral genome via reverse transcriptase-mediated recombination. Thus, the great genetic diversity of retroviruses, as well as the complexity of the host cell's genome may be influenced by the ability of the retrovirus to select precisely its genome for assembly into virions.

2 Identification of *cis*-Acting Packaging Signals in the Retroviral Genome

2.1 Deletion Analysis of Avian Retroviruses

The specificity with which retroviral full-length genomic RNAs are encapsidated suggests that specific sequences are required for RNA selection. The first indication that the retroviral genome actually contains sequences important for recognition and encapsidation of genomic RNA came from studies of a spontaneous mutant of RSV, an avian retrovirus. A Japanese quail cell line containing a single integrated copy of this RSV, called SE21Q1b, was shown to produce particles deficient in genomic RNA (LINIAL et al. 1978). Viral particles are produced from the cells in numbers equivalent to those produced by wild-type RSV-infected cultures, but the particles are incapable of leading to productive infections. The SE21Q1b particles are composed of all the usual structural proteins and contain reverse transcriptase. Analysis of the provirus in SE21Q1b cells revealed a deletion of about 150 base pairs near the 5'-end of the genome (SHANK and LINIAL 1980). The region encompassing the deletion has been termed the leader (or L) sequence since it does not encode protein but, residing upstream of the RSV splice donor site, is present on the subgenomic mRNAs encoded by the virus. The deletion does not affect the ability of the virus to synthesize genomic or subgenomic RNAs or any of the virally encoded proteins. Recent sequence analysis (P. SHANK, K. LEVINE, O. YANG, S. SHAW, and M. LINIAL, unpublished data) has shown the deletion to be 181 nucleotides in length, starting within the inverted repeat in U5 and extending 3' into the untranslated region (Fig. 1a). The deletion completely removes the (−)strand primer binding site (PBS). The mutations in the SE21Q1b provirus appear to be more complex than this single deletion, since as discussed further in Sect. 5.4, SE21Q1b particles encapsidate significant amounts of cellular mRNA.

Another spontaneous mutant of RSV, called TK15, also fails to package genomic RNA efficiently and is poorly infectious (KAWAI and KOYAMA 1984; KOYAMA et al. 1984). This mutant also contains a deletion in the L region (Fig. 1A; NISHIZAWA et al. 1985). Based on the results with SE21Q1b and TK15, several groups have constructed deletions in vitro within the avian retroviral L sequence. One such deletion mutant, pd12, lacks 64 nucleotides in L, and pd12 RNA is encapsidated about one-tenth as efficiently as wild type (KATZ et al. 1986). Comparison of the pd12 mutation with other deletion mutants created in this study led to the inference that 31 nucleotides within the pd12-defined region are required for efficient genomic RNA packaging. However, the effect of the pd12 mutation is less severe than the decrease in packaging with larger deletions in this region. Thus, pd12 may define a core packaging region but probably does not define the entire sequence required.

Recently, ca. 150 base pairs were deleted from the L region of an avian leukosis virus (RAV-1) provirus (STOKER and BISSELL 1988). This deletion severely reduced the infectivity of virus produced after transfection of a continuous quail cell line, QT6. Although the amount of genomic RNA encapsidated by this mutant (RAV-1Ψ-) was not directly measured, the location of the deletion (Fig. 1A) suggests that it is defective in packaging. The RAV-1Ψ- provirus produces virions which are much less infectious than TK15, and it was proposed that the severity of the defect might be ascribed to the deletion of the PBS in RAV-1-. This explanation is likely to be correct since SE21Q1b cells rarely transfer the genome, and the SE21Q1b provirus lacks PBS (P. SHANK, K. LEVINE,

a   5' packaging region of RSV\RAV

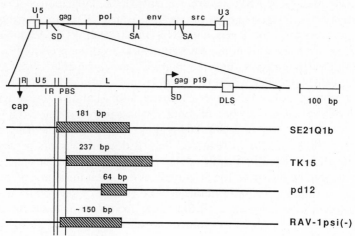

b packaging region (E) of SNV

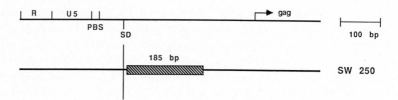

c   packaging region of MLV/MSV

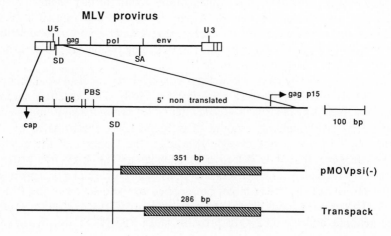

O. YANG, S. SHAW, and M. LINIAL, unpublished data). The RAV-1Ψ- provirus has been used to construct an avian retroviral packaging cell line in QT6 cells, similar to those in existence for MuLV or spleen necrosis virus (SNV or Rev; see Sect. 4).

The packaging region depicted in Fig. 1a may not comprise all the sequences required for the specific recognition of avian retroviral RNA since this region is insufficient to explain the ability of RSV to distinguish its genome from its subgenomic RNAs. As shown in Fig. 1a, the packaging region is positioned upstream of the splice donor site (SD) and therefore is present on the subgenomic mRNAs (env and src in the case of RSV, and env in the case of avian leukosis virus, ALV). Yet genomic RNA is packaged at least 20-fold more efficiently than env mRNA (STOLTZFUS and KUHNERT 1979; KATZ et al. 1986). One possible explanation is that a sequence in gag or pol (which is part of the env intron and thus excluded from env RNA) is also required for optimal packaging. Work with RSV indicates that a 28-nucleotide region in gag containing 22 self-complementary bases might be required for packaging. This 28-base sequence is located about 140 bases 3' of the start site for translation of gag (PUGATSCH and STACEY 1983). This region has been implicated in dimer linkage of two genomic RNA molecules to form the 70S complex which is found in virions. If involved in packaging, the position of this region would neatly explain differentiation between the packaging of genomic and mRNA. However, further experiments have not confirmed the original observations, and this region does not appear to be absolutely required for efficient packaging of either RSV or heterologous RNAs. Deletion of as many as 10 of the 22 self-complementary nucleotides did not greatly affect packaging (DeGUDICIBUS et al. 1986; NORTON and COFFIN 1985). RNA size could play a role in preferential packaging of genomic rather than mRNA. RNAs as small as 2.2 kilobases (BIEGALKE and LINIAL 1987) or as large as 11 kilobases (HERMAN and COFFIN 1987) can be packaged into particles, although the efficiencies have not been directly measured.

Another region of the RSV genome has been demonstrated to be indispensable for efficient genomic RNA packaging. During the construction of an RSV cloning vector, it was shown that deletion of both copies of a 115-nucleotide direct repeat flanking the src gene eliminated efficient viral replication. Virions produced from cells transiently transfected with the mutant genome lacked genomic RNA. One copy of the direct repeat appeared to be sufficient for packaging (SORGE et al. 1983). This cis-acting sequence is an absolute requirement

◄ ───

Fig. 1a–c. Location of packaging signals at the 5'-ends of retroviruses as determined by deletion analysis. The locations of deletion mutants have been drawn to scale with the 5'-ends of the proviral sequences. The 5'-end of the viral mRNAs are denoted by the vertical arrow at the cap; the start of translation in the gag gene is denoted by the horizontal arrow. U5, unique 5' sequences; U3, unique 3' sequences; SD, splice donor; SA, splice acceptor; IR, inverted repeat; PBS, minus strand primer binding site; DLS, putative dimer linkage site; bp, base pairs. Location of the deletions are from the following references: **a** SE21Q1b, P. SHANK, K. LEVINE, O. YANG, SHAH, M. LINIAL, unpublished results; TK15, NISHIZAWA et al. 1985; pd12, KATZ et al. 1986; RAV-1psi(−), STOKER and BISSELL 1988. **b** SW 250, WATANABE TEMIN 1979; EMBRETSON and TEMIN 1987, **c** pMOVpsi(−), MANN et al. 1983; Transpack, SORGE et al. 1984 for RSV genomic packaging; however, an analogous sequence near the 3'-end of MuLV or SNV has not been described. The RSV sequence could have a role in folding of the RNA molecule into a structure which is efficiently packaged. However, since the 115 nucleotides are present on both genomic and subgenomic RSV RNAs, they cannot explain the preferential packaging of genomic RNA. It will be of interest to determine whether heterologous RNAs must contain both 5' and 3' cis-packaging sequences for encapsidation into avian particles released from packaging lines, or whether the 3' sequence is specific for viral RNA.

The region required for genomic RNA packaging has also been determined for a second group of avian retroviruses, the spleen necrosis-reticuloendotheliosis viruses (SNV or Rev; Fig. 1b). An in vitro-constructed deletion mutant of SNV, SW250 (WATANABE and TEMIN 1979), containing a 185-nucleotide deletion near the 5'-end of the genome was shown to be replication defective because viral particles encoded by the SW250 genome lack genomic RNA. Further deletion analysis narrowed the encapsidation region (referred to as E in the case of Rev) to the 5'-most 144 nucleotides of the SW250-defined deletion. This region maps just downstream of the splice donor site for *env* mRNA (EMBRETSON and TEMIN 1987). Thus, Rev subgenomic mRNAs do not contain the E region. Although Rev was recovered from an avian species, it is more highly related to MuLV than ALV. It is interesting in this regard that the location of the packaging region relative to SD is more similar to MuLV than the other avian viruses (see Sect. 2.2).

2.2 Deletion Analysis of Murine Retroviruses

Based on information generated from the study of RSV mutants, deletions of sequences at similar locations in the Mo-MuLV provirus allowed definition of a signal required for packaging of MuLV (Fig. 1c). Deletion of 350 base pairs from an infectious MuLV clone allowed construction of a mutant called pMOVΨ which encodes virions lacking genomic MuLV RNA. Like the avian packaging mutants, cells containing pMOVΨ- produce large numbers of noninfectious virions which have reverse transcriptase activity. The pMOVΨ- deletion is considerably larger than that described for RSV, ALV, or Rev. Further deletion mutants in this region suggest that the packaging region is actually smaller than 350 base pairs because several deletions (32-83 nucleotides) in the 3'-end of Ψ do not appear to impair packaging of MuLV RNA greatly (SCHWARTZBERG et al. 1983). Deletion of a similarly located region from the closely related amphotropic murine virus 4070A (Fig. 1c) has identified a packaging signal of 280 base pairs which is similar in function to the Ψ signal defined for MoMuLV (SORGE et al. 1984).

As in the case of Rev, the MuLV Ψ signal resides in the *env* mRNA intron. If the Ψ sequence is placed downstream of the *env* gene (in the MuLV U3 region) in the proper orientation, there is only a small negative effect (fivefold) on encapsidation of viral RNA. However, in such a virus (SVX-ΨC), both genomic and subgenomic *env* RNAs are packaged, and upon subsequent infection, reverse transcribed, and integrated into the host cell genome (MANN and BALTIMORE 1984). Packaging of the two RNAs appeared to be roughly in proportion to their intracellular concentration, although the genomic length RNA may be en-capsidated preferentially. This is in contrast to RSV, where *env* RNA is not efficiently packaged despite the presence of the Ψ equivalent on the mRNA. In addition, the Ψ signal only directs encapsidation of RNA when inserted in the proper orientation (MANN and BALTIMORE 1984; also see Sect. 2.3).

There are also other regions in the Mo-MuLV genome which are required for efficient packaging of genomic RNA. Deletion of as little as 12 bp from the 5' portion of the U5 region of Mo-MuLV results in a 25-fold reduction in genomic RNA found in virions, and larger deletions result in up to a 100-fold decrease (MURPHY and GOFF, submitted for publication). This phenotype is similar to that observed for deletions of the classic Ψ signal from Mo-MuLV. No systematic analysis has been done to determine whether or not deletion of other small regions of MoMuLV results in a similar phenotype. Retroviral vectors in which the *gag*, *pol*, and *env* regions of MoMuLV are deleted and replaced with nonviral sequences can be encapsidated relatively efficiently, suggesting that the internal region of MoMuLV is not required for packaging of genomic RNA. However, this result does not provide a direct answer to the question because packaging of retroviral vectors, which are generally <5 kilobases in size, may be less constrained than packaging of the 8.3-kilobase MoMuLV genome.

The retroviral particle appears to be unable to package genomic RNA that is being actively translated. This conclusion is based on work with MuLV-infected cells treated with actinomycin D. Under these conditions, viral proteins continue to be synthesized and particles shed for at least 8 h, although the particles are devoid of genomic RNA after 3–4 h (LEVIN et al. 1974; LEVIN and ROSENAK 1976). The relative amounts of all of the viral structural proteins in the actinomycin D particles are unchanged from normal, making it unlikely that *trans*-acting factors (see Sect. 3) are responsible for the failure to encapsidate genomic RNA. Since genomic RNA and *gag* mRNA are structurally indistinguishable (VARMUS and SWANSTROM 1984), these data are consistent with a sequestered pool of genomic RNA which is associated with polyribosomes and hence unavailable for packaging.

2.3 Sequences That Are Sufficient for Heterologous RNA Packaging Into Virions

Deletion analysis of replication-competent helper viruses allows definition of sequences that are required for packaging of viral RNA but does not define sequences that are sufficient for packaging. Use of retroviral vectors allows partial definition of these sequences. Both SNV- and Mo-MuLV-based vectors constructed by deletion of most of the internal protein coding regions are packaged into virions with good efficiency. However, evidence has been obtained for the contribution of some internal regions in the helper virus for optimal vector

RNA packaging (BENDER et al. 1987; ARMENTANO et al. 1987). Since retroviral LTRs and other *cis*-acting sequences are required for the replication of retroviral vectors, an approach based on the behavior of retroviral vectors cannot define the minimal sequences required for RNA packaging.

Recently, the minimal sequences sufficient for packaging were defined for MuLV by the insertion of fragments of a Mo-MuLV-based retroviral vector into a nonretroviral transcription unit consisting of a cytomegalovirus (CMV) promoter, the *neo* gene, and a polyadenylation signal from simian virus 40 (SV40). Insertion of some MuLV sequences allowed packaging of the nonretroviral transcripts into virions, and this effect was dependent on the proper orientation of the insert. A fragment corresponding to Mo-MuLV bases 215–1038 allowed packaging of the nonretroviral RNAs at rates equivalent to those of Mo-MuLV genomic RNA (ADAM and MILLER 1988). This 823-base pair fragment is larger than the Ψ signal defined by deletion analysis an includes part of the *gag* region of Mo-MuLV. While the 350-base pair Ψ signal directs packaging of both nonretroviral RNA and retroviral vector RNA, the rate of packaging of both is clearly increased by addition of some *gag* sequences (BENDER et al. 1987; ARMENTANO et al. 1987; ADAM and MILLER 1988).

While deletion of portions of the U5 region of Mo-MuLV caused a marked reduction in packaging of its genomic RNA (MURPHY and GOFF, submitted for publication), it was not necessary to include this region in nonretroviral transcripts to effect packaging. Indeed, inclusion of this region in a construct containing the Ψ + signal had no effect on the packaging of RNA transcribed from the construct (ADAM and MILLER 1988). This apparent contradiction might be explained by the need for precise folding of an RNA as large as that of Mo-MuLV (8.3 kilobases) to allow encapsidation, while the overall structure of the short nonretroviral transcripts (< 4 kilobases) is less critical. Thus, the U5 region may not be directly involved in the process of selective packaging of viral RNA but is required to maintain the correct overall structure of the Mo-MuLV genome.

Recently, LEVER et al. (1989) reported the construction of a deletion mutant in HIV lacking 19 bases between the 5′ splice donor site and the start of *gag*. The mutant provirus is capable of producing particles containing viral proteins, but which contain less than 2% of the RNA of wild type virions. Thus, this mutation appears to delineate a cis-acting sequence required for HIV RNA packaging.

3 Search for *trans*-Acting Proteins Involved in Genomic RNA Packaging

The existence of a specific *cis*-acting genomic segment required for high efficiency RNA encapsidation suggests that it is a recognition site for a *trans*-acting factor, possibly a viral protein. The retroviral genome encodes three genes, *gag*, *pol*, and *env*. It has been known for some time that the gene products of both *pol* (reverse transcriptase) and *env* (envelope glycoproteins) are not required for assembly of particles containing genomic RNA. Conversely, viral particles are not produced in the absence of the *gag* gene proteins (reviewed in DICKSON et al. 1984). Thus, if a *trans*-acting factor is necessary for RNA recognition and assembly, it is likely to be part of the *gag* gene. All retroviral *gag* genes encode a precursor polyprotein which is subsequently cleaved by a virally encoded protease into three or four proteins. The current nomenclature for the three proteins which are highly conserved is MA (matrix), CA (capsid), and NC (nucleocapsid) (LEIS et al. 1988). Only the NC protein has been unequivocally shown to bind to RNA (FU et al. 1985; MERIC et al. 1984); however, no sequence specificity of binding has ever been demonstrated. Although the nonspecific RNA binding domain of Gag resides in NC, it is possible that sequence-specific binding is a component of a more complex structure such as the Gag precursor protein, which is thought to be cleaved only during or after virion release (reviewed in DICKSON et al. 1984; LINIAL and BLAIR 1984). For instance, NC could interact with another Gag domain to allow specific binding to the genomic packaging region and drive encapsidation. Later, cleavage of the Gag precursor could release NC, which would then nonspecifically coat the RNA.

Genetic evidence for the existence of a *trans*-acting factor required for proper RNA packaging comes from work with the avian retroviral mutant *SE21Q1b* (LINIAL et al. 1978). This mutant fails to package RSV genomic RNA. However, cells containing the defective provirus shed particles which contain cellular mRNA (LINIAL et al. 1978; GALLIS et al. 1979). If *SE21Q1b* cells are superinfected with a wild-type retrovirus, 90% of the encapsidated RNA is still of cellular origin, although the superinfecting virus can replicate. Thus, the packaging of cellular RNA appears to be *trans*-dominant. This result is most consistent with a second mutation in the RSV provirus which might affect a *trans*-acting packaging factor. In fact, recent sequence analysis of the *SE21Q1b* provirus reveals that in addition to the deletion in the L region, there is a cluster of nonconservative mutations in the NC portion of *gag* (P. SHANK, S. SHAH, O. WANG, K. LEVINE, M. LINIAL, unpublished observation). Whether the NC mutation is involved in the packaging of cellular RNA remains to be determined. However, several groups have found that mutations in NC lead to interesting phenotypes. One such mutant (constructed in vitro) led to the production of particles which lack dimeric genomic RNA but appear to contain 35S monomers (MERIC and SPAHR 1986). In other studies, an NC protein with two lysine residues replaced by isoleucine had a lowered binding affinity for RNA, and particles produced after transfection lacked viral RNA (FU et al. 1985, 1988). The most tantalizing evidence that the NC domain is involved in specific RNA recognition is recent work (GORELICK et al. 1989) demonstrating that mutations in NC "cys-his" motif (thought to be involved in RNA binding) lead to the production of noninfectious particles lacking genomic RNA but containing detectable levels of some cellular RNA. Similar (but not identical) MuLV NC mutations leading to noninfectious particle production have also been constructed by others (C. MERIC and S. GOFF, 1989).

In these latter experiments, the nucleic acid packaged into the mutant particles was examined. Cellular mRNA for β-actin was not detected in any mutant particles examined. Many of the mutations decreased the packaging of both MuLV and endogenous VL30 sequences into particles (see Sect. 5.3), although several led to decreased packaging of MuLV RNA without depressing VL30 RNA packaging. Taken together, these results strongly suggest that the NC domain is an important component of RNA packaging. However, much remains to be learned about specific vs nonspecific RNA binding of NC and the actual protein-RNA interaction that leads to genomic encapsidation.

4 Retrovirus Packaging Cell Lines

Knowledge of the sequences required for RNA encapsidation has led to the development of retroviral packaging cell lines, which have emerged as powerful reagents for gene transfer studies. Packaging cells are designed to synthesize all retroviral proteins necessary in *trans* for the production of infectious (but replication-defective) retrovirus. Introduction of a retroviral vector containing *cis*-acting retroviral signals into packaging cells results in the production of virus which can infect cells but which cannot spread to other cells. This feature is particularly important when using retrovirus vectors to mark cells in cell fusion studies, in cell lineage analysis, or in potential applications to human gene therapy.

The utility of such a gene transfer system stems from unique features of the retroviral life cycle, particularly the integration of a nonrearranged copy of the viral DNA into the genomic DNA of infected cells, resulting in the stable inheritance of transferred genes. Such vectors can be used to infect cells that are refractory to other techniques, including cells in intact animals. Retroviral vectors can be generated at high titer by using packaging cells and can infect a wide range of cell types from different vertebrate species.

4.1 Packaging Cell Line Construction

Packaging cell lines should be capable of synthesizing all the retroviral proteins required for the assembly of high titer infectious virus but should not release replication-competent virus. Several reported packaging cell lines meet these criteria and are capable of producing retroviral vectors at high titer (10^6 to 10^7 infectious units per ml) in the absence of helper virus production (< 1 unit per ml). However, packaging cells which are initially helper virus-free can convert to helper virus-positive during prolonged passage (BOSSELMAN et al. 1987), presumably due to recombination between the deleted proviral sequences used to make the packaging cells and endogenous retroviral-like elements found in the cells of most eukaryotes. In addition, the introduction of some retroviral vectors into packaging cells can result in helper virus production, most likely by recombination between homologous regions of the vector and the defective virus used to make the packaging cells. Introduction of a retroviral vector containing sequences that overlap with sequences 3′ to the end of the deletion reproducibly yields helper virus after short-term passage of the cells (MILLER et al. 1986; STOKER and BISSELL 1988).

The first packaging cell lines were made by using murine helper viruses from which the 350-base pair retroviral packaging signal had been deleted (Fig. 2B) (MANN et al. 1983; CONE and MULLIGAN 1984; MILLER et al. 1985). While packaging cells of this type have been used with success in a number of studies, these lines suffer from some important defects. First, although deletion of the packaging signal reduces the amount of helper virus RNA that is packaged into virions, the block is far from complete. Should the deleted helper genome be packaged, there are no further blocks to infection of other cells, as the signals for reverse transcription and integration are intact. Indeed, virus from this type of packaging cell is capable of rescuing retroviral vectors in the absence of overt helper virus production presumably because of transfer of the Ψ- helper virus (CONE and MULLIGAN 1984; MILLER and BUTTIMORE 1986). Further evidence that deletion of the packaging signal is not sufficient to prevent packaging comes from studying a Ψ- retroviral vector. Although the rate of packaging and transfer of this vector was reduced 3000-fold relative to a vector containing the packaging signal, it was easily detectable (MANN and BALTIMORE 1985). Thus, deletion of only the packaging signal from a helper virus does not completely prevent spread of the virus, which occurs at a greatly reduced rate. The other problem with packaging cell lines based on Ψ- helper viruses is the ease with which the Ψ signal can be restored (Fig. 2b).

These problems have been reduced by employing packaging cells made with helper virus genomes containing further deletions. An example is the PA317 cell line (MILLER and BUTTIMORE 1986). PA317 cells contain a helper virus in which the packaging signal was deleted, the 3′ LTR and plus strand PBS were replaced with a polyadenylation site from SV40, and the 5′-end of the 5′ LTR was deleted (Fig. 2c). Thus, in the event that RNA from this construct is packaged, it cannot be reverse transcribed, and sites in the LTRs required for integration of the virus are missing. Indeed, while rescue of a retroviral vector was observed by using virus from packaging lines containing Ψ- helper virus, no rescue was observed with virus from PA317 cells (MILLER and BUTTIMORE 1986). Helper virus production from PA317 cells was not detected after introduction of a vector which contained sequences capable of complementing the packaging genome by homologous recombination. Recombination must occur at two different regions of homology to generate helper virus (Fig. 2c), and the frequency of this is lower than that of the single recombination necessary to generate helper virus in cells containing the Ψ- helper virus (Fig. 2b).

Packaging cells have also been constructed by separating the *gag-pol* and *env* genes into two separate transcriptional units. In principle, the advantage of this

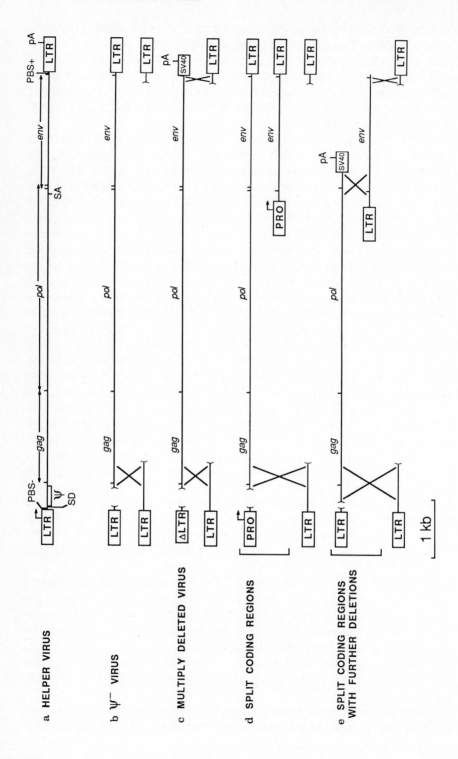

technique is that an additional site of recombination between these elements is required to produce helper virus. Unfortunately, early packaging lines generated via this strategy utilized a nearly complete retroviral genome for synthesis of *gag-pol* proteins (WATANABE and TEMIN 1983; BOSSELMAN et al. 1987) so that only one recombination event between the *gag-pol* transcriptional unit and endogenous retroviral elemets, or an introduced vector, is necessary to generate helper virus (Fig. 2d). Thus, in terms of recombination, these cell lines are functionally similar to packaging cells made with the helper virus depicted in Fig. 2b. More recently, a packaging line containing further deletions of the *gag-pol* and *env* transcriptional units was made such that three recombination events in separate regions would be required to generate helper virus (MARKOWITZ et al. 1988; Fig. 2E). However, the *pol* gene partially overlaps the *env* gene in the parental helper virus (Mo-MuLV), and so homologous recombination is potentially possible between the *gag-pol* and *env* transcripts.

Efforts to improve packaging cell lines involve attempts to reduce the generation of replication-competent virus, to alter the cell type and host range of virions produced by the cells, and to improve the viral titer. Potential production of helper virus from packaging cells remains a concern which can never be entirely excluded. Since helper virus production is a function of the packaging cells and the retroviral vectors used, much of the problem can be prevented by the elimination of homologous overlaps between vector and the defective helper virus. Although it is not known what role endogenous retroviral-like sequences in the packaging cells have on helper virus production, several of the available packaging cell lines have been grown for long periods of time in culture without detectable helper virus production, suggesting that the contribution of these sequences is minor. For many practical purposes, the problem of helper virus production has been solved with the currently available packaging cell lines.

4.2 Packaging Cell Host Range

The ability of virus from packaging cells to infect cells from different species and different tissues is dependent primarily upon the *env* gene product, which interacts with specific cell surface receptors during virus infection, and upon minor determinants in other viral proteins (reviewed in WEISS 1984; HUNTER and SWANSTROM, this volume). Packaging cell lines have been constructed by using

◄ ───────────────────────────────────────

Fig. 2a–e. Strategies for packaging cell line construction. A generic helper virus (modeled on Mo-MuLV) is shown in **a**. Possible strategies used to generate deleted viruses that provide all the proteins required for viral replication but which cannot themselves replicate are shown. The *bottom line* of each set of constructs depicts the regions of a generic retroviral vector (or other endogenous retrovirus-like element present in packaging cells) which contain sequence homology to the deleted viruses. The *large Xs* indicate potential areas of homologous recombination which could lead to helper virus production. *LTR*, viral long terminal repeat; *PRO*, second promoter (LTR, WATANABE and TEMIN 1983; or metallothionine promoter. BOSSELMAN et al. 1987); *pA*, polyadenylation signal; *SD*, splice donor; *SA*, splice acceptor; *PBS* − and *PBS* +, minus and plus strand primer binding sites

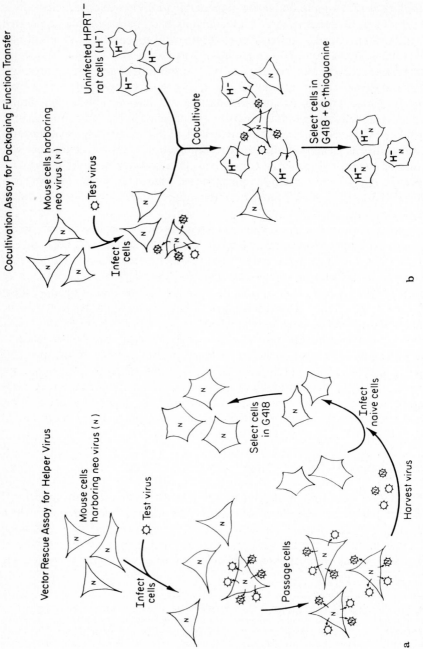

Fig. 3 a, b. Methods for detection of helper virus (**a**) and for detection of packaging function transfer (**b**)

ecotropic MuLV, amphotropic MuLV, SNV, and ALV. By far the widest host range can be obtained by using amphotropic packaging cells, which produce particles capable of infecting many vertebrate species including mouse, rat, dog, cat, monkey, chicken , mink, and human.

4.3 Helper Virus Detection

Helper virus or helper virus function can be detected by a number of techniques, with widely varying sensitivities and specificities (reviewed in WEISS 1984). Standard plaque formation or focus formation assays generally depend on rapid virus spread and can miss partially defective viruses which are in fact replication competent. For example, a single base change in Mo-MuLV is sufficient to make the virus undetectable by the XC plaque assay, although the virus is still infectious (MILLER and VERMA 1984). In addition, these techniques are capable of detecting virus with specific host ranges but might not detect retroviruses with an altered host range, which could arise by recombination events involving endogenous retroviruses present in the packaging cells.

A sensitive assay for helper virus production relies on the rescue of a replication-defective retrovirus vector carrying a selectable marker from cells that are nonproductively infected with the vector (Fig. 3a). The vector is not released by the cells unless helper virus is present. Medium to be tested for the presence of helper virus is incubated with the cells for 24 h, and the infected cells are passaged for 2–4 weeks to allow for virus spread. Medium harvested from the cells is then assayed for the presence of virus containing the selectable marker by infection of drug-sensitive cells. Production of drug-resistant colonies confirms the presence of helper virus. This assay will only detect viruses that are capable of infecting the nonproducer cells and the cells used for assay of drug-resistant virus, so these cells must be carefully chosen to enable measurement of all possible helper viruses. For example, mouse cells can release xenotropic viruses, but as these do not replicate in mouse cells, they would not be detected in an assay involving mouse cell infection.

Transfer to other cells of the genome containing the packaging region deletion is more difficult to detect than helper virus production because this genome is not rapidly spread to other cells, and low-level rescue of a retroviral vector may be difficult to detect. For example, infrequent transfer of a Ψ- helper virus to cells harboring a neo-vector can result in cells that secrete neo + virus, but because these cells constitute only a minor proportion of the population, little if any neo vector can be found in medium harvested from the cell population. In this case, the assay used for helper virus detection is modified to screen for production of the vector by isolated cells in a population. This is done by cocultivating the infected nonproducer cells with another cell line carrying a different marker (Fig. 3b). Following cocultivation, detection of cells that carry both selectable markers indicate transfer of the retroviral vector and thus transfer of packaging function from the packaging cells.

5 Packaging of Nongenomic RNAs

Although retroviral packaging of genomic RNA is a fairly precise process, other types of RNAs are also included in the particles, some by design, such as the minus-strand primer tRNA, others by accident (reviewed in COFFIN 1984a).

5.1 tRNAs and Other Small RNAs

It has been estimated that only half the RNA by weight encapsidated into retroviral particles is genomic; the rest is of smaller species. The primary type of small encapsidated RNA is host tRNA including, but not limited to, the specific tRNA which is utilized as the negative strand primer by reverse transcriptase. In addition, virions contain small amounts of 18S and 28S ribosomal RNAs, as well as 5S and 7S RNAs. Specific encapsidation of the primer tRNA appears to require association with reverse transcriptase, rather than with genomic RNA (LEVIN and SEIDMAN 1979; SAWYER and HANAFUSA 1979; PETERS and HU 1980).

Except for the primer tRNA, there is no evidence that any of the small RNAs which are encapsidated have a function in the retroviral life cycle. Interesting data have been obtained relating to the possible role of 7S L RNAs which are packaged into virions (TAYLOR and CYWINSKI 1984; CHEN et al. 1985). 7S RNAs are RNA polymerase III transcripts and share sequence homology with the abundant DNA repeat family, Alu (JAGADEESWARAN et al. 1981; ULLU et al. 1982). 7S L RNA is the RNA component of the signal recognition particle, which mediates the translocation of secretory proteins across the endoplasmic reticulum (WALTER and BLOBEL 1982). It has been suggested that the large Alu family of pseudogenes may have arisen by retrotransposition (JAGADEESWARAN et al. 1981; VAN ARSDELL et al. 1981). Since 7S is packaged into retroviruses, is it possible that retroviral-mediated reverse transcription and integration of a 7S-like sequence could account for the Alu repeats in the eukaryotic genome? In fact, a detectable endogenous reverse transcription product from SE21Q1b virions [which encapsidate cellular rather than viral RNAs (LINIAL et al. 1978); see Sect. 5.4] is a cDNA copy of 7S RNA (CHEN et al. 1985). This cDNA product is made using random tRNA-like primers (CHEN et al. 1985; TAYLOR and CYWINSKI 1984). Thus, a mechanism exists which could link retroviruses and Alu-like sequences. However, SE21Q1b virions are shed from quail cells, a species which does not contain highly repetitive Alu-like DNA (J.M. TAYLOR, personal communication), and conversely, the reverse transcription of 7S RNAs has not been examined in retroviruses of mammalian origin.

5.2 Subgenomic Viral mRNAs

Wild-type retroviruses can also encapsidate viral mRNAs which are less than genomic length. Efficient encapsidation of subgenomic mRNAs could have profound effects on the ability of a virus to replicate. Subgenomic mRNAs contain both minus- and plus-strand primer sites for reverse transcriptase, as well as the sequences at the ends of U5 and U3 thought to be important for high-efficiency integration. Thus, packaged *env* or other subgenomic mRNAs would be efficiently integrated into the infected cell genome and might preclude productive infection. The subgenomic RNAs of mammalian retroviruses do not contain Ψ sequences and thus are excluded from encapsidation. While the subgenomic mRNAs of avian retroviruses such as RSV or ALV do contain leader-region packaging sequences, they are not packaged as efficiently as genomic RNA for unknown reasons (KATZ et al. 1986), although size could be a factor.

There are examples of infection by avian retroviruses leading to the rapid disappearance of full-length provirus and the concomitant appearance of proviruses similar in structure to subgenomic RNA. One dramatic case is that of the defective transforming avian retrovirus MH2. The genomic RNA is 5.4 kb and is comprised of a portion of the *gag* gene, as well as the oncogenes v-*mil* and v-*myc*. The *mil* gene product is encoded as a Gag polyprotein from the genomic length RNA. In addition, a 2.5 kb subgenomic RNA is transcribed which serves as the mRNA for the *myc* gene product (reviewed in BISTER and JANSEN 1986). MH2 virus does not encode *gag*, *pol*, or *env* gene products and thus requires a nondefective helper virus for the production of particles containing the MH2 genome. Several groups have found proviruses in MH2-transformed cells, whose sizes and sequences indicate that they were derived from subgenomic *myc* mRNA (MARTIN et al. 1986; PATSCHINSKY et al. 1986; BIEGALKE and LINIAL 1987). In one study (BIEGALKE and LINIAL 1987), it was found that greater than 90% of the transformed cells obtained after infection with MH2 lacked detectable full-length provirus, although all cells contained a provirus of a size compatible with reverse transcription and integration of the subgenomic RNA (BIEGALKE and LINIAL 1987). In fact, stocks of MH2 virus were found to encapsidate significant amounts of the MH2 subgenomic RNA (B. BIEGALKE and M. LINIAL, unpublished observations). Passage of MH2 leads to decreased titers of transforming virus, since the presence of both *myc* and *mil* is required for efficient transformation. It is not known why MH2 has a propensity to encapsidate more subgenomic RNAs than other avian retroviruses such as RSV.

Analysis of a RSV mutant, TK15, also clearly demonstrates the genetic transfer of subgenomic viral mRNAs to infected cells. TK15 is poorly infectious, due in part to a deletion in the leader region packaging signal (KAWAI and KOYAMA 1984; KOYAMA et al. 1984). TK15 infection gives rise to transformed cell clones which do not produce infectious virus. Sequence analysis of the proviruses from the nonproducer cells demonstrated that many of them have structures which are consistent with reverse transcription and integration of subgenomic *src* mRNA. Such an event presumably occurs in wild-type RSV infection as well but is masked by the more efficient spread of wild-type proviruses. Evidence for this comes from experiments in which transformants were obtained via rescue of RSV from RSV-transformed nonproducer mammalian cells after cell fusion with avian cells. Despite the presence of packaging sequences in the original RSV provirus, rescued virus particles induced transformants containing a proviral structure consistent with reverse transcription and subsequent integration of *src* mRNA (SVOBODA et al. 1986; GERYK et al. 1986; J. BODOR and J. SVOBODA et al., personal communication). The reverse transcription and integration of RSV *env* mRNA has also been inferred from genetic analysis after microinjection of *env* mRNA, although the structure of the provirus was not directly analyzed (WANG and STACEY 1982).

5.3 Heterologous Retroviral RNAs

Replication competent retroviruses (such as MLV) are not the only retroviral genomes found in eukaryotic cells. Cell lines derived from many species contain large numbers of endogenous retroviruses with diverse structures and patterns of transcription (reviewed in COFFIN 1984b). Many of these are expressed to high levels; others are transcriptionally inactive. Many endogenous viral genomes are related to their exogenous counterparts, and their gene products could be encapsidated into particles encoded by related proviruses. For instance, it has been shown that particles produced from a Rev packaging line can package viral RNAs lacking encapsidation (E) sequences, if no RNAs containing the encapsidation signal are present (EMBRETSON and TEMIN 1987). Both E- Rev RNAs and MLV RNAs are packaged with an efficiency of about 20% relative to E + Rev RNA. Thus, retroviral genomes may contain sequences and/or structures other than the defined packaging signals which facilitate their encapsidation.

An example of a highly transcribed endogenous retroviral family are the VL30s. These elements are found in both mouse and rat cells. Some VL30s are transcribed into RNAs of about 5 kb; however, these transcripts do not encode any viral proteins. VL30 RNA is efficiently encapsidated into both murine and other mammalian retroviral particles, even in the presence of Ψ + RNAs (SHERWIN et al. 1978; BESMER et al. 1979; SCOLNICK et al. 1979), indicating that the VL30 genome may contain a packaging sequence related to that of exogenous retroviruses. In fact, mouse VL30 genomes have been deliberately introduced into tissue culture cells via infection by particles released from wild-type infected cells, as well as from the packaging cell line Ψ-2 (SHERWIN et al. 1978; RODLAND et al. 1987). Particles produced from Ψ-2 and PA317 packaging cell lines (in the presence or absence of packageable retroviral vector RNAs) contain easily detectable amounts of VL30 RNA (R. ARONOFF and M. LINIAL, unpublished observations). Mutations in the NC domain of *gag* can affect packaging of MLV and VL30 RNAs independently (C. MERIC and S. GOFF, personal communication; see Sect. 3). The ability of diverse retroviruses to package endogenous retroviral-like RNAs has implications for some potential uses of retroviral vectors in gene therapy (see Sect. 4).

5.4 Cellular mRNAs

Packaging, reverse transcription, and integration of cellular RNAs by retroviruses could have profound effects on the structure of the eukaryotic genome. In fact, it has been known for some time that wild-type retroviruses do occasionally encapsidate cellular mRNAs. One example is the packaging of a specific cellular mRNA encoding a 36 K protein into RSV particles (ADKINS and HUNTER 1981). The 36 K protein appears to be related to glyceraldehyde phosphate dehydrogenase (J. COOPER, personal communication). In this case, there may be a specific association of the mRNA with the particular viral strain used, since the RNA is packaged disproportionately to its representation in the cell. Another example of cellular RNA packaging is the incorporation of globin mRNA into Friend leukemia virus particles released from erythroid cells (IKAWA et al. 1974). This probably represents the amplified detection of a rare random event, since globin mRNA is the major mRNA in these cells. In neither of these cases were the consequences of cellular RNA packaging examined. Indeed, in order to study the transfer of cellular RNAs by retroviral infection, a selectable marker is required, since the event is predicted to be rare.

Several mutants of RSV package cellular mRNAs to a greater extent than wild-type virus. TK15 contains a deletion in the leader packaging site (NISHIZAWA et al. 1985; see Fig. 1A). Although TK15 particles contain little genomic RSV RNA, it has been inferred that they do contain RNAs, possibly including cellular mRNAs. TK15 particles induce virus-nonproducing transformants at high frequency. Sequence analysis has revealed that many of these transformants contain proviruses in which portions of the viral genome have been replaced by cellular sequences, probably derived from mRNAs (NISHIZAWA et al. 1987). These recombinants might arise because the mutant packages cellular mRNA. Retroviruses are known to undergo high frequency recombination (reviewed in LINIAL and BLAIR 1984). Although not directly demonstrated, recombination is thought to occur during reverse transcription. Because retroviruses are diploid, both templates could participate in the generation of a single provirus, and template switching by reverse transcription could generate recombinants. Both "copy-choice" and "strand-invasion" recombination models have been proposed (COFFIN 1979, HUNTER 1978). Structures compatible with a strand displacement model have been visualized under the electron microscope (JUNGHANS et al. 1982). Copackaging of cellular and viral RNAs into a single retroviral particle could lead to rare recombinants through a similar reverse transcriptase-mediated mechanism, and this has been proposed for TK15 viral-cell recombinants (NISHIZAWA et al. 1987). Since the flanking regions of the inserted sequences in the TK15 proviruses have not been sequenced, it is not known whether recombination occurs through small regions of homology or at heterologous sequences.

It has been shown that competent transforming virus can be generated in vitro from a nontransforming MLV and a transforming virus (HaSV) deleted at the 3' end. The transforming viruses regained the 3'-end by recombination with the MLV genome at a region in which no sequence homology exists between the two genomes and hence occurred through illegitimate recombination (GOLDFARB and WEINBERG 1981). It should be noted, however, that illegitimate recombination mediated by reverse transcriptase has not been directly demonstrated.

In the HaSV studies, it was suggested that transcripts originating in the genomes with 3′ deletions continued through into the flanking genomic sequences. The existence of such readthrough RNAs suggests a general mechanism by which cellular sequences could be incorporated into retroviral genomes. Readthrough RNAs which initiate from retroviral transcriptional signals in the 5′ LTR and continue through the genome into cellular flanking sequences comprise a large fraction of the retroviral RNA in ALV-infected fibroblasts (HERMAN and COFFIN 1986). Packaging of such readthrough RNAs into retroviral particles has been shown to occur if the retroviral polyadenylation signal is mutated (HERMAN and COFFIN 1987) and could presumably also occur at lower levels in wild-type retroviral infections. Encapsidation of downstream cellular RNA sequences via transcriptional readthrough and subsequent deletion of viral sequences and/or recombination with helper virus during reverse transcription could generate chimeric genomes characteristic of acute transforming viruses. In fact, recent experiments with additional mutants which have no functional U3 polyadenylation signals suggest that the actual sequences at the 3′-end of the RNA are irrelevant to packaging (M. SWAIN and J. COFFIN, personal communication).

The mutant cell line SE21Q1b produces particles containing predominantly poly-A + cellular RNA (LINIAL et al. 1978). When the RNA isolated from SE21Q1b virions is translated in vitro, the protein profile is similar to that of in vivo-labelled quail fibroblasts (GALLIS et al. 1979). Thus, cellular RNAs appear to be randomly packaged, in rough proportion to their intracellular concentration. Interestingly, the cellular RNA is encapsidated as a complex, since the average sedimentation coefficient of the RNA decreases from greater than 35S to less than 28S upon heat denaturation (LINIAL et al. 1978). Viral genomic and mRNAs are randomly packaged into virions in proportion to their intracellular concentration as well. However, virions are rarely infectious, since even if genomic RNA is encapsidated, it lacks a (−) strand PBS (see Sect. 2.1 and Fig. 1a). As discussed in Sect. 3, cellular RNA packaging may be a consequence of mutations in the *gag* gene. This is supported by the finding that some packaging cell lines produce particles lacking the specific cellular mRNAs which can be readily detected in SE21Q1b virions (R. ARONOFF and M. LINIAL, unpublished results).

6 Retroviruses and Genetic Flux

Processed pseudogenes are abundant genetic elements, comprising at least 5% of the mammalian cell genome. These pseudogenes lack introns and often contain poly-A rich 3′-ends, suggestive of an mRNA intermediate in their genesis (reviewed in TEMIN 1985; WEINER et al. 1986). Since retroviral particles encapsidate reverse transcriptase and are ubiquitous, encapsidation of cellular mRNAs into viral particles could be a mechanism (among others) by which processed pseudogenes are generated (BALTIMORE 1985). Packaging cell lines have provided an opportunity to examine whether RNAs which do not contain retroviral sequences normally used by the virus for reverse transcription and integration can nonetheless be stably transferred by retroviral infection. Selectable genes which are transcribed from DNAs lacking most retroviral sequences can be introduced into packaging cells. If the selectable genes are packaged into retroviral particles, the ability of retroviral infection to confer the selectable phenotype to other cells can then be assessed.

The following three strategies have been utilized to transfer nonretroviral genes by viral infection. (a) Some avian packaging cell lines such as $SE21Q1b$ and TK15 release retroviral particles containing cellular RNAs. This has been exploited by transfection of $SE21Q1b$ cells with plasmids containing the neomycin phosphotransferase gene of Tn5 (neo). Other quail cells are then infected with the neo + particles (LINIAL 1987). In this case neo sequences are randomly packaged into virions in proportion to their intracellular concentration along with other cellular RNAs. (b) An encapsidation signal ($\Psi+$; BENDER et al. 1987) has been inserted into a neo plasmid lacking retroviral sequences and transfected into a packaging cell line. Particles specifically encapsidate the neo RNA (ADAM and MILLER 1988) and can transfer the neo marker upon infection (R. ARONOFF and M. LINIAL, unpublished results). (c) A transcriptional unit containing the selectable marker hygro driven by an SV40 promoter and including an additional upstream MLV promoter was introduced into SNV packaging cells. In this case the upstream promoter was included so that reverse transcription and integration of a transcript starting in this promoter would result in a hygro gene with an intact SV40 promoter. Transfer of the hygromycin resistance phenotype from the packaging cells into recipients by viral infection was dependent upon reverse transcription and integration of an RNA lacking all retroviral sequences (DORNBURG and TEMIN 1988). These three strategies are outlined in Fig. 4. To date, there are no examples of retrotransposition of cellular sequences by retrotransposons, such as mammalian IAP particles, L1 elements, or yeast Ty elements, unless the cellular sequences are incorporated between retrotransposon sequences.

Analysis of the mechanism of the transfer of nonretroviral sequences by infection with $SE21Q1b$ particles (termed retrofection; Fig. 4a) has shown that the acquisition of neo^R is RNA mediated and requires no retroviral sequences. The neo allele is inherited as a single integrated copy (LINIAL 1987). Thus, the retroviral particle is capable of reverse transcribing RNA lacking retroviral primer binding signals. The enzymatic requirements for integration of the cDNAs into the cell genome are not known. The efficiency of gene transfer via retrofection to quail cells by $SE21Q1b$ is surprisingly high. It is estimated that 0.1%–1.0% of the particles which encapsidate neo mRNA are capable of converting infected cells to the neo^R phenotype (G418 resistance). Thus, despite the lack of specific

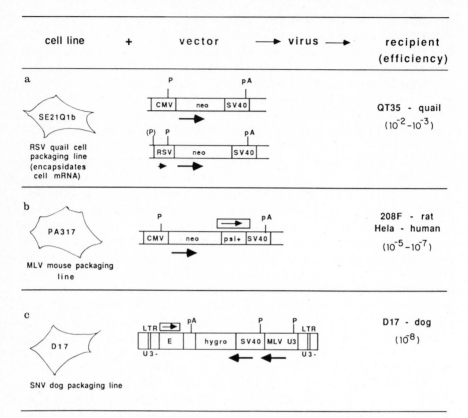

Fig. 4a–c. Strategies to examine retroviral transfer of nonretroviral sequences encapsidated into particles. Indicated vectors were transfected into the cell lines shown in **a** and **b**. In **c**, D17 cells were infected with a viral vector which led ultimately to the formation of the indicated vector structure. Vectors, cell lines, and efficiencies of transfer were taken from the following references: **a** LINIAL 1987; **b** R. ARONOFF and M. LINIAL, unpublished data; **c** DORNBURG and TEMIN 1988. *CMV*, cytomegalovirus; *RSV*, Rous sarcoma virus; *neo*, neomycin resistance gene; *hygro*, hygromycin resistance gene; *psi*, MLV packaging region; *E*, SNV(packaging region; *MLV U3*, 3′ unique sequences of murine leukemia virus; *LTR*, SNV long terminal repeat with U3 deletion; *P*, promoter; *pA*, polyadenylation signal. *Arrows below the plasmid* indicate the direction and extent of transcription from the promoters; *boxed arrows above the plasmid* indicate the direction of the packaging signal in the vector. Efficiencies are based on a wild-type virus or wild-type vector efficiency of 1.0

primers for reverse transcription and of sequences and structures necessary for retroviral-mediated integration, these events are accomplished with a high efficiency. However, this may be a unique feature of the avian cell. In dog cells the efficiency of retroviral-mediated stable transfer of hygromycin resistance in the absence of retroviral sequences is much lower (estimated at 10^{-8}-fold) than with retroviral vectors (DORNBURG and TEMIN 1988). A low efficiency of retrofection is also seen in rat and human cells, where only about 0.0001% of the particles lead to G418 resistance (decreased about 10^6-fold from wild-type vector infection; R. ARONOFF and M. LINIAL, unpublished results). Interestingly, in all of the infected mammalian cell cultures, it was noted that many antibiotic-resistant clones appeared, which were only transiently resistant and did not grow into cultures (DORNBURG and TEMIN 1988; R. ARONOFF and M. LINIAL, unpublished data). This is not seen with infected quail cells (LINIAL 1987; R. ARONOFF and M. LINIAL, unpublished data). One possibility for the decreased gene transfer in mammalian cells is that integration is less efficient (DORNBURG and TEMIN 1988).

It is important to emphasize that the acquisition of natural processed pseudogenes are germ-line events, while the systems amenable to genetic analysis involve infection of established cell lines. It is likely that the enzymatic apparatus of meiotic and mitotic cells is different, particularly with regard to enzymes involved in recombination. Thus, if retroviruses are involved in natural processed pseudogene formation, the cellular factors, and hence the resulting genetic structures, could be quite different from those observed in tissue culture systems. There are classes of endogenous retroviruses and retrotransposons which are transcribed during early embryogenesis (BICZYSKO et al. 1973; HUANG et al. 1981) and are capable of retrotransposition within the germ line (COPELAND et al. 1983). Such elements could perhaps mediate processed pseudogene formation. Natural processed pseudogene formation could also occur completely intracellularly without a requirement for exogenously infectious virions. In fact, genetic events consistent with retrotransposition of a defective MLV provirus have been detected in mouse cells in culture, at an extremely low frequency (HEIDMANN et al. 1988). Despite the inability to detect infectious particles in this system, the participation of some retroviral-like particle in retrotransposition events cannot be ruled out. However, these data are consistent with intracellular retrotransposition, akin to that seen with the Ty elements of yeast, which involves intracellular rather than extracellular virus-like particles (GARFINKEL et al. 1985).

Processed pseudogenes often share structural features such as short stretches of poly-A at the 3' end and direct repeats of 8–40 bp in the flanking cellular DNA. Thus, it is of interest to determine whether the "processed genes" created by retroviral infection have these features as well, despite the inherent weaknesses of a tissue culture system as a model for pseudogene formation. Molecular cloning and sequencing of the *neo* sequences which have been retrofected into quail cells have provided some information as to possible mechanisms of reverse transcription and integration of the nonretroviral sequences (B. STEINER, K. JOHNSON, K. LEVINE, and M. LINIAL, unpublished results). Three independently derived *neo*[R] clones have been analyzed in some detail. In each case a single copy of the *neo* gene has integrated at a different chromosomal location. The structure of the integrated *neo* genes suggests that the priming site for reverse transcription of the *neo* RNA is likely to be at the 3'-end at or near the poly-A tail on the mRNA. The 3' ends are just downstream of a consensus polyadenylation site, but there is no poly-A tract. In two cases, direct repeats of the *neo* gene have been created during the gene transfer process. These might have arisen as a consequence of formation of "snap-back" cDNA during reverse transcription of the 5'-end of the mRNA. Such structures are often seen in vitro during cDNA synthesis reactions employing reverse transcriptase and in vivo reverse transcription of the cauliflower mosaic virus genome (COVEY and TURNER 1986). Integration of the cDNAs appears to have occurred at or near direct repeats that preexisted in the quail DNA, and integration is concomitant with deletion of some quail sequences. In one case a direct repeat of 7 nucleotides is found at the site of *neo* integration. However, this small repeat is a vestige of a 40-nucleotide perfect direct repeat that was present at the preintegration site. Integration of *neo* led to a ca. 900-bp deletion, including most of the direct repeat. It will be of interest to determine whether such deletion events accompany cDNA integration in other artificially processed genes as well as natural polymorphic processed pseudo-genes. The sequence data which have been obtained to date are consistent with integration of a cDNA molecule into a break in the chromosomal DNA, perhaps as part of a DNA repair mechanism. Such breaks could have occurred as a result of homologous recombination between direct repeats.

7 Conclusions

The sequences involved in genomic RNA packaging have been localized for three classes of retroviruses, the murine oncoviruses MLV and MSV, the avian oncoviruses RSV and ALV, and the avian retroviruses Rev and SNV. In all of them, a major component of the genomic RNA recognition is localized near the 5′-end of the virion RNA. Deletion of small stretches of this region (ca. 100–300 nucleotides) prevents specific encapsidation of the viral RNA into virions. The packaging region has been termed psi (Ψ) for MLV/MSV and RSV, and E for SNV. Deletion of the packaging region has allowed construction of cell lines (packaging cell lines) which produce particles lacking parental genomic RNA. Similar regions of the genome can be added to retroviral or nonretroviral vectors to ensure their efficient encapsidation into the particles produced from packaging cell lines. The details of the sequence specificity of the *cis*-acting RNA sequences which are required for efficient encapsidation are not as yet known. Even less is known about the virally coded factor(s) which interact with the Ψ sequences. Recent data suggest that the nucleocapsid (NC) protein component of the *gag* gene is an important component of specific retroviral RNA packaging. The packaging of retroviral RNA should provide an excellent system in which to study the details of specific RNA-protein interactions, since the system is highly amenable to mutation and genetic analysis, and the end product (infectious virions) is easily assayed. Understanding of the specifics of the encapsidation should prove useful in designing the optimal vectors and packaging lines for future gene therapy applications.

Acknowledgements. We thank numerous colleagues who contributed unpublished results and preprints which added to the completeness of this chapter. We are indebted to Jon Cooper, Bob Eisenman, Kate Levine, and Rachel Aronoff for their critiques. Work from our laboratories was supported by grants from the National Cancer Institute and the National Heart, Lung, and Blood Institute.

References

Adam MA, Miller AD (1988) Identification of a signal in a murine retrovirus that is sufficient for packaging of non-retroviral RNA into virions. J Virol 62: 3802–3806

Adkins B, Hunter T (1981) Identification of a packaged cellular mRNA in virions of Rous sarcoma virus. J Virol 39: 471–481

Armentano D, Yu S-F, Kantoff PW, von Ruden T, Anderson WF, Gilboa E (1987) Effect of internal viral sequences on the utility of retroviral vectors. J Virol 61: 1647–1650

Baltimore D (1985) Retroviruses and retrotransposons: the role of reverse transcriptase in shaping the eukaryotic genome. Cell 40: 481–482

Bender MA, Palmer TD, Gelinas RE, Miller AD (1987) Evidence that the packaging signal of Moloney murine leukemia virus extends into the *gag* region. J Virol 61: 1639–1646

Besmer P, Olshevsky D, Baltimore D, Dolberg D, Fan H (1979) Virus-like 30S RNA in mouse cells. J Virol 29: 1168–1176

Biczysko W, Pienkowski M, Solter D, Koprowski H (1973) Virus particles in early mouse embryos. JNCI 51: 1041–1959

Biegalke B, Linial M (1987) Retention or loss of v-*mil* sequences after propagation of MH2 virus in vivo or in vitro. J Virol 61: 1949–1956

Bister K, Jansen HW (1986) Oncogenes in retroviruses and cells: biochemistry and molecular genetics. Adv Cancer Res 47: 99–188

Bosselman RA, Hsu R-Y, Bruszewski J, Hu S, Martin F, Nicholson M (1987) Replication-defective chimeric helper proviruses and factors affecting generation of competent virus: expression of Moloney murine leukemia virus structural genes via the metallothionein promoter. Mol Cell Biol 7: 1797–1806

Canaani E, von der Helm K, Duesberg P (1973) Evidence for 30–40S RNA as precursor of the 60–70S RNA of Rous sarcoma virus. Proc Natl Acad Sci USA 70: 401–405

Chen P-J, Cywinski A, Taylor JM (1985) Reverse transcription of 7S-L RNA by an avian retrovirus. J Virol 54: 278–284

Cheung K–S, Smith RE, Stone MP, Joklik WK (1972) Comparison of immature (rapid) and mature Rous sarcoma virus particles. Virology 50: 851–864

Coffin JM (1979) Structure, replication and recombination of retrovirus genomes. J Gen Virol 42: 1–26

Coffin JM (1984a) Structure of the retroviral genome. In: Weiss R, Teich N, Varmus H, Coffin J (eds) 2nd edn, Part 1, Cold Spring Harbor Laboratory, Cold Spring Harbor, pp 261–368

Coffin JM (1984b) Endogenous viruses. In: Weiss R, Teich N, Varmus H, Coffin J (eds) RNA tumor viruses. 2nd edn, Part 2. Cold Spring Harbor Laboratory, Cold Spring Harbor, pp 1110–1202

Coffin JM (1985) Genome structure. In: Weiss R, Teich N, Varmus H, Coffin J (eds) RNA tumor viruses. 2nd edn, Part 2. Cold Spring Harbor Laboratory, Cold Spring Harbor, pp 17–74

Cone RD, Mulligan RC (1984) High-efficiency gene transfer into mammalian cells: generation of helper-free recombinant retrovirus with broad mammalian host range. Proc Natl Acad Sci USA 81: 6349–6353

Copeland NG, Hutchison KW, Jenkins NA (1983) Excision of the DBA ecotropic provirus in dilute coat-color revertants of mice occurs by homologous recombination involving the viral LTRs. Cell 33: 379–387

Covey SN, Turner DS (1986) Hairpin DNAs of cauliflower mosaic virus generated by reverse transcription in vivo. EMBO J 5: 2763–2768

DeGudicibus SJ, Gentile B, Bhatt RS, Poonian MS, Stacey DW (1986) Studies of retroviral packaging. In: Celis JE, Graessmann A, Loyter A (eds) Microinjection and organelle transplantation techniques. Academic, London, pp 59–65

Dickson C, Eisenman R, Fan H, Hunter E, Teich N (1984) Protein biosynthesis and assembly. In: Weiss R, Teich N, Varmus H, Coffin J (eds) RNA tumor viruses 2nd edn, Part I. Cold Spring Harbor Laboratory, Cold Spring Harbor, pp 785–998

Dornburg R, Temin HM (1988) Retroviral vector system for the study of cDNA gene formation. Mol Cell Biol 8: 2329–2334

Embretson JE, Temin HM (1987) Lack of competition results in efficient packaging of heterologous murine retroviral RNAs and reticuloendotheliosis virus encapsidation-minus RNAs by the reticuloendotheliosis virus helper cell line. J Virol 61: 2675–2683

Fu X, Phillips N, Jentoft J, Tuazon PT, Traugh JA, Leis J (1985) Site-specific phosphorylation of avian retrovirus nucleocapsid protein pp 12 regulates binding to RNA. J Biol Chem 260: 9941–9947

Fu X, Katz RA, Skalka AM, Leis J (1988) Site-directed mutagenesis of the avian retrovirus nucleocapsid protein pp 12: mutation which affects RNA binding in vitro blocks viral replication. J Biol Chem 263: 2134–2139

Gallis B, Linial M, Eisenman R (1979) An avian oncovirus mutant deficient in genomic RNA: characterization of the packaged RNA as cellular messenger RNA. Virology 94: 146–161

Garfinkel DJ, Boeke JD, Fink GR (1985) Ty element transposition: reverse transcriptase and virus-like particles. Cell 42: 507–517

Geryk J, Pichrtova J, Guntaka RV, Gowda S, Svoboda J (1986) Characterization of transforming viruses rescued from a hamster tumour cell line harbouring the v-src gene flanked by long terminal repeats. J Gen Virol 67: 2395–2404

Gerwin BI, Levin JG (1977) Interactions of murine leukemia virus core components: characterization of reverse transcriptase packaged in the absence of 70S genomic RNA. J Virol 24: 478–488

Goldfarb MP, Weinberg RA (1981) Generation of novel, biologically active Harvey sarcoma viruses via apparent illegitimate recombination. J Virol 38: 136–150

Gorelick RJ, Henderson LE, Hanser JP, Rein A Point mutants of Moloney murine leukemia virus that fail to package viral RNA: evidence for specific RNA recognition by a "zinc finger-like" protein sequence. Proc Nat Acad Sci USA 85: 8420–8424

Heidmann T, Heidmann O, Nicolas J-F (1988) An indicator gene to demonstrate intracellular transposition of defective retroviruses. Proc Natl Acad Sci USA 85: 2219–2223

Herman SA, Coffin JM (1986) Differential transcription from the long terminal repeats of integrated avian leukosis virus. J Virol 60: 497–505

Herman SA, Coffin JM (1987) Efficient packaging of readthrough RNA in ALV: implications for oncogene transduction. Science 236: 845–848

Huang TTF, Calarco PG (1981) Evidence of cell surface expression of intracisternal A particle-associated antigens during early mouse development. Dev Biol 82: 388–392

Hunter E (1978) The mechanism for genetic recombination in the avian retroviruses. Curr Top Microbiol Immunol 79: 295–309

Ikawa Y, Ross J, Leder P (1974) An association between globin messenger RNA and 60S RNA derived from Friend leukemia virus. Proc Natl Acad Sci USA 71: 1154–1158

Jagadeeswaran P, Forget BG, Weissman SM (1981) Short interspersed repetitive DNA elements in eukaryotes: transposable NA elements generated by reverse transcription of RNA pol III transcripts? Cell 26: 141–142

Junghans RP, Boone LR, Skalka AM (1982) Retroviral DNA H structures: displacement-assimilation model of recombination. Cell 30: 53–62

Katz RA, Terry RW, Skalka AM (1986) A conserved cis-acting sequence in the 5′ leader of avian sarcoma virus RNA is required for packaging. J Virol 59: 163–167

Kawai S, Koyama T (1984) Characterization of a Rous sarcoma virus mutant defective in packaging its own genomic RNA: biological properties of mutant TK15 and mutant-induced transformants. J Virol 51: 147–153

Kiessling A, Crowell R, Connell R (1987) Sperm-associated retrovirus in the mouse epididymus. Proc Natl Acad Sci 84: 8667–8671

Koyama T, Harada F, Kawai S (1984) Characterization of a Rous sarcoma virus mutant defective in packaging its own genomic RNA: biochemical properties of mutant TK15 and mutant-induced'transformants. J Virol 51: 154–162

Leis J, Baltimore D, Bishop JM, Coffin J, Fleissner E, Goff SP, Oroszlan S, Robinson H, Skalka AM, Temin HM, Vogt VM (1988) Standardized and simplified nomenclature for proteins common to all retroviruses. J Virol 62: 1808–1809

Lever A, Gottlinger H, Haseltine W and Sodroski J (1989) Identification of a sequence required for efficient packaging of human immunodeficiency virus type 1 RNA into virions. J Vir 63: 4085–4087

Levin JG, Rosenak MJ (1976) Synthesis of murine leukemia virus proteins associated with virions assemble in actinomycin D-treated cells: evidence for persistence of viral messenger RNA. Proc Natl Acad Sci USA 73: 1154–1158

Levin JG, Seidman JG (1979) Selective packaging of host tRNAs by murine leukemia virus particles does not require genomic RNA. J Virol 29: 328–335

Levin JG, Grimley PM, Ramseur JM, Berezesky IK (1974) Deficiency on 60 to 70S RNA in murine leukemia virus particles assembled in cells treated with Actinomycin D. J Virol 14: 152–161

Linial M (1981) Transfer of defective avian tumor virus genomes by a Rous sarcoma virus RNA packaging mutant. J Virol 38: 380–382

Linial M (1987) Creation of a processed pseudogene by retroviral infection. Cell 49: 93–102
Linial M, Blair D (1984) Genetics of Retroviruses. In: Weiss R, Teich N, Varmus H, Coffin J (eds) RNA tumor viruses. Cold Spring Harbor Laboratory, Cold Spring Harbor, pp 650–783
Linial M, Medeiros E, Hayward WS (1978) An avian oncovirus mutant (*SE21Q1b*) deficient in genomic RNA: biological and biochemical characterization. Cell 15: 1371–1381
Mann R, Baltimore D (1985) Varying the position of a retrovirus packaging sequence results in the encapsidation of both unspliced RNAs. J Virol 54: 401–407
Mann R, Mulligan RC, Baltimore D (1983) Construction of a retrovirus packaging mutant and its use to produce helper-free defective retrovirus. Cell 33: 153–159
Markowitz D, Goff S, Bank A (1988) A safe packaging line for gene transfer: separating viral genes on two different plasmids. J Virol 62: 1120–1124
Martin P, Henry C, Ferre F, Bechade C, Begue A, Calothy G, Debuire B, Stehelin D, Saule S (1986) Characterization of a *myc*-containing avian retrovirus generated by the propagation of an MH2 viral subgenomic RNA. J Virol 57: 1191–1194
Meric C, Darlix JL, Spahr PF (1984) It is Rous sarcoma virus p12 and not p19 that binds tightly to Rous sarcoma virus RNA. J Mol Biol 173: 531–538
Meric C, Goff SP (1989) Characterization of Moloney murine leukemia virus mutants with single-amino-acid substitutions in the Cys-his box of the nucleocapsid protein. J Vir 63: 1558–1568
Meric C, Spahr P-F (1986) Rous sarcoma virus nucleic acid-binding protein p12 is necessary for viral 70S RNA dimer formation and packaging. J Virol 60: 450–459
Miller AD, Buttimore C (1986) Redesign of retrovirus packaging cell lines to avoid recombination to helper virus production. Mol Cell Biol 6: 2895–2902
Miller AD, Verma IM (1984) Two base changes restore infectivity to a noninfectious molecular clone of Moloney murine leukemia virus (pMLV-1). J Virol 49: 214–222
Miller AD, Law MF, Verma IM (1985) Generation of helper-free amphotropic retroviruses that transduce a dominant-acting methotrexate-resistant DHFR gene. Mol Cell Biol 5: 431–437
Miller AD, Trauber DR, Buttimore C (1986) Factors involved in the production of helper virus-free retrovirus vectors. Somatic Cell Mol Genet 12: 175–183
Murphy J, Goff SP Construction and analysis of deletion mutations in the U5 region of Moloney murine leukemia virus: effects on RNA packaging and reverse transcription. J Vir 63: 319–327
Nishizawa M, Koyama T, Kawai S (1985) Unusual feature of the leader sequence of Rous sarcoma virus packaging mutant TK15. J Virol 55: 881–885
Nishizawa M, Koyama T, Kawai S (1987) Frequent segregation of more defective variants from a Rous sarcoma virus packaging mutant TK15. J Virol 61: 3208–3213
Norton PA, Coffin JM (1985) Bacterial β-galactosidase as a marker of Rous sarcoma virus gene expression and replication. Mol Cell Biol 5: 281–290
Patschinsky T, Jansen HW, Blocker H, Frank R, Bister K (1986) Structure and transforming function of transduced mutant alleles of the chicken c-*myc* gene. J Virol 59: 341–353
Peters GG, Hu J (1980) Reverse transcriptase as the major determinant for selected packaging of tRNAs into avian sarcoma virus particles. J Virol 36: 692–700
Pugatsch T, Stacey DW (1983) Identification of a sequence likely to be required for avian retroviral packaging. Virology 128: 505–511
Rodland KD, Brown AMC, Magun B (1987) Individual mouse VL30 elements transferred to rat cells by viral pseudotypes retain their responsiveness to activators of protein kinase C. Mol Cell Biol 7: 2296–2298
Sawyer RC, Hanafusa H (1979) Comparison of the small RNAs of polymerase-deficient and polymerase-positive Rous sarcoma virus and another species of avian retrovirus. J Virol 29: 863–871
Schwartzberg P, Colicelli J, Goff SP (1983) Deletion mutants of Moloney murine leukemia virus which lack glycosylated *gag* protein are replication competent. J Virol 46: 538–546
Scolnick EM, Vass WC, Howk RS, Duesberg PH (1979) Defective retrovirus-like 30S RNA species of rat and mouse cells are infectious if packaged by type C helper virus. J Virol 29: 964–972
Shank PR, Linial M (1980) Avian oncovirus mutant (SE21Q1b) deficient in genomic RNA: characterization of a deletion in the provirus. J Virol 36: 450–456
Sherwin SA, Rapp UR, Benveniste RE, Sen A, Todaro GJ (1978) Rescue of endogenous 30S retroviral sequences from mouse cells by baboon type C virus. J Virol 26: 257–264
Shimotohno K, Mizutani S, Temin HM (1980) Sequence of retrovirus provirus resembles that of bacterial transposable elements. Nature 285: 550–554

Shinnick TM, Lerner RA, Sutcliffe JG (1981) Nucleotide sequence of Moloney murine leukemia virus. Nature 293: 543–548

Sorge JD, Ricci W, Hughes SH (1983) cis-Acting RNA packaging locus in the 115-nucleotide direct repeat of Rous sarcoma virus. J Virol 48: 667–675

Sorge JD, Wright D, Erdman VD, Cutting AE (1984) Amphotropic retrovirus vector system for human cell gene transfer. Mol Cell Biol 4: 1730–1737

Stoker AW, Bissell MJ (1988) Development of avian sarcoma and leukosis virus-based vector-packaging cell lines. J Virol 62: 1008–1015

Stoltzfus CM, Kuhnert LK (1979) Evidence for the identity of shared 5'-terminal sequences between genomic RNA and subgenomic mRNAs of B77 avian sarcoma virus. J Virol 32: 536–545

Svoboda J, Dvorak M, Guntaka R, Geryk J (1986) Transmission of (LTR, v-src, LTR) without recombination with a helper virus. Virology 153: 314–317

Taylor JM, Cywinski A (1984) A defective retrovirus particle (SE21Q1b) packages and reverse transcribes cellular RNA, utilizing tRNA-like primers. J Virol 51: 267–271

Temin H (1985) Reverse transcription in the eukaryotic genome: retroviruses, pararetroviruses, retrotransposons and retranscripts. Mol Biol Evol 2: 455–468

Ullu E, Murphy S, Melli M (1982) Human 7SL RNA consists of a 140 nucleotide middle-repetitive sequence inserted in an Alu sequence. Cell 29: 195–202

Van Arsdell SW, Denison RA, Bernstein LB, Weiner AM Manser T, Gesteland RF (1981) Direct repeats flank three small nuclear RNA pseudogenes in the human genome. Cell 26: 11–17

Varmus H, Swanstrom R (1984) Replication of Retroviruses. In: Weiss R, Teich N, Varmus H, Coffin J (eds) RNA tumor viruses. Cold Spring Harbor Laboratory, Cold Spring Harbor, pp 369–512

Voynow S, Coffin JM (1985) Truncated gag-related proteins are produced by large deletion mutants of Rous sarcoma virus and form virus particles. J Virol 55: 79–85

Walter P, Blobel G (1982) Signal recognition particle contains a 7S RNA essential for protein translocation across the endoplasmic reticulum. Nature 288: 691–698

Wang L-H, Stacey DW (1982) Participation of subgenomic retroviral mRNAs in recombination. J Virol 41: 919–930

Watanabe S, Temin HM (1979) Encapsidation sequences for spleen necrosis virus, an avian retrovirus, are between the 5' long terminal repeat and the start of the gag gene. Proc Natl Acad Sci USA 79: 5986–5990

Watanabe S, Temin HM (1983) Construction of a helper cell line for avian reticuloendotheliosis virus cloning vectors. Mol Cell Biol 3: 2241–2249

Weiner AM, Deininger PL, Efstratiadis A (1986) Nonviral retroposons: genes, pseudogenes, and transposable elements generated by the reverse flow of genetic information. Annu Rev Biochem 55: 631–661

Weiss R (1984) Experimental biology and assay of RNA tumor viruses. In: Weiss R, Teich N, Varmus H, Coffin J (eds) RNA tumor viruses. Cold Spring Harbor Laboratory, Cold Spring Harbor, pp 209–260

Retroviral Proteinases

S. Oroszlan and R. B. Luftig

1 Introduction and Historical Perspective

Limited proteolysis is a well-established posttranslational mechanism by which cellular and viral precursor proteins are cleaved by specific proteinases into functional species (KOCH and RICHTER 1980). Examples of such cellular proteins are the neuropolypeptide prohormones (MAINS et al. 1983) and propiocortin, while the best known viral polyproteins are the polio (SUMMERS and MAIZEL 1968; JACOBSON and BALTIMORE 1968) and retroviral *gag* and *gag-pol* encoded polyproteins (DICKSON et al. 1984). Two recent reviews during the past year have focused on viral proteinases coded for by positive-strand RNA viruses e.g., picorna and toga-flavivirus families (KRÄUSSLICH and WIMMER 1988), or by plant viruses (WELLINK and VAN KAMMEN 1988). The focus of this review will be on a

Research sponsored by the National Cancer Institute, DHHS under contract No. NO1-CO-74101 with Bionetics Research, Inc. and Grant 5RO1-CA-37380-06. The contents of this publication do not necessarily reflect the views or policies of the Department of Health and Human Services, nor does mention of trade names, commercial products, or organization imply endorsement by the U.S. Government

[1] Laboratory of Molecular Virology and Carcinogenesis, BRI-Basic Research Program, NCI-Frederick Cancer Research Facility, Frederick, MD 21701, USA

[2] Department of Microbiology, Immunology and Parasitology, Louisiana State Medical School, 1901 Perdido St., New Orleans, LA 70112-1393, USA

discussion of the biochemical properties as well as functions of retroviral proteinases (PR). These enzymes cleave both *gag* and *gag-pol* encoded polyproteins (cleavage of the *env* encoded polyprotein occurs via a cellular Golgi-localized enzyme).

The first evidence for the existence of proteolysis in retroviral Gag polyprotein processing came from pulse-chase radioactive labeling studies (VOGT et al. 1975) with avian myeloblastosis virus (AMV)-infected chick embryo fibroblasts (CEF). A polyprotein precursor, pr76^{gag}, which was radiolabeled, chased into the virus Gag structural proteins, p19 (MA), p10, p27 (CA), p12 (NC), p15 (PR) (nomenclature is that of LEIS et al. 1988). Similar immunoprecipitation studies with Rauscher (Ra) or Moloney (Mo) murine leukemia virus (MuLV)-infected mouse fibroblasts using monospecific MuLV Gag sera showed the presence of a Pr65^{gag} polyprotein precursor (called P65, p70, or Pr70 at various times) (BARBACID et al. 1976; ARCEMENT et al. 1976) which was then cleaved into the murine tumor virus Gag structural proteins: p15 (MA), p12, p30 (CA), p10 (NC) (JAMJOOM et al. 1976, 1977). Further, in both the MuLV and avian Rous sarcoma virus (RSV) systems an additional, higher Mr polyprotein Pr180$^{gag-pol}$ was also detected, albeit only at 1/20th the level of Pr65^{gag} and Pr76^{gag} (JAMJOOM et al 1977; OPPERMANN et al. 1977; see also reviews by EISENMAN and VOGT 1978 and DICKSON et al. 1984, 1985). The above pulse-chase experiments with avian and murine retrovirus-infected cells strongly suggested that a proteinase was involved in cleavage of the Gag and probably Gag-Pol polyproteins. Further, the knowledge that identical N-terminal amino acids of MuLV p30 (Pro-Leu-Arg) occurred in the p30s of several murine retroviruses and that Pro was found as the invariant N-terminus of the CA protein of other retroviruses suggested that such a proteinase has a high degree of specificity (OROSZLAN et al. 1975; OROSZLAN et al. 1978; OROSZLAN and GILDEN 1979; OROSZLAN and GILDEN 1980).

The observation that the retroviral polyproteins undergo proteolytic processing was followed by reports that both avian and murine retroviruses contain a proteolytic factor as part of the virus particle. VON DER HELM (1977) reported cleavage of avian Pr76^{gag} (labeled in vitro as a substrate) by the p15 *gag*-encoded proteinase fraction obtained from gel filtration of virion proteins in the presence of 6*M* guanidine-HC1, while YOSHINAKA and LUFTIG (1977a, b) reported a similar specific cleavage of murine Pr65^{gag} by a proteolytic factor present in detergent-treated extracts of MuLV. Further, with MuLV, it was noted that this cleavage was accompanied by a morphological transformation of "immature" to "mature" particles (YOSHINAKA and LUFTIG 1977a, c), which, as later observed, paralleled the production of infectious virus (LU et al. 1979; WITTE and BALTIMORE 1978; KATOH et al. 1985). Both of the above in vitro polyprotein cleavages appeared specific in that for each case the Gag proteins generated were the same size as those found in virions. Also the cleavage appeared to have fidelity since the N-terminal amino acids of MuLV p30 generated in vitro were the same as that of p30 purified from virions (YOSHINAKA et al. 1985c). A puzzle that arose at this time, however, was the finding that although the avian PR appeared to be an abundant virion protein encoded in *gag*, this was not the case for the murine PR (YOSHINAKA and LUFTIG

1980). It was not until several years later, when sufficient quantities of the MuLV PR could be obtained for sequencing, that this dilemma was resolved. MuLV PR was found in fact not to be encoded by *gag* but by *gag-pol*, and synthesis of PR occurred through suppression of the amber termination codon found at the end of the *gag* gene (YOSHINAKA et al. 1985a).

During the next few years, additional retroviral proteinases were isolated and either completely or partially sequenced, and the complete sequences inferred from the known nucleotide sequence data. The feline leukemia virus (FeLV) proteinase was purified in the same manner as MuLV PR, based on an assay utilizing the MuLV Pr65^{gag} as substrate for protease activity. When the N-terminal sequence of FeLV PR was aligned with the known nucleotide sequence (LAPREVOTTE et al. 1984), it was seen to be encoded at the 5'-end of the *pol* gene and, like MuLV PR, synthesized through in-frame suppression (rather than by splicing or frameshift as suggested by the nucleotide sequence) of the *gag* gene amber termination codon by insertion of a glutamine residue at the fifth position of the protein, with the first four amino acids being derived from the *gag* gene (YOSHINAKA et al. 1985a, b). As with MuLV and FeLV, the bovine leukemia virus (BLV) PR was purified to homogeneity and was found to have the same Mr (14 000) as the MuLV and FeLV PRs; however, it was synthesized in a different manner. It was suggested that in BLV the translation of the *gag-pro* gene occurs via a (-1) ribosomal frameshift at the end of the *gag* gene, where a characteristic AAAA AA sequence is found (RICE et al. 1985; YOSHINAKA et al. 1986). The molecular basis of this novel translational mechanism, which has been shown to occur for several retroviruses, e.g., RSV (JACKS and VARMUS 1985), MMTV (HIZI et al. 1987), HTLV-I (NAM and HATANAKA 1986), and HIV (JACKS et al. 1988a), will be discussed elsewhere (JACKS, this volume).

In the early 1980s, HIV was isolated from a large number of AIDS and ARC patients by cocultivation of infected lymphocytes with permissive T cells (BARRÉ-SINOUSSI et al. 1983; POPOVIC et al. 1984; GALLO et al. 1984; LEVY et al. 1984). Several of the proviruses obtained from established cell lines were sequenced (RATNER et al. 1985; MUESING et al. 1985; WAIN-HOBSON et al. 1985; SANCHEZ-PESCADOR et al. 1985), and based on similarities of inferred amino acid sequences, it was concluded that the translation of a second open reading frame, as with RSV and BLV by ribosomal frameshifting, yielded a Gag-Pol polyprotein which contained both the HIV PR as well as reverse transcriptase (RT). In the case of HIV, the Pr55^{gag} polyprotein precursor is cleaved by PR into p17 (MA), p24 (CA), p7 (NC), and p9/6 Gag proteins (HENDERSON et al. 1988b; VERONESE et al. 1988). Since the cleavage of Gag and Gag-Pol polyproteins is essential for infectious progeny virus function (CRAWFORD and GOFF 1985; KATOH et al. 1985; KOHL et al. 1988; SEELMEIER et al. 1988), it is hoped that by inhibiting the HIV PR one could thereby inhibit virus replication and spread within an infected individual.

In order to obtain sufficient amounts of HIV PR for biochemical and structural studies, recombinant DNA technology has been used to express the cloned gene in a variety of vector systems, e.g., bacteria (FARMERIE et al. 1987; DEBOUCK et al. 1987; LE GRICE et al. 1988; GRAVES et al. 1988; HANSEN et al. 1988) and yeast (KRAMER et al. 1986). Also, it has been chemically synthesized (COPELAND and OROSZLAN 1988; SCHNEIDER and KENT 1988; NUTT et al. 1988) to yield substantial amounts of proteolytically active material. Use of these materials led to several recent important findings about PR structure that has helped answer some intriguing questions. For example, in 1985 when several PR sequences become available, TOH et al. (1985) showed that there was sequence homology between retrovirus and retrotransposon PRs as well as a strong correlation with known aspartyc proteinases. A dilemma, however, was the low molecular weight (11 000–14 000) for the retroviral PRs compared with 32 000–36 000 for the aspartyc proteinases. One possible way to account for this difference was the finding that MuLV PR exhibits an apparent molecular size on Sephadex columns of 22K, suggesting that it is a dimer (YOSHINAKA and LUFTIG 1980). A model of the retroviral PR (PEARL and TAYLOR 1987b) supported the dimer structure. More recently, determination of the crystallographic structures of RSV PR (MILLER et al. 1989) and HIV PR (NAVIA et al. 1989) has confirmed the dimeric model. Furthermore, the recombinant HIV-1 PR was found to be active in the dimeric form (MEEK et al. 1989).

Several compounds have been found to inhibit RSV and HIV PR activity, i.e., pepstatin A, fusidic acid, cerulenin, and its analogues (DITTMAR and MOELLING 1978; KATOH et al. 1987; SEELMEIER et al. 1988; SCHNEIDER and KENT 1988; HANSEN et al. 1988; BU et al. 1989). Also, now that the 3-dimensional crystal structure is available for RSV and HIV PR, rational drug design to develop inhibitors of therapeutic value becomes a possibility. Use of PR inhibitors will also provide insight into the detailed molecular steps whereby retroviral PRs cause conversion of "immature" precursor polyprotein-containing particles into "mature" virions. Based on the potential for developing drugs to treat AIDS patients, the study of inhibitors of the HIV PR has become an area of research drawing considerable attention over the past 2 years (for example, see KRÄUSSLICH et al. 1989b).

In this review, we intend to outline briefly the role of protease in viral replication. Then, we will individually discuss several of the most well-characterized retroviral proteinases, including a description of their biochemical properties and 3-dimensional structure, where available. Finally, we will present in an appendix the known cleavage sites for the retroviral PRs.

2 Biosynthesis of Proteinase and Its Role in Virus Replication

The genome of all replication competent retroviruses consists of at least three genes required for viral infection and replication. They are arranged in the order 5'-*gag-pol-env*-3'. Soon after a retrovirus enters the cell by receptor-mediated endocytosis or direct fusion with the cell membrane, the viral genome is transcribed by the RT to generate the DNA which integrates into the host chromosomes to form the provirus. Next, the proviral DNA is transcribed by cellular RNA polymerase II into genome size RNA. The *gag* gene-encoded internal structural proteins, the RT and endonuclease or integration protein (IN) that are coded for by the *pol* gene, and the viral PR are synthesized by the translation of genome size mRNA. A smaller spliced mRNA codes for the viral envelope proteins. The primary translational product of the *env* gene is a polyprotein that is first glycosylated and then proteolytically processed into the surface glycoprotein and transmembrane protein by a cellular enzyme during transport to the plasma membrane. The primary translational products of the *gag* and *gag-pol* genes are polyproteins that first assemble with genomic RNA to form a characteristic doughnut-shaped core structure of immature particles encapsulated by the viral envelope. The immature particles that are initially formed through the budding process are not infectious. To produce mature infectious progeny virus, the cleavage of the polyproteins of the immature core into the smaller mature structural proteins and replication enzymes RT and IN is also necessary. This cleavage is accomplished by the viral PR, product of the *pro* gene (see Fig. 1). The sequence of events of retrovirus replication is depicted in the scheme below.

Phase I:	Adsorption-penetration	Receptor	
Phase II:	Synthesis of viral DNA	Reverse transcriptase, RNase H	Early events
Phase III:	Integration of viral DNA (provirus)	Integration protein	
Phase IV:	Transcription of proviral DNA (genomic and mRNAs)	RNA polymerase II	
Phase V:	Translation Genome-size mRNA Polyproteins: Gag Gag-Pol Gag-Pro-Pol Spliced mRNA Env polyprotein	Translational control Cleavage by cell protease	
Phase VI:	Assembly and budding (immature virion)	Extracellular	
Phase VII:	Virus maturation Processing of core proteins Infectious progeny virus	Viral proteinase	Late events

The *pol* gene of all retroviruses is located downstream of the *gag* gene. In mammalian type C viruses (Mo-MuLV is a prototype) the *gag* and *pol* genes are separated by an amber termination codon (UAG) and are translated in the same reading frame. The polyprotein containing both *gag* and *pol* sequences (Pr180$^{gag-pol}$) in MuLV, FeLV, and other mammalian type C viruses is synthesized by the inframe suppression (read through) of the *gag* terminator, most likely accomplished by normal tRNA^{Gln} (YOSHINAKA et al. 1985a, b).

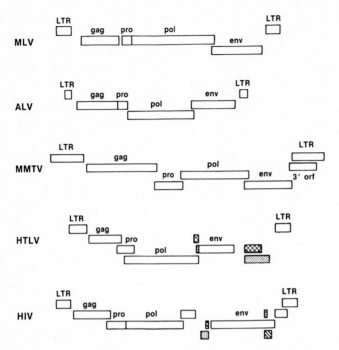

Fig. 1. Genomic organization and reading frames. The long terminal repeats (LTR) and open reading frames are indicated by boxes. MLV, mouse leukemia virus, a prototype mammalian type C retrovirus; ALV, avian leukosis virus; MMTV, mouse mammary tumor virus, a prototype type B virus (the gene organization of type D retroviruses is similar); HTLV, human T-cell leukemia virus (two strains have been identified, HTLV-1 and HTLV-2). Simian T-cell leukemia virus(es) (STLV) as well as the bovine leukemia virus have a similar gene organization. HIV, human immunodeficiency virus representing two major groups, HIV-1 and HIV-2. Simian immunodeficiency virus(es) show similar gene organization. Hatched and shaded boxes show coding regions for regulatory proteins

In all other retroviruses for which nucleotide sequences have been determined, the *gag* and *pol* genes are read in different frames which overlap (Fig. 1). In these viruses the Gag-Pol polyprotein is expressed through ribosomal frameshifting. The exact site of shifting the reading frame has been determined by protein sequencing of transframe proteins made in vivo (HIZI et al. 1987) or in vitro (JACKS and VARMUS 1985; JACKS et al. 1988a, b).

The most direct way of identifying processing sites in polyproteins is to determine the N- and C-terminal sequences of the fully processed protein products and compare the results with nucleotide sequences of the viral genome. When the amino acid sequences of all the viral proteins are taken together with the complete nucleotide sequence of the proviral DNA, the data provide a complete biosynthetic pathway and allow the proteolytic processing events to be accurately delineated as shown for Mo-MuLV (Fig. 2a) and for HIV (Fig. 2b).

The mechanism of activation of the viral PR is not known at present. It is, however, believed to be an autocatalytic process. The involvement of cellular enzyme(s) is unlikely in most cases, although that of some unknown cellular

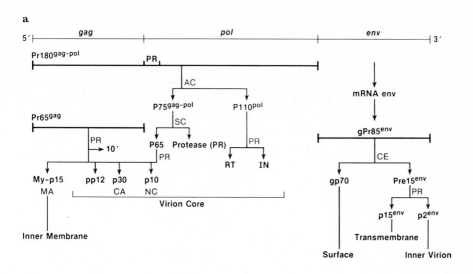

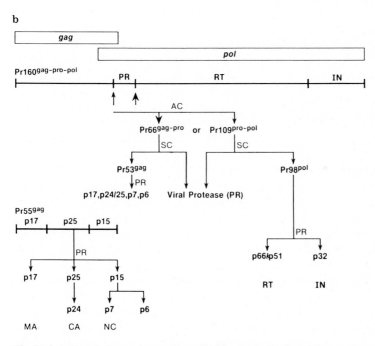

Fig. 2 a, b. a Translation and processing of Moloney murine leukemia virus Gag (Pr65), Gag-Pol (Pr180), and Env (gPr85) polyproteins. *AC*, Autocatalysis, the first cleavage occurring between PR and RT; *SC*, self-cleavage; *CE*, cellular enzyme; *PR*, viral protease; *RT*, reverse transcriptase; *IN*, integration protein. (Taken from OROSZLAN et al. 1987b.) **b** Translation and processing of human immunodeficiency virus (HIV-1) Gag (Pr55) and Gag-Pol (Pr160) polyproteins. The first cleavage could occur either at the N-terminus (↑) or at the C-terminus (▲) of viral protease (PR) *AC*, autocatalysis; *SC*, self-cleavage; *RT*, reverse transcriptase; *IN*, integration protein

factors has not been entirely ruled out. The autocatalytic mechanism is supported by recent genetic studies in which autoprocessing of recombinant polyproteins containing the wild-type PR domain could be demonstrated while appropriate mutations in the PR active site region abolished such activity (LOEB et al. 1989, and references therein). Early experiments of WITTE and BALTIMORE (1978) indicated that processing of viral proteins does not take place until the time of virion formation, and accumulating evidence suggests that activation and subsequent processing occur in the extracellular immature virion. Based on crystal structure (MILLER et al. 1989, NAVIA et al. 1989) the PR can be active only in the dimeric form. Thus, the polyprotein zymogen must first dimerize to form an active enzyme as originally suggested by PEARL and TAYLOR (1987b). The extent of dimerization is not known. Theoretically, a single dimer would be sufficient to start the autocatalytic process. The first cleavage(s) could occur in *cis* (intramolecular cleavage) to release the PR dimer or in *trans* (intermolecular cleavage), in which case the activated polyprotein dimer would first cleave an inactive polyprotein monomer, and the released PR monomers would dimerize to complete the processing event necessary for virus maturation. The study of the activation process in virus-producing cells is one of the most important areas of contemporary retroviral proteinase research to be pursued. Such studies will facilitate the development of inhibitors of viral maturation.

Very recently, a novel function of retroviral proteinase was suggested by ROBERTS and OROSZLAN (1989). They reported the purification of equine infectious anemia virus (EIAV) capsids to a homogenous preparation using detergent treatment to dissociate envelope components and zonal rate centrifugation in a Ficoll density gradient. Since extensive sequence homology has been demonstrated between the Gag structural proteins and the *pol*-encoded enzymes of EIAV and HIV (STEPHEN et al. 1986), and both viruses have similar morphology (GONDA 1988), this was intended to be a model study for HIV. The purified capsids appeared under the electron microscope as cone-shaped particles 120 nm in length, 60 nm in width at the wide end, and 25 nm at the narrow end (Fig. 3). They have been shown to contain RNA and RT. In addition, they have topoisomerase activity (PRIEL et al. 1990). The major protein components are the structural proteins p11 (NC) and p26 (CA) in a 1:1 molar ratio. When purified capsids were incubated at room temperature or at 37°C a pH-dependent cleavage of the NC protein, p11, into smaller polypeptides, p6 and p4, was observed. The p11 cleavage was shown to be due to the presence of viral proteinase packaged in the capsid. It was inhibited by pepstatin A, a known inhibitor of cellular and retroviral aspartic proteinases, but not by Phenyl Methyl Sulfonyl Fluorid (PMSF), a serine protease inhibitor. It is conceivable that the proteinase packaged in the capsid is involved through the NC protein cleavage in a critical step in the early phases of replication including reverse transcription and integration of viral DNA into the host cell. Such involvement in the early events, before the infectious state is established, would make the proteinase a very· attractive and probably a more readily accessible target in the cytoplasm for drug therapy than the proteinase functioning in the very late phase of virus replication, i.e., maturation.

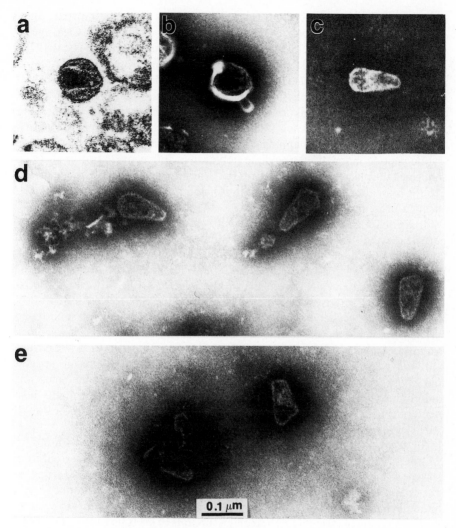

Fig. 3 a–e. Electron micrographs of intact equine infectious anemia virus and capsids: **a** thin section and **b** negative-stained intact virus; **c** negative-stained capsid pelleted through 30% sucrose; **d** capsids obtained after first and **e** second banding through Ficoll. (Reproduced in part from ROBERTS and OROSZLAN 1989)

3 Avian Proteinase

As noted in the Introduction, the earliest evidence for proteolysis in retroviral polyprotein processing came from studies of avian tumor viruses; specifically, the assembly and maturation of avian tumor viruses in CEF was shown to proceed through synthesis of the high M_r polyprotein, Pr76^{gag} [NH$_2$-p19(MA)-p10-

p27(CA)-p12(NC)-p15(PR)-COOH], followed by its cleavage into individual *gag*-encoded proteins (VOGT et al. 1975; EISENMAN et al. 1975). Cleavage is mediated by p15(PR), the C-terminal *gag* gene product (VON DER HELM 1977). Further support for the role of p15 as a proteinase came from studies (DITTMAR and MOELLING 1978; MOELLING et al. 1980) in which PR was purified and partially characterized in physicochemical terms. Also, when avian Pr76^{gag} was expressed in *E. coli*, it was found to be rapidly processed into specific Gag proteins, e.g., p27(CA), unless a PR deletion mutant was present in p15 (MERMER et al. 1983). Pactamycin mapping experiments (SHEALY et al. 1980) as well as tryptic peptide maps of intermediate polyprotein fragments (VOGT et al. 1979) confirmed the placement of p15(PR) at the C-terminus of Pr76^{gag}. This means the p15 PR is an abundant protein made in stoichiometric amounts with other *gag*-encoded proteins.

It is not yet clear how the first p15 PR is produced in an avian tumor virus particle. Several years ago, it was noted that when Rous sarcoma virus (RSV) infected mammalian cells instead of CEF (EISENMAN et al. 1975), a block in cleavage of Pr76^{gag} occurred. This block, however, could be overcome if the infected mammalian cells were fused with uninfected CEF. However, if the N-terminal pp60^{src} myristylation signal is placed at the N-terminus of Pr76^{gag} (which is normally acetylated) and *gag* expressed using an SV40 plasmid-based system in mammalian cells transfected with the modified plasmid, then the block is almost completely overcome, i.e., a fivefold enhancement in Pr76^{gag} cleavage and virus particles is produced (WILLS et al. 1989). These above results suggest that Pr76^{gag} may need to be attached to a specific site on the plasma membrane and/or the polyprotein needs a certain intracellular environment at the host membrane to permit proper folding and packaging so that it can be autocatalytically cleaved.

In addition to cleavage of Pr76^{gag}, avian p15 PR also cleaves Pr180$^{gag-pol}$ (MOELLING et al. 1980), the precursor to RT and IN, which is synthesized from genome size mRNA via a ribosomal frameshift near the end of the *gag* sequence (JACKS and VARMUS 1985). Avian Pr180$^{gag-pol}$ is present in smaller (about 1/20th) amounts than Pr76^{gag} in avian-infected cells, and its cleavage appears to occur in viral particles, generating both the α and β subunits of RT (OPPERMAN et al. 1977) as well as IN. Thus, virus harvested at short (3 h) intervals contains significantly more uncleaved polyprotein precursors than later (24 h) harvested virions (MOELLING et al. 1980). Further, in vitro cleavage of Pr180$^{gag-pol}$ initially shows an increase of the larger, β subunit of RT Pr180$^{gag-pol}$, followed by cleavage of β to α + IN.

As noted earlier avian p15 PR has been purified by ion exchange chromatography and gel filtration and characterized (DITTMAR and MOELLING 1978). It has a pH optimum of about 5.7 and shows only one band at 15K on SDS-PAGE. Several observations initially suggested a thiol protease activity, i.e., it yielded similar cleavage patterns to those found for papain with a variety of substrates, such as bovine serum albumin, ovalbumin, and concanavalin A; and it was inhibited by iodoacetamide (50 mM) and NEM (10 mM). However, we now know from sequence homology (TOH et al. 1985) and X-ray crystallography studies (MILLER et al. 1989) that avian PR, as do all retrovirus PRs, belongs to the aspartic proteinase family. It is of interest to note in this regard that DITTMAR and MOELLING (1978) early on showed inhibition of p15 PR cleavage by pepstatin A. At this time, however, we do not understand how the thiol inhibitors also block p15 PR activity. It may reflect blockage of p15 PR at its cysteine residue. Avian PR appears to be relatively inefficient compared with papain, because about 20 times more PR is needed to initiate the same cleavage profile of BSA (68K) into 38K and 30K products (YOSHINAKA and LUFTIG 1981).

Another form of avian PR must exist. This could arise from the Gag-Pol polyprotein as the result of cleavage to generate the N-terminus of RT. Thus, $p15^{gag-\Delta pol}$ (p15^{gag} extended at the C-terminus by an additional seven amino acids) could also be an active protease. Its functional role in polyprotein processing remains to be determined.

As noted earlier, processing of the entire avian Pr76^{gag} by p15 PR can occur in *E. coli* expressing the Prague C RSV DNA genome cloned in pBR322. This is due to the fact that the viral long terminal repeat (LTR) contains a fortuitous bacterial promoter, and viral sequences near the *gag* initiation codon are similar to the prokaryote Shine-Dalgarno sequence (MERMER et al. 1983). These authors also noted that the half life of Pr76^{gag} in *E. coli* under the assay conditions used is less than 5 min, while it is 45 min in RSV-infected turkey cells (DICKSON et al. 1984), suggesting that *E. coli* presents a different, albeit still accurate cleavage environment. Cleavage of Pr76^{gag} in *E. coli* is clearly attributable to AMV PR in that: (a) the pattern of intermediate cleavage products is the same as that found in vitro with Pr76^{gag} and p15 PR and (b) using a plasmid with a C-terminal deletion of 55 amino acids in p15 yields a stable, uncleaved high molecular weight Gag-LacZ fusion protein in *E. coli* transfectants, which is cleaved to p27 (CA) when p15 PR is added to such extracts in vitro.

More recently, expression in *E. coli* of a portion of the *gag* gene fused to LacZ was accompanied by its accurate processing into the p15 PR (SEDLACEK et al. 1988). By separation of the expression product from inclusion bodies in *E. coli*, PR was obtained in high yield (SEDLÁCEK et al. 1988). In this system an initial cleavage takes place upstream of p15, within p12, and this cleavage precedes generation of the N-terminus of PR. It has also been shown that *E. coli*-produced p15 PR can accurately process to give RT and IN proteins from a 99K polyprotein precursor (KOTLER et al. 1988b). Furthermore, KOTLER et al. (1988a) have found that small synthetic peptides containing Tyr-Pro as the cleavage site can be utilized both as a model substrate and to develop inhibitors of the avian PR reaction. For example, the peptide Thr-Phe-Gln-Ala-Tyr/Pro-Leu-Arg-Glu-Ala that extends five amino acids in both directions from the cleavage site is accurately hydrolyzed. Such studies extend those reported a number of years ago by COPELAND and OROSZLAN (1981) in which a synthetic dodecapeptide containing the cleavage site at the avian p12/p15 junction was found to be accurately hydrolyzed by p15 PR. KOTLER et al. (1988a) not only demonstrated that the above peptide representing the site between RT and IN was hydrolyzed but also found that if Tyr was substituted with Ile, the Ile/Pro peptide was inhibitory. Recently, STROP and colleagues (personal communication) have shown that substitution of Tyr-Pro with Phe-statine also shows inhibitory activity. Statine is contained within the molecular structure of pepstatin A, an inhibitor of aspartic proteinases.

Such studies as above with synthetic peptides of the avian system and previous comparisons of natural cleavage sites found in precursor proteins have led to the proposals for a "consensus" cleavage sequence (at P4 to P1 of the site positions) of retroviral PRs (OROSZLAN and COPELAND 1985; PEARL and TAYLOR 1987a; KOTLER et al. 1988a). It is also of interest to note that although Tyr-Pro or Phe-Pro cleavage sites are found frequently in MuLV, HIV, and other retroviral precursors, they are present only once among avian polyprotein cleavage sites and not at all in BLV or HTLV Gag which do contain Leu-Pro. Thus, there is specificity for more than one cleavage site built into retroviral PRs (see Appendix). Assay conditions appear to influence cleavage site specificity. For example, VOGT et al. (1979) had observed earlier that cleavage of $Pr76^{gag}$ was stimulated by high salt. Also, high ionic strength ($\geqslant 1M$ NaCl) at pH 5.5 showed optimal activity for the above Tyr-Pro decapeptide as well as with the Ala-Pro decapeptide; the latter is not cleaved at low salt concentrations (KOTLER et al. 1989). In contrast, murine PR activity is inhibited by high salt concentrations in vitro, and processing of $Pr65^{gag}$ is reduced in cells exposed to higher salt concentrations (YOSHINAKA and LUFTIG 1981). Thus, careful attention needs to be paid not only to the substrates used but also to the specific conditions of assay, when one tries to develop inhibitors for the retroviral PRs.

4 Murine Leukemia Virus Proteinase

MuLVs are among the most well-characterized mammalian retroviruses and have become models for studying not only the cleavage of the polyprotein precursor, $Pr65^{gag}$, but also the morphogenesis of mammalian type C retroviruses. The pathway of assembly for MuLV proposed below is consistent with the following features of virus assembly: (a) the size and structure of an icosahedral core (BOLOGNESI 1974; BOLOGNESI et al. 1978; NERMUT et al. 1972); (b) $Pr180^{gag-pol}$ is a precursor to PR, RT, and IN (JAMJOOM et al. 1977); (c) the finding of about 70 molecules of RT per virion (PANET et al. 1975); (d) evidence that $Pr180^{gag-pol}$ alone is not sufficient for assembling the viral structure (FELSENSTEIN and GOFF 1988), although $Pr65^{gag}$ can make a particle alone (SHIELDS et al. 1978); (e) the indication above that PR functions as a dimer and observations that in vitro cleavage of $Pr65^{gag}$ by MuLV PR is accompanied by a morphological change of an "immature" to "mature" (YOSHINAKA and LUFTIG 1978) virus particle, occurring apparently from vertex to vertex (Fig. 4) to yield infectious particles (LU et al. 1979; WITTE and BALTIMORE 1978; KATOH et al. 1985). Our assembly model

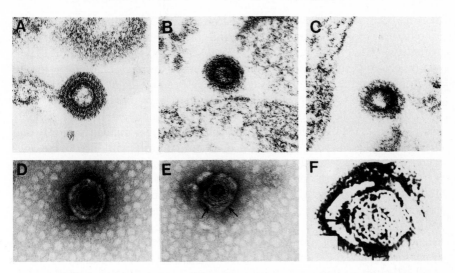

Fig. 4 a–f. Stages in murine leukemia virus morphogenesis as seen by thin section (**a–c**) and negative stain electron microscopy (**d–f**). *First*. Budding or released "immature" virus particles are seen to exhibit a characteristic concentric coiling of the (Pr65^{gag}-RNA) complex. Note an electronlucent (**a**) or stain-penetrated (**d**) region, respectively, dependent on the EM technique used. Also the outline of the particle appears spherical. *Second*. Partial cleavage by the retroviral protease results in a shift to more of an angular pattern on the core where two edges can now be discerned (**e**, *arrows*). There is also some proteinaceous material appearing in the center of the particle (**b, e**). *Third*. Complete cleavage yields a mature particle in which the concentric coil of RNA has collapsed to a single-stranded appearance, showing a hexagonal outline (*arrows*, **f**). The darkly stained nature of the inner coils seen in thin sections of (**a**) and (**b**) (presumably uranyl acetate staining of RNA) is no longer visualized (**c**). Magnification of **a–e** is ×120000; f ×200000

proposes that about 1500 Pr65^{gag} and 60 Pr180$^{gag-pol}$ molecules, together with two genomic RNA strands, are brought as a nucleoprotein complex to the membrane surface of infected cells, leading through budding to the formation of an "immature" particle. This may occur in dimeric complexes of Pr65^{gag} molecules (PEPINSKY 1983) that are relatively underphosphorylated (YOSHINAKA et al. 1984). Then, just as the particle is released from the cell membrane or soon thereafter, the proteinase is activated from perhaps similar dimeric Pr180$^{gag-pol}$ molecules to cleave itself as well as Pr65^{gag} into the proteins needed for a mature, infectious virus. The roles of RNA, polyprotein phosphorylation, and the pH of the particle microenvironment in triggering cleavage have to be considered. The morphological change from a spherical to the hexagonal, centrally located core exhibited in Fig. 4 accompanies the action of the protease. A somewhat similar change can also be demonstrated in vitro when MuLV PR is added to detergent-treated immature particles (YOSHINAKA and LUFTIG 1980).

One of the interesting features of MuLV and other retroviral proteinases is their uniqueness in cleaving specific substrates, such as those that contain Tyr-Pro or Phe-Pro (OROSZLAN et al. 1978). These are hydrophobic amino acids, and the cleavage occurs at the imino function of Pro. Such a cleavage site, while frequent in retroviral polyproteins, is rarely and inefficiently hydrolyzed by other proteinases (HILL 1965); for example, KÖNIGSBERG and HILL (1962) showed that pepsin could cleave Phe-Pro bonds in human hemoglobin under certain conditions, and the efficient cleavage of a Tyr/Pro peptide by pepsin at a high salt concentration was reported recently (KOTLER et al. 1989).

It should also be noted that MuLV PR is made in extremely small amounts relative to the AMV/RSV p15 PR, and this has made it difficult to purify and characterize this enzyme. MuLV PR does not copurify with any of the *gag*-encoded proteins, using several different chromatographic techniques (YOSHINAKA and LUFTIG 1980). As noted earlier, it was not until YOSHINAKA et al. (1985a), utilizing relatively large amounts of virus to isolate the proteinase and N-terminal sequencing, that its location was found to be at the N-terminus of the MuLV *pol* gene, but its first 4 amino acids are derived from *gag*. MuLV PR thus extends through the *gag* terminator translated as Gln into the N-terminal protein of *pol* for a total of 125 amino acids.

The limited availability of MuLV PR when isolated from virus particles has made it difficult to perform many studies. From the initial studies the following observations have been made: (a) MuLV PRs purified from Mo-MuLV or Ra-MuLV both elute on Sephadex columns as a dimer of ~ 22K (YOSHINAKA and LUFTIG 1980); (b) in vitro cleavage of Ra- or Mo-MuLV Pr65^{gag} by Mo-MuLV PR gives rise to the Ra-MuLV Pr40^{gag} and Mo-MuLV Pr41.5^{gag} intermediate cleavage products, respectively, confirming that the initial cleavage at the Phe-Pro site of MuLV Pr65^{gag} occurs between p12 and p30 in both Gag polyproteins; (c) the final stage in Env protein maturation involving cleavage of the TM intermediate protein Pr15(E) to p15(E) and p2(E) requires the virally encoded PR since mutants in PR fail to cleave Pr15(E) or Pr65^{gag} (KATOH et al. 1985; CRAWFORD and GOFF 1985; SCHULTZ and REIN 1985). This is consistent with immunofluorescence studies of SATAKE and LUFTIG (1983) showing overlapping fluorescence of p15 (presumably Pr65^{gag}) and p15E [presumably Pr15(E)] antigenic determinants at the cell membrane, suggesting that the two interact during assembly; (d) MuLV production was greatly inhibited, and normal cleavage of both Pr65^{gag} and Pr80^{env} was simultaneously blocked by addition of 20 µg/ml cerulenin (KATOH et al. 1986; IKUTA and LUFTIG 1986), in part due to specific inhibition of MuLV PR (LUFTIG et al. 1988).

Recent unpublished studies utilizing *E. coli* expressing a recombinant plasmid containing MuLV PR have shown that a band at 14K is produced after expression of a 50K *trp*E-PR fusion protein, presumably due to autocatalytic cleavage of the 50K precursor (CALKINS and LUFTIG, unpublished). This PR can cleave MuLV Pr65^{gag} in vitro to a Pr40^{gag} intermediate and p30(CA). In an attempt to increase production so as to obtain enough PR for crystallographic studies, another plasmid was constructed in which the glutamine codon (CAG) was inserted in place of the *gag* termination codon UAG. Although cleavage of active PR occurred, the yield of PR in *E. coli* was not significantly increased (CALKINS and LUFTIG, unpublished).

5 Bovine Leukemia Virus and Human T-Cell Leukemia Virus Proteinases

Soon after the initial isolation of the first bona fide human retrovirus (POIESZ et al. 1980), the human T-cell leukemia virus (HTLV), it was shown by protein sequencing of the CA proteins that HTLV is genetically more closely related to bovine leukemia virus (BLV) than to any other retrovirus (OROSZLAN et al. 1982). This relationship has been confirmed by DNA sequencing of the entire genome of both HTLV-1 and BLV (SEIKI et al. 1983; RICE et al. 1985). The initial DNA sequence of HTLV-1 as determined by SEIKI et al. (1983) indicated the presence of numerous termination codons in the *pro* reading frame overlapping the 3'-end of the *gag* and the 5'-end of the *pol* gene where, based on the primary structure in MuLV (YOSHINAKA et al. 1985), the proteinase was expected to be located. This initially suggested that HTLV-1 does not code for a viral proteinase. However, the cleavage sites determined in HTLV $Pr55^{gag}$ were found to be very similar to those occurring in MuLV $Pr65^{gag}$, and thus based on these observations, OROSZLAN and COPELAND (1985) predicted that the *pro* gene from a replication competent genome of HTLV-1 would also encode a viral proteinase. These predictions have been confirmed by NAM and HATANAKA (1986), who sequenced a DNA clone of a replication competent genome of HTLV-1 and found an open reading frame (ORF) encoding the entire PR protein. These results were similar to the DNA sequence of HTLV-2 previously reported by SHIMOTOHNO et al. (1985). At about the same time BLV PR was isolated and characterized (YOSHINAKA et al. 1986). BLV proteinase, which like other retroviral PRs was shown to be inhibited by pepstatin A in vitro (KATOH et al. 1987), shows higher homology to the PR of both HTLV-1 and HTLV-2 (NAM and HATANAKA 1986) than to other retroviral PRs. HTLV-1 PR has been studied by expressing the *gag-pro* coding sequence in a vaccinia virus expression vector (NAM et al. 1988). The proteinase expressed in the form of a fusion protein through ribosomal frame shifting was capable of processing the $Pr53^{gag}$ precursor polyprotein. An autoc talytic cleavage was suggested to be responsible for the release of active proteinase from the *gag-pro* precursor, presumably acting in *cis* (i.e., intra-molecular cleavage). A mutation introduced by changing the putative active site sequence Asp-Thr-Gly to Gly-Thr-Gly by site-directed mutagenesis abolished the activity.

6 Human Immunodeficiency Virus Proteinase

As with other retroviral proteinases, HIV PR is a virally encoded enzyme that cleaves both $Pr55^{gag}$ and $Pr160^{gag-pol}$ polyproteins, the primary translational products of genome size mRNA. Their cleavage is also temporally linked to virus·

instead of an MuLV-icosahedral-like core, the HIV mature core has a "cone-shaped" morphology similar to that of EIAV (Fig. 3) and other members of the lentivirus family. The size of the HIV PR is drastically smaller (99aa) than that of MuLV (125aa).

HIV PR, like other retroviral PRs, exhibits a high homology to a conserved region (LVDTGA) that is present in the active site region of aspartic proteinases such as pepsin and renin. In support of this, pepstatin A has been shown to inhibit activity of the HIV PR in vitro (SEELMEIER et al. 1988; KOHL et al. 1988; HANSEN et al. 1988; SCHNEIDER and KENT 1988; KRÄUSSLICH et al. 1988; BU et al. 1989; KRÄUSSLICH et al. 1989a). Recent studies using site-specific mutagenesis in and around the DTG site, viz., changing the Asp or other nearby amino acids (LE GRICE et al. 198; KOHL et al. 1988; SEELMEIER et al. 1988; LOEB et al. 1989), have shown the importance of the aspartyl and other conserved residues for activity.

Due to the importance of developing potential chemotherapeutic agents for treating ARC or AIDS patients, research on HIV PR has vastly accelerated relative to the other proteinases. In the next three sections, we will detail research on HIV PR that has taken place during the past few years.

6.1 Recombinant DNA-Derived Human Immunodeficiency Virus Proteinase

Several laboratories have recently cloned and expressed the HIV proteinase gene in bacteria or yeast. FARMERIE et al. (1987) constructed a plasmid in which the HIV *pol* gene sequences were placed into an inducible expression vector system. This plasmid, called pBRT-1 prt$^+$, contained a 2586 bp *Bgl*II to *Eco*RI *pol* fragment, starting at the 5' end of the *pol* gene and ended just inside the IN gene. The products expressed in *E. coli* were a doublet of 66/51K, characteristic of RT (VERONESE et al. 1986), as well as an 11K PR band (LOEB et al. 1989; BU et al. 1989). Crude bacterial extracts displayed both RT and proteinase activity in in vitro assays. A PR deletion plasmid was also constructed which contained the 2126 bp *Hind*III-*Eco*-RI HIV *pol* fragment. *E. coli* transformed with this mutant did not exhibit the appropriate cleavage of RT from a larger 84K precursor. These results suggest that HIV PR can be expressed in *E. coli* and further that its activity is required in order to process itself autocatalytically as well as HIV RT.

KRAMER et al. (1986) had earlier provided evidence showing that an active HIV PR gene could be expressed in yeast cells transformed with a plasmid containing all the *gag* and a portion of *pol* restriction fragment. In a pulse-chase experiment, the HIV Pr55^{gag} precursor was seen to be processed into *gag*-encoded proteins, such as p24 (CA). A similar expression of the HIV Pr55^{gag} polyprotein precursor and its cleavage by a coexpressed HIV PR gene in *E. coli* has also been reported (DEBOUCK et al. 1987). Two constructs used in the latter study expressed HIV PR as truncated polyproteins of 20K and 25K. Upon expression in *E. coli* both constructs gave rise to a 10K protein seen by Western blot with PR-specific antisera, consistent with an autocatalytic event at the Phe-

Pro cleavage sites on either side of the HIV PR domain. Also, an insertion *pol* mutant containing four internal amino acids in the PR domain gave rise to an unprocessed 25K product, supporting the idea that HIV PR is autocatalytic.

In order to define the limits for activity, HANSEN et al. (1988) constructed a PR mutant in *E. coli* in which 17 amino acids at the C-terminus were deleted. This mutant showed loss of activity. Also, partial purification of HIV PR by solubilization with acetone as well as passage over ultragel suggested a higher M_r form for HIV PR than the 11K monomer (HANSEN et al. 1988; BILLICH et al. 1988). Further, based on a kinetic analysis, it appears that HIV autocatalysis from the *pol*-encoded product occurs first at the C- and then at the N-terminus of HIV PR. A similar conclusion was reached by MOUS et al. (1988): Using an *E. coli* CAT-HIV *pol* fusion product, an initial 34K protein corresponding to CAT plus PR is formed, prior to the release of PR.

Another approach was used by GRAVES et al. (1988) who showed that by constructing a plasmid containing only DNA encoding the 99aa HIV PR sequence and expressing it in *E. coli*, an active product was obtained. This bypassed the need for autoprocessing. The PR product thus obtained could cleave HIV *gag* as well as *pol*-specific polyprotein substrates in vitro. This supports the idea that the same processing of Gag-Pol sequences can occur whether the cleavage PR is in *cis* (intramolecular) or *trans* (intermolecular). In confirmation of its size in *E. coli*, a 11K species in HIV virions was shown to be recognized by serum against peptides in the PR domain. LILLEHOJ et al. (1988) also showed that HIV PR purified from extracellular virus and *E. coli* extracts had the same size and sequence. The proteinase of 99 residues starts at the 69th position of the *pol* ORF. Their evidence also supports observations mentioned above that HIV PR is initially processed auto-catalytically from a larger Gag-Pol precursor.

Recently, LOUIS et al. (1989) reported on the chemical synthesis of the HIV PR gene and its subsequent expression in *E. coli*. It was demonstrated that the polypeptide product of the synthetic gene corresponds in molecular weight to the 11.5K PR found in virions and that the 99 aa protein is an active proteinase. Since synthesis of the gene was in five discrete fragments, the effect of mutations in any region of the gene can be easily tested. The recent extensive mutational analysis of HIV PR by LOEB et al. (1989) has also confirmed that the above sequence is HIV PR. Furthermore, in support of DTG sequence homology with the aspartyc proteinases, they showed that missense mutations within an 11 aa domain containing the DTG homology abolished processing of a *pol* precursor. They also provided evidence of a minimal sequence requirement of 4 aa to define the left hand cleavage site of the scissile bond and suggested like HANSEN et al. (1988) that the PR-RT site is cleaved first, before the RT-IN site.

6.2 Chemically Synthesized Human Immunodeficiency Virus Proteinase

Knowledge of the chemical structure of any biologically active natural product is a prerequisite for its production by synthetic methods of chemistry. Advances in peptide synthesis have made possible the successful synthesis of several biologically active proteins including enzymes for which the complete amino acid sequences have been determined. The total chemical synthesis of active HIV PR has recently been accomplished by three laboratories (COPELAND and OROSZLAN 1988; SCHNEIDER and KENT 1988; NUTT et al. 1988). As with all other biologically active proteins, knowledge of the primary structure of HIV PR was crucial for the synthetic approach. This structure has been accurately determined by chemical and immunochemical analysis of the protein (OROSZLAN et al. 1987a; HENDERSON et al. 1988b; COPELAND and OROSZLAN 1988; LILLEJOH et al. 1988) and comparison of the protein data with known nucleotide sequences (RATNER et al. 1985; WAIN-HOBSON et al. 1985). These studies established that the proteinase protein is composed of 99 aa and showed that the PR reading frame is located in the HIV genome immediately upstream of the RT N-terminus (VERONESE et al. 1986; LIGHTFOOTE et al. 1986) in the *pol* ORF encompassing 297 nucleotides (RATNER et al. 1985; WAIN-HOBSON et al. 1985). These results reveal a surprisingly small size for a proteolytic enzyme and have stimulated interest in the biogenetic expression of the HIV proteinase (see above) and in its chemical synthesis. Evidence that the 99 aa synthetic polypeptide can be refolded into an active molecule capable of proteolysis was reported first in 1987 (OROSZLAN et al. 1987a). Its specificity was demonstrated by cleavage of synthetic peptide substrates corresponding to natural cleavage sites, as previously done with avian retroviral PR (COPELAND and OROSZLAN 1981). These initial results have now been fully confirmed, and synthetic proteinases of both HIV-1 and HIV-2 are available, which, due to refined methods of synthesis and refolding, exhibit a much higher specific activity (COPELAND and OROSZLAN 1988; SCHNEIDER and KENT 1988; NUTT et al. 1988).

Assembly of the 99 aa polypeptide chain was accomplished by the stepwise solid-phase peptide synthesis method of MERRIFIED (1963) on phenylacetomidomethyl (PAM) resin (MITCHELL et al. 1976). The deprotected unfolded proteins were refolded under reducing conditions for HIV-1 proteinase (contains two half-cysteines) from guanidine-HCL (COPELAND and OROSZLAN 1988; SCHNEIDER and KENT 1988) or 50% acetic acid (NUTT et al. 1988) by dialysis against appropriate buffers. Refolding of HIV-2 PR (contains no cysteines) from guanidine-HC1 occurred either by dialysis or quick dilution into an appropriate buffer in the absence of reducing agents (COPELAND and OROSZLAN 1988).

7 Three-Dimensional Structure

Recently the three-dimensional structure of the PR from two retroviruses has been determined. MILLER et al. (1989) described the crystal structure of avian RSV PR at high resolution (2 Å) and NAVIA et al. (1989) provided a structure of

HIV-1 PR at medium (3 Å) resolution. In general, both analyses confirmed a dimeric structure predicted by PEARL and TAYLOR (1987b) and BLUNDELL et al. (1988). These authors examined the amino acid sequences of cellular aspartic proteinase and retroviral proteinase families, using pattern reognition, structure prediction, and molecular modeling techniques and concluded that the retroviral PRs which are shorter (SAUER et al. 1981; YOSHINAKA et al. 1985a, b, 1986) correspond to a single domain of an aspartic proteinase and probably function in a dimeric form that has the folding and active sites resembling those of pepsin-like proteinase.

The retroviral PR monomers contain β-sheet, turn, and α-helix structural elements. A schematic illustration of the three-dimensional structure of RSV PR in shown in Fig. 5. The arrangements of all the well-defined structural elements in pepsins and in the dimeric retroviral PRs of RSV and HIV-1 have been compared by BLUNDELL and PEARL (1989). In this analysis each subunit of the dimeric retroviral enzymes as for the bilobal pepsin contains a mixed β-pleated sheet of two intertwined motifs of four strands (a, b, c, d and a', b', c', d') related by a pseudo dyad. The active-site Asp-Thr-Gly or Asp-Ser-Gly sequence occurs on the wide loop (c, d) which is crossed by strand d' to give a Ψ-like structure. Although only the RSV, and not the HIV-1 structure has been reported at resolution high enough reliably to indicate the side-chain conformations, it

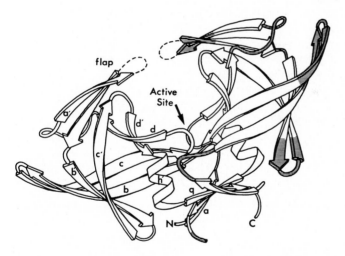

Fig. 5. Structure of RSV PR homodimer. This figure is a modification of the one drawn by Jane Richardson based on the results of Miller et al. (1989) and modified by Irene Weber. The subunit on the *left* shows the nomenclature for the secondary structure, with β strands a to d and a' to d', and helix h' (BLUNDELL et al. 1985). The amino- and carboxyl-termini are indicated by N and C. The corresponding sequence alignment is given in Fig. 7. The subunit on the *right* is shaded where the structure of HIV PR differs from that of RSV, usually due to shorter surface turns. The active site is indicated by an *arrow*, and the *dashed lines* represent the residues of the flap which were not visible in the electron density map for RSV PR (courtesy of Irene Weber)

appears that both enzymes have the characteristic aspartates hydrogen bonded together at the center of the active-site cleft (MILLER et al. 1989; NAVIA et al. 1989) as shown in Fig. 6, taken from BLUNDELL and PEARL (1989). The serine and threonine next to the catalytically active Asp stabilizes the symmetrical dimer in an exactly analogous way to pepsin by forming a buried "fireman's grip" between the subunits (PEARL and BLUNDELL, 1984). BLUNDELL and PEARL (1989) also pointed out the significant differences they have observed between the reported structures of RSV and HIV-1 PRs. These occurred mainly in the topology of the dimer interface region.

The determination of RSV PR crystal structure at high resolution (MILLER et al. 1989) allowed WEBER et al. (1989) to construct a three-dimensional model of HIV-1 PR. To build the model, they aligned the 99 residue HIV-1 PR sequence with the much longer (124 residues) RSV PR sequence by permitting deletions only at the large surface loops. The alignment is shown in Fig. 7, where the active-site triplet Asp-Thr-Gly and a second most highly conserved sequence in all retroviral PRs (Gly-Arg-Asp/Asn) are marked with asterisks. In this alignment the secondary structural elements of the RSV PR are indicated over the amino acid sequences and labelled according to the scheme proposed for pepsin (BLUNDELL et al. 1985). The designations a-d and a'-d' represent β strands, h represents α-helix with a single turn and h' is a longer α-helix. The flexible "flap'" lies between a' and b'.

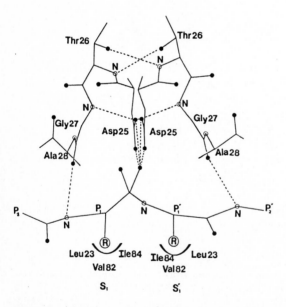

Fig. 6. Arrangements of the active-site residues Asp-Thr-Gly-Ala at the active site of retroviral proteinases, together with a model of the transition state of the substrate. *Dashed lines* indicate possible hydrogen bonds. The scissile bond lies between P_1 and P_1'. (From BLUNDELL and PEARL 1989)

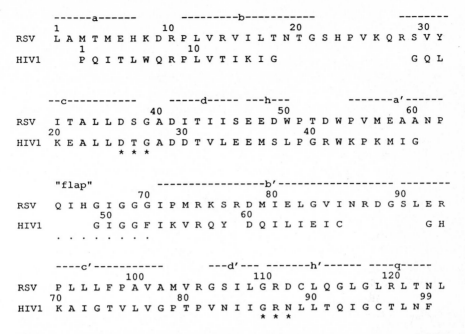

Fig. 7. Amino acid sequence alignment of the PRs from RSV and HIV-1. The secondary structural elements are indicated on top of the amino acid sequences (single letter code). The flexible "flap" lies between β strands a' and b'. The active site triad, Asp-Thr/Ser-Gly is indicated by *asterisks*. Another highly conserved region Gly-Arg-Asp/Asn also indicated by *asterisks* is located at the start of helix h' (courtesy of WEBER et al. 1989).

This model showed that the residues of the shorter HIV-1 PR could be accommodated in a conformation very similar to that of the longer RSV PR. The major difference between the three dimensional structure of RSV PR determined by MILLER et al. (1989) and HIV-1 proteinase determined by NAVIA et al. (1989) was the absence in the HIV-1 PR of an α-helix in a relatively well-conserved region, h', and the lack of participation of the N-terminal amino acids of HIV-1 PR in intermolecular contacts with the other subunits of the dimer. Most recently these discrepancies have been resolved by WLODAWER et al. (1989) who determined the crystal structure of chemically synthesized HIV-1 proteinase. This structure of HIV-1 PR was very similar to the structure of RSV PR as previously suggested by the model of WEBER (1989) and corrected the previously reported experimentally determined structure of NAVIA et al. (1989). The C_α backbone tracing of the fully refined model of the HIV-1 proteinase dimer is shown in Fig. 8. In the electron density maps the presence of helix (h'), residues 86–94, was confirmed in very good agreement with Weber's model (WEBER et al. 1989), and residues 1–5 at the N-terminus, which were previously reported to be disordered (NAVIA et al. 1989) were clearly visible. They are arranged into a four-stranded antiparallel β-sheet at the dimer interface. As for the RSV PR structure, several hydrogen-bond interactions stabilize the β-sheet conformation and the

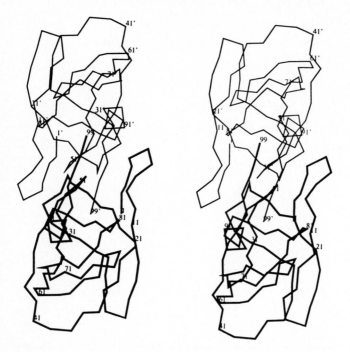

Fig. 8. Stereo view of the α-carbon structure of HIV-1 PR dimer (From Wlodawer et al. 1989)

N-terminus of one subunit is held tightly in place by ionic interaction with the C-terminus of the other subunit. On the basis of this arrangement of the subunit termini at the dimer interface WLODAWER et al. (1989) suggested that only intermolecular catalysis can be responsible for the release of the proteinase in both RSV and HIV-1. All the known retroviral proteinase sequences ranging from 99 to 125 residues in length can be accommodated into the structural alignment of the RSV and HIV-1 proteases. Such an alignment by WEBER (1989) is shown in Fig. 9. It should be pointed out that in addition to the active site, a second highly conserved region (Gly-Arg-Asp/Asn) occurs in the retroviral

▶

Fig. 9. The structural alignment of retroviral PRs. Amino acid sequences, shown in the single letter code were taken from the Protein Sequence Database (PIR). The proteinases are from: HIV-1, human immunodeficiency virus type 1 (SF2 isolate); HIV-2, human immunodeficiency virus type 2 (ROD isolate); SIV, simian immunodeficiency virus (MAC isolate); EIAV, equine infectious anemia virus; VISNA, visna lentivirus (strain 1514); MMLV, Moloney murine leukemia virus; FELV, feline leukemia virus; BEV, M7 baboon endogenous virus; HTLV-1, human T cell leukemia virus type I; HTLV-2, human T cell leukemia virus type II; BLV, bovine leukemia virus; RSV, Rous sarcoma virus (Prague C strain). N or C termini that are longer, or undetermined, are indicated by *terminal hyphens*. The sequence numbering is shown for HIV-1 PR and for RSV PR. The secondary structure of HIV-1 PR (WLOCAWER et al. 1989) and of RSV PR (MILLER et al. 1989) is indicated by *dashed lines* and *letters* which represent β strands, except for h which designates helical conformation. The *"flap"* is indicated, and the *dotted line* shows residues which are not visible in the RSV PR structure. (From WEBER 1989)

Retroviral Protease Sequences

```
        ----a----              -----b---------                    -----
        1                      10
HIV1    P Q I T L W      Q R P L V T I R I G                      G Q L
HIV2    P Q F S L W      K R P V V T A H I E                      G Q P
SIV     P Q F S L W      R R P V V T A H I E                      G Q P
EIAV    -V T Y N L E     K R P T T I V L I N                      D T P
VISNA-A P Y V V T E      A P P K I E I K V G                      T R W
MMLV    -Q G G Q G Q DPP P E P R I T L K V G                      G Q P
FELV    -Q E T Q G Q DPP P E P R I T L R I G                      G Q P
BEV     -Q G C Q G S GAP P E P R L T L S V G                      G H P
HTLV1-P V I P L D P A R R P V I K A Q V D T Q T        S H P K T
HTLV2-P L I P L R Q Q Q Q P I L G V R I S V M G        Q T P Q P
BLV     L S I P L A    R S R P S V A V Y L S G P W L      Q P S Q N Q
RSV     L A M T M E H K D R P L V R V I L T N T G S H P V K Q R S V Y
        1                      10                  20                  30
        ----a----              ---------b----------        --------
```

```
        ---c----------        -----d------                    ---a'---
        20                    30                    40
HIV1    K E S L L D T G A D D D T V L E E      M N    L P G K W K P K M
HIV2    V E V L L D T G A D D S I V A G        I E    L G N N Y S P K I
SIV     V E V L L D T G A D D S I V T G        I E    L G P H Y T P K I
EIAV    L N V L L D T G A D T S V L T T A H Y N R L K Y R G R K Y Q G T
VISNA   K K L L V D T G A D K T I V T S        H D    M G I P K G R I I
MMLV    V T F L V D T G A Q H S V L T Q        N P    G P L S D K S A W
FELV    V T F L V D T G A Q H S V L T R        P D    G P L S D R T A L
BEV     T T F L V D T G A Q H S V L T K        A N    G P L S S R T S W
HTLV1   I E A L L D T G A D M T V L P I A L F S S N T P    L K N T S
HTLV2   T Q A L L D T G A D L T V I P Q T L V P G P V K    L H D T L
BLV     A L M L V D T G A E N T V L P Q N W L V R D Y P    R I P A A
RSV     I T A L L D S G A D I T I I S E E D W P T D W P    V M E A A N P
        40                    50                         60
        --c----------        --d--- ----h---        --------a'------....
```

```
        -------      -----------------b'-----------------       ---
        50                    60
HIV1    I G G I G G F I K V R Q Y    D Q I P V E I C          G H
HIV2    V G G I G G F I N T K E Y    K N V E I E V L          N K
SIV     V G G I G G F I N T K E Y    K N V E I E V L          G K
EIAV    G I I G V G G N V E T F S T    P V T I K K K          G R
VISNA   L Q G I G G I I E G E K W    E Q V H L Q Y K          D K
MMLV    V Q G A T G G K R Y R W T T    D R K V H L A T        G K
FELV    V Q G A T G S K N Y R W T T    D R R V Q L A T        G K
BEV     V Q G A T G R K M H K W T N    R R T V N L G Q        G M
HTLV1   V L G A G G Q T Q D H F K L T S L P V L I R L P F R T T P I
HTLV2   I L G A S G Q T N T Q F K L L Q T P L H I F L P F R R S P V
BLV     V L G A G G V S R N R Y N W L Q G P L T L A L K P E G P F I
RSV     Q I H G I G G G I P M R K S R D M I E L G V I N R D G S L E R
        70                    80                    90
        "flap".......        ----------b'-----------------      ---------
```

```
        --c'--------------      --d'--- -------h'-------- ----q----
        70                    80                    90                  99
HIV1    K A I G T V L V G P T P V N I I G R N L L T Q I G C T L N F
HIV2    K V R A T I M T G D T P I N I F G R N I L T A L G M S L N L
SIV     R I K G T I M T G D T P I N I F G R N I L T A L G M S L N L
EIAV    H I K T R M L V A D I P V T I L G R D I L Q D L G A K L V L-
VISNA   M I K G T I V V L A TSP V E V L G R D N M R E L G I G L I M-
MMLV    V T H S F L H V P D C P Y P L L G R D L L T K L K A Q I H F E G S G
FELV    V T H S F L Y V P E C P Y P L L G R D L L T K L K A Q I H F T G E G
BEV     V T H S F L V V P E C P Y P L L G R D L L T K L G A Q I H F S E A G
HTLV1   V L T S C L V D T K N N W A I I G R D A L Q Q C Q G V L Y L P E A K
HTLV2   I L S S C L L D T H N K W T I I G R D A L Q Q C Q G L L Y L P D D P
BLV     T I P K I L V D T F D K W Q I L G R D V L S R L Q A S I S I P E E V
RSV     P L L L F P A V A M V R G S I L G R D C L Q G L G L R L T N L
        100                   110                   120
        --c'--------------      --d'--- -------h'-------- ---q---
```

PRs which is not present in any of the cellular aspartic proteinases. Arg 87 of the HIV PR is located in the helix (h') and forms an ion pair with Asp 29 that is also highly conserved. Conservative substitution of Lys for Arg 87 produced inactive proteinase (LOUIS et al. 1989b), which is consistent with a conserved conformation.

Less information is available about the flap extending over the active-site cleft. In RSV the flaps are disordered and not resolved. In HIV-1, the positions of the flaps are fixed by intermolecular packing interactions in the crystal. Mutational analysis has revealed that the amino acids in the flap of the HIV-1 proteinase are crucial for protease activity, and there is some evidence that amino acids in the flap interact with the substrate (R. SWANSTROM, personal communication), as is the case for other aspartic proteinases.

Processing of retroviral proteins has been studied for less than 15 years. There are now two crystal structures available with more structural information sure to follow. The viral proteinase is receiving attention from many quarters and is providing a ready target for the design of potentially important antiviral compounds.

Acknowledgements. We thank T. Blundell, L. Pearl, J. Richardson, I. Weber, and A. Wlodawer for permission to use their figures. We also thank Cheri Rhoderick for the preparation of the manuscript. Work in the authors laboratory was supported by contract No. NO1-CO-74104 with BRI and by Public Health Service Grant 5RO1-CA-37380-06 from the National Institutes of Health.

References

Arcement LJ, Karshin WL, Naso RB, Jamjoom GA, Arlinghaus RB (1976) Biosynthesis of Rauscher leukemia viral proteins: presence of p30 and envelope p15 sequences in precursor polyproteins. Virology 69: 763–774

Barbacid M, Stephenson JR, Aaronson SA (1976) *Gag* gene of mammalian type C RNA tumor viruses. Nature 262: 554–559

Barré-Sinoussi F, Chermann J-C, Rey F, Nugeyre MT, Chamaret S, Gruest J, Dauguet C, Axler-Blin C, Brun-Vézinet F, Rouzious C, Rozenbaum W, Montagnier L (1983) Isolation of a T-lymphotropic retrovirus from a patient at risk for acquired immune deficiency. Science 220: 868–871

Berger A, Schechter I (1970) Mapping the active site of papain with the aid of peptide substrate and inhibitors. Philos Trans R Soc Lond [Biol] 257: 249–264

Billich S, Knoop M-T, Hansen J, Strop P, Sedlacek J, Mertz R, Moelling K (1988) Synthetic peptides as substrates and inhibitors of human immunodeficiency virus-1 protease. J Biol Chem 263: 17905–17908

Blundell T, Pearl L (1989) Retroviral proteinases—a second front against AIDS. Nature 337: 596–597

Blundell T, Jenkins J, Pearl L, Sewell T, Pedersen V (1985) The high resolution structure of endothiapepsin. In: Kostka V (ed) Aspartic proteinases and their inhibitors. de Gruyter, Berlin, pp 151–161

Blundell T, Carney D, Gardner S, Hayes F et al. (1988) 18th Sir Hans Krebs lecture. Knowledge-based protein modelling and design. Eur J Biochem 172: 513–520

Bolognesi DP (1974) Structural components of RNA tumor viruses. Adv Virus Res 19: 315–359

Bolognesi DP, Montelaro RC, Frank H, Schafer W (1978) Assembly of type C oncornaviruses: a model. Science 199: 183–186

Bu M, Oroszlan S, Luftig RB (1989) Inhibition of bacterially expressed HIV protease activity as determined by an in vitro cleavage assay with MuLV Pr65^{gag}. AIDS Res Hum Retroviruses 5: 259–268

Copeland TD, Oroszlan S (1981) Chemical synthesis of a retroviral nucleic acid binding protein. In: Rich DH, Gross E (eds) Peptides: synthesis, structure and function. Pierce, Rockford, pp 497–500

Copeland TD, Oroszlan S (1988) Genetic locus, primary structure and chemical synthesis of HIV protease. Gen Anal Tech 5: 109–115

Copeland TD, Oroszlan S, Kalyanaraman VS, Sarngadharan MG, Gallo RC (1983) Complete amino acid sequence of human T-cell leukemia virus structural protein p 15. FEBS Lett 162: 390–395

Crawford S, Goff SP (1985) A deletion mutant in the 5' part of the *pol* gene of Moloney murine leukemia virus blocks proteolytic processing of the *gag* and *pol* polyproteins. J Virol 53: 899–907

Debouck C, Gorniak JG, Strickler JE, Meek TD, Metcalf BW, Rosenberg M (1987) Human immunodeficiency virus protease expressed in *Escherichia coli* exhibits autoprocessing and specific maturation of the *gag* precursor. Proc Natl Acad Sci USA 84: 8903–8906

Dickson C, Eisenman R, Fan H, Hunter E, Teich N (1984) Protein biosynthesis and assembly. In: Weiss R, Teich N, Varmus H (eds) RNA tumor viruses, molecular biology of tumor viruses, 1st ed. Cold Spring Harbor Laboratory, Cold Spring Harbor, pp 528–547

Dickson C, Eisenman R, Fan H (1985) Supplement. Protein biosynthesis and assembly. In: Weiss R, Teich N, Varmus H, Coffin J (eds) RNA tumor viruses, molecular biology of tumor viruses, 2nd ed. Cold Spring Harbor Laboratory, Cold Spring Harbor, pp 135–143

Dittmar KJ, Moelling K (1978) Biochemical properties of p15-associated protease in an avian RNA tumor virus. J Virol 28: 106–118

Eisenman RN, Vogt VM (1978) The biosynthesis of oncovirus proteins. Biochem Biophys Acta 473: 187–239

Eisenman RN, Vogt VM, Diggelman H (1975) Synthesis of avian RNA tumor virus structural proteins. Cold Spring Harbor Symp Quant Biol 39: 1067–1075

Farmerie WG, Loeb DD, Casavant NC, Hutchison CA III, Edgell MH, Swanstrom R (1987) Expression and processing of the AIDS virus reverse transcriptase in *Escherichia coli*. Science 236: 305–308

Felsenstein KM, Goff SP (1988) Expression of the *gag-pol* fusion protein of Moloney murine leukemia virus without *gag* protein does not induce virion formation of proteolytic processing. J Virol 62: 2179–2182

Gallo RC, Salahuddin SZ, Popovic M, Shearer GM, Kaplan M, Haynes BF, Palker TJ, Redfield R, Oleske J, Safai B, White G, Foster P, Markham PD (1984) Frequent detection and isolation of cytopathic retrovirus (HTLV-III) from patients with AIDS and at risk for AIDS. Science 224: 500–503

Gonda MA (1988) Molecular genetics and structure of the human immunodeficiency virus. J Electron Microsc Tech 8: 17–40

Graves MC, Lim JJ, Heimer EP, Kramer RA (1988) An 11-kDa form of human immunodeficiency virus protease expressed in Escherichia coli is sufficient for enzymatic activity. Proc Natl Acad Sci USA 85: 2449–2453

Hafenrichter R, Thiel HJ (1985) Simian sarcoma virus-encoded *gag*-related protein: in vitro cleavage by Friend leukemia virus-associated proteolytic activity. Virology 143: 143–152

Hansen J, Billich S, Schulze T, Sukrow S, Moelling K (1988) Partial purification and substrate analysis of bacterially expressed HIV protease by means of monoclonal antibody. EMBO J 7: 1785–1791

Henderson LE, Sowder RC, Smythers G, Benveniste RE, Oroszlan S (1985) Purification and N-terminal amino acid sequence comparisons of structural proteins from retrovirus-D/Washington and Mason-Pfizer monkey virus. J Virol 55: 778–787

Henderson LE, Benveniste RE, Sowder R, Copeland TD, Schultz AM, Oroszlan S (1988a) Molecular characterization of *gag* proteins from simian immunodeficiency virus (SIV$_{Mne}$). J Virol 62: 2587–2595

Henderson LE, Copeland TD, Sowder RC, Schultz AM, Oroszlan S (1988b) Analysis of proteins and peptides purified from sucrose gradient banded HTLV-III. In: Bolognesi D (ed) Human retroviruses, cancer and AIDS: approaches to prevention and therapy, Liss, New York, pp 135–147

Hill RL (1965) Hydrolysis of proteins. Adv Protein Chem 20: 37–107

Hizi A, Henderson LE, Copeland TD, Sowder RC, Hixson CV, Oroszlan S (1987) Characterization of mouse mammary tumor virus *gag-pro* gene products and the ribosomal fremeshift site by protein sequencing. Proc Natl Acad Sci USA 84: 7041–7045

Hizi A, Henderson LE, Copeland TD, Sowder RC, Krutzsh HC, Oroszlan S (1989) Analysis of *gag* proteins from mouse mammary tumor virus. J Virol 63: 2543–2549

Ikuta K, Luftig RB (1986) Inhibition of cleavage of Moloney murine leukemia virus *gag* and *env* coded precursor polyproteins by cerulenin. Virology 154: 195–206

Jacks T, Varmus HE (1985) Expression of the Rous sarcoma virus *pol* gene by ribosomal frameshifting. Science 230: 1237–1242

Jacks T, Townsley K, Varmus HE, Majors J (1987) Two efficient ribosomal frameshifting events are required for synthesis of mouse mammary tumor virus *gag*-related polyproteins. Proc Natl Acad Sci USA 84: 4298–4302

Jacks T, Power MD, Masiarz FR, Luciw PA, Barr PJ, Varmus HE (1988a) Characterization of ribosomal frameshifting in HIV-1 *gag-pol* expression. Nature 331: 280–283

Jacks T, Madhani HD, Masiarz FR, Varmus HE (1988b) Signals for ribosomal frameshifting in the Rous sarcoma virus *gag-pol* region. Cell 55: 447–458

Jacobson MF, Baltimore D (1968) Polypeptide cleavages in the formation of poliovirus proteins. Proc Natl Acad Sci USA 61: 77–84

Jamjoom GA, Naso RB, Arlinghaus RB (1976) Selective decrease in the rate of cleavage of an intracellular precursor to Rauscher leukemai virus p30 by treatment of infected cells with Actinomycin D. J Virol 19: 1054–1072

Jamjoom GA, Naso RB Arlinghaus RB (1977) Further characterization of intracellular precursor polyproteins of Rauscher leukemia virus. Virology 78: 11–34

Katoh I, Yoshinaka Y, Rein A, Shibuya M, Odaka T, Oroszlan S (1985) Murine leukemia virus maturation: protease region required for conversion from "immature" to "mature" core form and for virus infectivity. Virology 145: 280–292

Katoh I, Yoshinaka Y, Luftig RB (1986) The effect of cerulenin on Moloney murine leukemia virus morphogenesis. Virus Res 5: 265–276

Katoh I, Yasunaga T, Ikawa Y, Yoshinaka Y (1987) Inhibition of retroviral protease activity by an aspartyl proteinase inhibitor. Nature 329: 654–656

Katz RA, Fu XD, Skalka AM, Leis J (1986) Avian retrovirus nucleocapsid protein, pp12, produced in Escherichia coli has biochemical properties identical to unphosphorylated viral protein. Gene 50: 361–369

Koch G, Richter D (eds) (1980) Biosynthesis modifications and processing of cellular and viral polyproteins. Academic, New York

Kohl NE, Emini EA, Schleif WA, Davis LJ, Heimbach JC, Dixon RA, Scolnick EM, Sigal IS (1988) Active human immunodeficiency virus protease is required for viral infectivity. Proc Natl Acad Sci USA 85: 4686–4690

Königsberg W, Hill RJ (1962) The structure of human hemoglobin V. The digestion of the α chain of human hemoglobin with pepsin. J Biol Chem 237: 3157–3162

Konze-Thomas B, von der Helm K (1981) Proteolytic processing of avian and simian sarcoma and leukemia viral proteins. Hamatol Bluttransfus 26: 409–413

Korant BD, Longberg-Holm KK (1981) Viral proteins and site-specific cleavage. Acta Biol Med Ger 40: 1481–1488

Kotler M, Katz RA, Danho W, Leis J, Skalka AM (1988a) Synthetic peptides as substrates and inhibitors of a retroviral protease. Proc Natl Acad Sci USA 85: 4185–4189

Kotler M, Katz RA, Skalka AM (1988b) Activity of avian retroviral protease expressed in Escherichia coli. J Virol 62: 2696–2700

Kotler M, Danho W, Katz RA, Leis J, Skalka AM (1989) Avian retroviral proteases and cellular aspartic proteases are distinguished by activities on peptide substrates. J Biol Chem 264: 3428–3435

Kramer RA, Schaber MD, Skalka AM, Ganguly K, Wong-Staal F, Reddy EP (1986) HTLV-III *gag* protein is processed in yeast cells by the virus *pol*-protease. Science 231: 1580–1584

Kräusslich HG, Wimmer E (1988) Viral proteinases. Annu Rev Biochem 57: 701–754

Kräusslich HG, Schneider H, Zybarth G, Carter CA, Wimmer E (1988) Processing of in vitro-synthesized *gag* precursor proteins of human immunodeficiency virus (HIV) type 1 by HIV proteinase generated in Escherichia coli. J Virol 62: 4393–4397

Kräusslich HG, Ingraham RH, Skoog MT, Wimmer E, Pallai PV, Carter CA (1989a) Activity of purified biosynthetic proteinase of human immunodeficiency virus on natural substrates and synthetic peptides. Proc Natl Acad Sci USA 86: 807–811

Kräusslich HG, Oroszlan S, Wimmer E (1989b) Viral proteinases as targets for Chemotherapy. Current communications in molecular biology. Cold Spring Harbor Laboratory, Cold Spring Harbor

Laprevotte I, Hampe A, Sherr CJ, Galibert F (1984) Nucleotide sequence of *gag* gene and *gag-pol* junction of feline leukemia virus. J Virol 50: 884–894

Le Grice SFJ, Mills J, Mous J (1988) Active site mutagenesis of the AIDS virus protease and its alleviation by *trans* complementation. EMBO J 7: 2547–2553

Leis J, Baltimore D, Bishop JM, Coffin J, Fleissner E, Goff SP, Oroszlan S, Robinson H, Skalka AM, Temin HM, Vogt V (1988) Standardized and simplified nomenclature for proteins common to all retroviruses. J. Virol 62: 1808–1809

Levy JA, Hoffman AD, Kramer SM, Landis JA, Shimabukuro JM, Oshiro LS (1984) Isolation of lymphocytopathic retroviruses from San Francisco patients with AIDS. Science 225: 840–842

Lightfoote MM, Coligan JE, Folks TM, Fauci AS, Martin MA, Venkatesan S (1986) Structural characterization of reverse transcriptase and endonuclease polypeptides of the acquired immunodeficiency syndrome retrovirus. J Virol 60: 771–775

Lillehoj EP, Salazar FHR, Mervis RJ, Raum MG, Chan HW, Ahmad N, Venkatesan S (1988) Purification and characterization of the putative *gag-pol* protease of human immunodeficiency virus. J Virol 62: 3053–3058

Loeb DD, Hutchinson CA III, Edgell MH, Farmerie WG, Swanstrom R (1989) Mutational analysis of human immunodeficiency virus type I protease suggests functional homology with aspartic proteinases. J Virol 63: 111–121

Louis JM, Wondrak EM, Copeland TD, Dale Smith CA, Mora PT, Oroszlan S (1989a) Chemical synthesis and expression of the HIV-I protease gene in *E. coli*. Biochem Biophys Res Commun 159: 87–94

Louis JM, Smith CAD, Wondrak EM, Mora PT, Oroszlan S (1989b) Substitution mutations of the highly conserved arginine 87 of HIV-1 protease result in loss of proteolytic activity. Biochem Biophys Res Commun 164: 30–38

Lu AH, Soong MM, Wong PKY (1979) Maturation of Moloney murine leukemia virus. Virology 93: 269–274

Luftig RB, Bu M, Ikuta K (1989) In: Kostka V (ed) Proteases of Retroviruses de Gruytr. Morphogenesis of retroviruses in the presence and absence of protease inhibitors. Berlin, pp 11–14

Mains RE, Eipper BA, Glembotski CC, Dores RM (1983) Strategies for the biosynthesis of bioactive peptides. Trends Neurosci 4: 229–235

Meek TD, Dayton BD, Metcalf BW, Dreyer GB, Strickler JE, Gorniak JG, Rosenberg M, Moore ML, Magaard VW, Debouck C (1989) Human immunodeficiency virus 1 protease expressed in *Escherichia Coli* behaves as a dimeric aspartic protease. Proc Natl Acad Sci USA 86: 1841–1845

Merrifield RB (1963) Solid phase peptide synthesis. I. The synthesis of a tetrapeptide. J Am Chem Soc 85: 2149–2154

Mermer B, Malamy M, Coffin JM (1983) Rous sarcoma virus contains sequences which permit expression of the *gag* gene in *Escherichia coli*. Mol Cell Biol 3: 1746–1758

Miller M, Jaskólski M, Rao JKM, Leis J, Wlodawer A (1989) Crystal structure of a retroviral protease proves relationship to aspartic protease family. Nature 337: 576–579

Mitchell AR, Erickson BW, Ryabstey MN, Hodges RS, Merrifield RB (1976) Tert-butoxycarbonyl-aminoacyl-4-(oxymethyl)-phenylacetamidomethyl-resin, a more acid-resistant support for solid-phase peptide synthesis. J Am Chem Soc 98: 7357–7362

Moelling K, Scott A, Dittmar KEJ, Owada M (1980) Effect of p15-associated protease from an avian RNA tumor virus on avian virus-specific polyprotein precursors. J Virol 33: 680–688

Mous J, Heimer EP, LeGrice SFJ (1988) Processing protease and reverse transcriptase from HIV-1 polyprotein in *E. coli*. J Virol 62: 1433–1436

Muesing MA, Smith DH, Cabradilla CD, Benton CV, Lasky LA, Capon DJ (1985) Nucleic acid structure and expression of the human AIDS/lymphadenopathy retrovirus. Nature 313: 450–458

Nam SH, Hatanaka M (1986) Identification of protease gene of human T-cell leukemia virus type I (HTLV-I) and its structural comparison. Biochem Biophys Res Commun 139: 129–135

Nam SH, Kidokoro M, Shida H, Hatanaka M (1988) Processing of *gag* precursor polyprotein of human T-cell leukemia virus type I by virus-encoded protease. J Virol 62: 3718–3728

Navia MA, Fitzgerald PMD, McKeever BM, Leu C-T, Heimbach JC, Herber WK, Sigal IS, Darke PL, Springer JP (1989) Three-dimensional structure of aspartyl protease from human immunodeficiency virus HIV-1. Nature 337: 615–620

Nermut MV, Frank H, Schafer W (1972) Properties of mouse leukemia viruses. III. Electron microscopic appearance as revealed after conventional preparation techniques as well as freeze-drying and freeze-etching. Virology 49: 345–358

Nutt RF, Brady SF, Darke PL, Ciccarone TM, Colton CD, Nutt EM, Rodkey JA, Bennett CD, Waxman LH, Sigal IS, Anderson PS, Veber DF (1988) Chemical synthesis and enzymatic activity of a 99-residue peptide with a sequence proposed for the human immunodeficiency virus protease. Proc Natl Acad Sci USA 85: 7129–7133

Oppermann H, Bishop JM, Varmus HE, Levintow L (1977) A joint product of the genes gag and pol of avian sarcoma virus: a possible precursor of reverse transcriptase. Cell 12: 993–1005

Oroszlan S, Copeland TD (1985) Primary structure and processing of gag and env gene products of human T-cell leukemia viruses HTLV-I$_{CR}$ and HTLV-I$_{ATK}$. Curr Top Microbiol Immunol 115: 221–233

Oroszlan S, Gilden RV (1979) Amino acid sequences of plant and animal viral proteins. In: Fraenkel-Conrat H, Wagner RW (eds) Comprehensive Virology. vol 13, Plenum, New York, pp 1–35

Oroszlan S, Gilden RV (1980) Primary structure analysis of retrovirus proteins. In: Stephenson JR (ed) Molecular biology of RNA tumor viruses. Academic, New York, pp 299–344

Oroszlan S, van Beveren C (1985) Appendix E: amino acid sequences of retroviral proteins. In: Weiss R, Teich N, Varmus H, Coffin J (eds) RNA tumor viruses. Molecular biology of tumor viruses, 2nd edn. vol 2, Cold Spring Harbor Laboratory, Cold Spring Harbor, pp 1209–1221

Oroszlan S, Copeland TD, Summers MR, Smythers G, Guilden RV (1975) Amino acid sequence homology of mammalian type C RNA virus major internal proteins. J Biol Chem 250: 6232–6239

Oroszlan S, Henderson LE, Stephenson JR, Copeland TD, Long CW, Ihle JN, Gilden RV (1978) Amino- and Carboxyl-terminal amino acid sequences of proteins coded by gag gene of murine leukemia virus. Proc Natl Acad Sci USA 75: 1404–1408

Oroszlan S, Sarngadharan MG, Copeland TD, Kalyanaraman VS, Gilden RV, Gallo RC (1982) Primary structure analysis of the major internal protein p24 of human type C T-cell leukemia virus. Proc Natl Acad Sci USA 79: 1291–1294

Oroszlan S, Copeland TD, Henderson LE (1987a) Human immunodeficiency virus protease. 3rd International Conference on AIDS, Washington, abstract M 9.3

Oroszlan S, Henderson LE, Hizi A, Copeland TD (1987b) Retroviral genes and gene products: Control of expression. In: Lapis K, Eckhardt S (eds) Lectures and Symposia, 14th International Cancer Congress, Budapest 1986, vol 4, Karger, Basel, pp 243–250

Pal R, Gallo RC, Sarngadharan MG (1988) Processing of the structural proteins of human immunodeficiency virus type 1 in the presence of monensin and cerulenin. Proc Natl Acad Sci USA 85: 9283–9286

Panet A, Baltimore D, Hanafusa T (1975) Quantitation of avian RNA tumor virus reverse transcriptase by radioimmunoassay. J Virol 16: 146–152

Pearl LH, Blundell T (1984) The active site of aspartic proteinases. FEBS Lett 174: 96–101

Pearl LH, Taylor WR (1987a) Sequence specificity of retroviral proteases. Nature 328: 482

Pearl LH, Taylor WR (1987b) A structural model for the retroviral proteases. Nature 329: 351–354

Pepinsky RB (1983) Localization of lipid-protein and protein-protein interactions within the murine retroviruses gag precursor by a novel peptide-mapping technique. J Biol Chem 258: 11229–11235

Pepinsky RB, Cappiello D, Wilkowski C, Vogt VM (1980) Chemical cross-linking of proteins in avian sarcoma and leukemia viruses. Virology 102: 205–210

Poiesz BJ, Ruscetti FW, Gazdar AF, Bunn PA, Minna JD, Gallo RC (1980) Isolation of type C retrovirus particles from cultured and fresh lymphocytes of a patient with cutaneous T-cell lymphoma. Proc Natl Acad Sci USA 77: 7415–7419

Popovic M, Sargadharan MG, Read E, Gallo RC (1984) Detection, isolation, and continuous production of cytopathic retroviruses (HTLV-III) from patients with AIDS and pre-AIDS. Science 224: 497–500

Priel E, Showalter SD, Roberts M, Yosef O, Segal S, Aboud M, Oroszlan S, Blair DG (1990) Topoisomerase I activity associated with human immunodeficiency virus (HIV) particles and equine infectious anemia virus core proteins. Virology (submitted)

Ratner L, Haseltine W, Patarca R, Livak J, Starcich B, Josephs SF, Doran ER, Rafalski JA et al. (1985) Complete nucleotide sequence of the AIDS virus, HTLV-III. Nature 313: 277–284

Rice NR, Stephens RM, Burny A, Gilden RV (1985) The gag and pol genes of bovine leukemia virus: nucleotide sequence and analysis. Virology 142: 357–377

Roberts MM, Oroszlan S (1989) The preparation and biochemical characterization of intact capsids of equine infectious anemia virus. Biochem Biophys Res Commun 160: 486–494

Sanchez-Pescador R, Power MD, Barr PJ, Steimer KS, Stempien MM, Brown-Shimer SL, Gee WW, Renard A et al. (1985) Nucleotide sequence and expression of an AIDS-associated retrovirus (ARV-2). Science 227: 484–492

Satake M, Luftig RB (1983) Comparative immunofluorescence of murine leukemia virus-derived membrane-associated antigens. Virology 124: 259–273

Sauer RT, Allen DW, Niall HD (1981) Amino acid sequence of p15 from avian myeloblastosis virus complex. Biochemistry 20: 3784–3791

Schneider J, Kent SBH (1988) Enzymatic activity on a synthetic 99 residue protein corresponding to the putative HIV-1 protease. Cell 54: 363–368

Schultz AM, Rein A (1985) Maturation of murine leukemia virus env proteins in the absence of other viral proteins. Virology 145: 335–339

Šedlácek J. Strop P, Kaprálek F, Pecenka V, Kostka V, Trávnicek M, Riman J (1988) Processed enzymatically active protease (p15^{gag}) of avian retrovirus obtained in an E. coli system expressing a recombinant precursor (Pr25^{lacΔgag}). FBES Lett 237: 187–190

Seelmeier S, Schmidt H, Turk V, von der Helm K (1988) Human immunodeficiency virus has an aspartic-type protease that can be inhibited by pepstatin A. Proc Natl Acad Sci USA 85: 6612–6616

Seiki M, Hattori S, Hirayama Y, Yoshida M (1983) Human adult T-cell leukemia virus: complete nucleotide sequence of the provirus genome integrated in leukemia cell DNA. Proc Natl Acad Sci USA 80: 3618–3622

Shealy DJ, Mosser AG, Rueckert RR (1980) Novel p19-related protein in Rous-associated virus type 61: implications for avian gag gene order J Virol 34: 431–437

Shields A, Witte ON, Rothenberg E, Baltimore D (1978) High frequency of an aberrant expression of Moloney murine leukemia virus in clonal infections. Cell 14: 601–609

Shimotohno K, Takahashi Y, Shimizu N, Gojobori T, Golde DW, Chen ISY, Miwa M, Sugimura T (1985) Complete nucleotide sequence of an infectious clone of human T-cell leukemia virus type II: an open reading frame for the protease gene. Proc Natl Acad Sci USA 82: 3101–3105

Skalka AM (1989) Retroviral proteases: first glimpse at the anatomy of a processing machine. Cell 56: 911–913

Stephens RM, Casey JW, Rice NR (1986) Equine infectious anemia virus gag and pol genes: Relatedness to Visna and AIDS virus. Science 231: 589–594

Summers DF, Maizel JV (1968) Evidence for large precursor proteins in poliovirus synthesis. Proc Natl Acad Sci USA 59: 966–971

Toh H, Ono M, Saigo K, Miyata T (1985) Retroviral protease-like sequence in the yeast transposon Ty1. Nature 315: 691

Veronese FD, Copeland TD, DeVico AL, Rahman R, Oroszlan S, Gallo RC, Sarngadharan MG (1986) Characterization of highly immunogenic p66/51 as the reverse transcriptase of HTLV-III/LAV. Science 231: 1289–1291

Veronese FD, Copeland TD, Oroszlan S, Gallo RC, Sarngadharan MG (1988) Biochemical and immunological analysis of human immunodeficiency virus gag gene products p17 and p24. J Virol 62: 795–801

Vogt VM, Eisenman R, Diggelmann H (1975) Generation of avian myeloblastosis virus structural proteins by proteolytic cleavage of a precursor polypeptide. J Mol Biol 96: 471–493

Vogt VM, Wight A, Eisenman R (1979) In vitro cleavage of avian retrovirus gag proteins by viral protease p15. Virology 98: 154–167

Von der Helm K (1977) Cleavage of Rous sarcoma viral polypeptide precursor into internal structural proteins in vitro involves viral protein p15. Proc Natl Acad Sci USA 74: 911–915

Wain-Hobson S, Sonigo P, Danos O, Cole S, Alizon M (1985) Nucleotide sequence of the AIDS Virus, LAV. Cell 40: 9–17

Weber IT (1989) Structural alignment of retroviral protease sequences. Gene (in press)

Weber IT, Miller M, Jaskolski M, Leis J, Skalka AM, Wlodawer A (1989) Molecular modelling of the HIV-1 protease and its substrate binding site. Science 243: 928–931

Wellink J, van Kammen A (1988) Proteases involved in the processing of viral polyproteins. Arch Virol 98: 1–26

Wills JW, Craven RC, Achacoso JA (1989) Creation and expression of myristylated forms of Rous sarcoma virus Gag protein in mammalian cells. J Virol 63: 4331–4343

Witte ON, Baltimore D (1978) Relationship of retrovirus polyprotein cleavages to virion maturation studied with temperature-sensitive murine leukemia virus mutants. J Virol 26: 750–761

Wlodawer A, Miller M, Jaskolski M, Sathyanarayana BK, Baldwin E, Weber IT, Selk LM, Clawson

L, Schneider J, Kent SBH (1989) Conserved folding in retroviral proteases: crystal structure of a synthetic HIV-1 protease. Science 245: 616–621

Yoshinaka Y, Luftig RB (1977a) Murine leukemia virus morphogenesis: Cleavage of P70 in vitro can be accompanied by a shift from a concentrically coiled internal strand ("immature") to a collapsed ("mature") form of the virus core. Proc Natl Acad Sci USA 74: 3446–3450

Yoshinaka Y, Luftig RB (1977b) Partial characterization of a P70 proteolytic factor that is present in purified virions of Rauscher leukemia virus (RLV). Biochem Biophys Res Commun 76: 54–63

Yoshinaka Y, Luftig RB (1977c) Properties of a P70 proteolytic factor of murine leukemia viruses. Cell 12: 709–719

Yoshinaka Y, Luftig RB (1978) Morphological conversion of "immature" Rauscher leukaemia virus cores to a "mature" form after addition of the P65–70 (gag gene product proteolytic factor). J Gen Virol 40: 151–160

Yoshinaka Y, Luftig RB (1980) Physiochemical characterization and specificity of the murine leukaemia virus Pr65^{gag} proteolytic factor. J Gen Virol 48: 329–340

Yoshinaka Y, Luftig RB (1981) Inhibition of murine leukemia virus Pr65^{gag} cleavage in vitro and in vivo by hypertonic medium. J Virol 37: 1066–1070

Yoshinaka Y, Katoh I, Luftig RB (1984) Murine retrovirus Pr65^{gag} forms a 130K dimer in the absence of disulfide reducing agents. Virology 136: 274–281

Yoshinaka Y, Katoh I, Copeland TD, Oroszlan S (1985a) Murine leukemia virus protease is encoded by the gag-pol gene and is synthesized through suppression of an amber termination codon. Proc Natl Acad Sci USA 82: 1618–1622

Yoshinaka Y, Katoh I, Copeland TD, Oroszlan S (1985b) Translational readthrough of an amber termination codon during synthesis of feline leukemia virus protease. J Virol 55: 870–873

Yoshinaka Y, Shames RB, Luftig RB, Smythers GW, Oroszlan S (1985c) In vitro cleavage of Pr65^{gag} by the Moloney murine leukaemia virus proteolytic activity yields p30 whose N-terminal sequence is identical to virion p30. J Gen Virol 66: 379–383

Yoshinaka Y, Katoh I, Copeland TD, Smythers GW, Oroszlan S (1986) Bovine leukemia virus protease: purification, chemical analysis and in vitro processing of the gag-precursor polyproteins. J Virol 57: 826–832

Appendix: Proteinase cleavage site sequences in retroviral polyproteins. The designation of amino acid residues spanning the cleavage site is according to BERGER and SCHECHTER (1970). Since the PR cleavage site sequences are highly variable, it is difficult to define a consensus sequence of cleavage. Residues in P_1 and P_1' are usually hydrophobic, but there are exceptions.

1. PR cleavage sites in RSV Gag and Gag-Pol polyproteins (SKALKA 1989). PR' is the transframe protein that is extended by 7aa at the C-terminus of PR p15^{gag}.

RSV

Schematic of Pr76^{gag} showing MA (p19, X$_1$, p10), CA (p27), X$_2$, NC (p12), PR (p15); and Pr180$^{gag-pol}$ showing RT p63(α) and IN p32.

P5	P4	P3	P2	P1	↓	P1'	P2'	P3'	P4'	P5'	
Gly	Thr	Ser	Cys	Tyr		His	Cys	Gly	Thr	Ala	MA/X$_1$
Pro	Pro	Tyr	Val	Gly		Ser	Gly	Leu	Tyr	Pro	X$_1$/p10
Pro	Val	Val	Ala	Met		Pro	Val	Val	Ile	Lys	p10/CA
Ile	Ala	Ala	Ala	Met		Ser	Ser	Ala	Ile	Gln	CA/X$_2$
Gln	Pro	Leu	Ile	Met		Ala	Val	Val	Asn	Arg	X$_2$/NC
Pro	Pro	Ala	Val	Ser		Leu	Ala	Met	Thr	Met	NC/PR
Arg	Ala	Thr	Val	Leu		Thr	Val	Ala	Leu	His	PR'/RT
Thr	Phe	Gln	Ala	Tyr		Pro	Leu	Arg	Glu	Ala	RT/IN
Ser	Pro	Leu	Phe	Ala		Gly	Ile	Ser	Asp	Trp	IN

2. PR cleavage sites in Mo-MuLV Gag and Gag-Pol polyproteins (OROSZLAN and VAN BEVEREN 1985).

Mo-MuLV

Schematic of Pr65^{gag} showing MA (p15, p12), CA (p30), NC (p10), PR; and Pr200$^{gag-pol}$ showing p14, RT p80, IN p46.

P5	P4	P3	P2	P1	↓	P1'	P2'	P3'	P4'	P5'	
Arg	Ser	Ser	Leu	Tyr		Pro	Ala	Leu	Thr	Pro	MA/p12
Thr	Ser	Gln	Ala	Phe		Pro	Leu	Arg	Ala	Gly	p12/CA
Met	Ser	Lys	Leu	Leu		Ala	Thr	Val	Val	Ser	CA/NC
Gln	Thr	Ser	Leu	Leu		Thr	Leu	Asp	Asp	Gln	NC/PR
Pro	Leu	Gln	Val	Leu		Thr	Leu	Gln	Ile	Glu	PR/RT
Thr	Ser	Thr	Leu	Leu		Ile	Glu	Asn	Ser	Ser	RT/IN

3. PR cleavage sites n MMTV Gag, Gag-Pro, and Gag-Pro-Pol polyproteins (HIZI et al. 1989). Several polypeptides derived from the Gag region originally designated p21 have been purified and sequenced. They are p3, p8, and n.

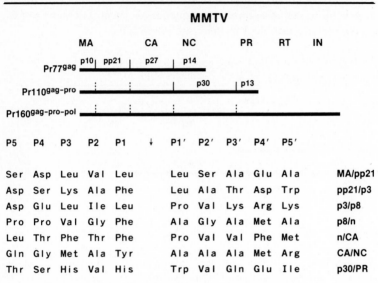

MMTV

P5	P4	P3	P2	P1	↓	P1'	P2'	P3'	P4'	P5'	
Ser	Asp	Leu	Val	Leu		Leu	Ser	Ala	Glu	Ala	MA/pp21
Asp	Ser	Lys	Ala	Phe		Leu	Ala	Thr	Asp	Trp	pp21/p3
Asp	Glu	Leu	Ile	Leu		Pro	Val	Lys	Arg	Lys	p3/p8
Pro	Pro	Val	Gly	Phe		Ala	Gly	Ala	Met	Ala	p8/n
Leu	Thr	Phe	Thr	Phe		Pro	Val	Val	Phe	Met	n/CA
Gln	Gly	Met	Ala	Tyr		Ala	Ala	Ala	Met	Arg	CA/NC
Thr	Ser	His	Val	His		Trp	Val	Gln	Glu	Ile	p30/PR

4. PR cleavage sites in BLV Gag, Gag-Pro, and Gag-Pro-Pol polyproteins (RICE et al. 1985; YOSHINAKA et al. 1986).

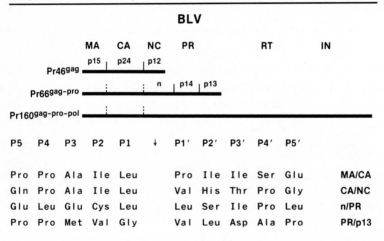

BLV

P5	P4	P3	P2	P1	↓	P1'	P2'	P3'	P4'	P5'	
Pro	Pro	Ala	Ile	Leu		Pro	Ile	Ile	Ser	Glu	MA/CA
Gln	Pro	Ala	Ile	Leu		Val	His	Thr	Pro	Gly	CA/NC
Glu	Leu	Glu	Cys	Leu		Leu	Ser	Ile	Pro	Leu	n/PR
Pro	Pro	Met	Val	Gly		Val	Leu	Asp	Ala	Pro	PR/p13

5. PR cleavage sites in HTLV-1 Gag, Gag-Pro, and Gag-Pro-Pol polyproteins (OROSZLAN et al. 1982; COPELAND et al. 1983).

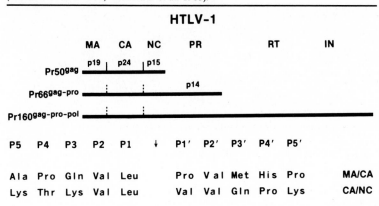

HTLV-1

P5	P4	P3	P2	P1	↓	P1′	P2′	P3′	P4′	P5′	
Ala	Pro	Gln	Val	Leu		Pro	Val	Met	His	Pro	MA/CA
Lys	Thr	Lys	Val	Leu		Val	Val	Gln	Pro	Lys	CA/NC

6. PR cleavage sites in HIV-1 Gag and Gag-Pol polyproteins. TF, transframe protein (HENDERSON et al. 1988a, b).

HIV-1

P5	P4	P3	P2	P1	↓	P1′	P2′	P3′	P4′	P5′	
Val	Ser	Gln	Asn	Tyr		Pro	Ile	Val	Gln	Asn	MA/CA
Lys	Ala	Arg	Val	Leu		Ala	Glu	Ala	Met	Ser	CA/X
Thr	Ala	Thr	Ile	Met		Met	Gln	Arg	Gly	Asn	X/NC
Arg	Pro	Gly	Asn	Phe		Leu	Gln	Ser	Arg	Pro	NC/p6
Val	Ser	Phe	Asn	Phe		Pro	Gln	Ile	Thr	Leu	TF/PR
Cys	Thr	Leu	Asn	Phe		Pro	Ile	Ser	Pro	Ile	PR/RT
Phe	Arg	Lys	Ile	Leu		Phe	Leu	Asp	Gly	Ile	RT/IN

Retrovirus Envelope Glycoproteins

E. Hunter[1] and R. Swanstrom[2]

[1] Department of Microbiology, University of Alabama at Birmingham, Birmingham, AL 35294, USA

[2] Department of Biochemistry and Lineberger Cancer Research Center, University of North Carolina at Chapel Hill, Chapel Hill, NC 27599, USA

Current Topics in Microbiology and Immunology, Vol. 157
© Springer-Verlag Berlin·Heidelberg 1990

1 Introduction

The envelope glycoprotein complex of replication competent retroviruses is comprised of two polypeptides, an external, glycosylated, hydrophilic polypeptide (SU) and a membrane-spanning protein (TM), that form a knob or knobbed spike on the surface of the virion. Both polypeptides are encoded in the *env* gene and are synthesized in the form of a polyprotein precursor that is proteolytically cleaved during its transport to the surface of the cell. While these proteins are not required for the assembly of enveloped virus particles, they do play a critical role in the virus replication cycle by recognizing and binding to specific receptors (SU) and by mediating the fusion of viral and cell membranes (TM): virus particles lacking envelope glycoproteins are thus noninfectious.

Although the sizes and amino acid composition of the SU and TM proteins from different retroviruses vary, as summarized in Fig. 1, there is an overall structural similarity between the different glycoproteins. The basic organization is defined by three hydrophobic or apolar regions that are arranged along the envelope molecule. At the N-terminus is the signal peptide, a short stretch of hydrophobic amino acids that directs the nascent *env* gene product into the secretory pathway of the infected cell. It is removed from the nascent *env* gene product during translation.

Near the C-terminus is a longer hydrophobic region that stops the translocation process, anchors the molecule in the membrane, and causes it to span the lipid bilayer. The molecule is thus oriented with its N-terminus outside and its C-terminus in the cytoplasm—a type 1 glycoprotein—and is therefore similar to that of the influenza virus hemagglutinin (HA; PORTER et al. 1979; GETHING et al. 1980), the vesicular stomatitis virus (VSV) G protein (GALLIONE and ROSE 1983), and several, membrane-spanning, cell-encoded glycoproteins.

A third apolar domain, postulated to be involved in the process of membrane fusion during virus entry, is located at the N-terminus of the TM protein and C-terminal to a conserved stretch of basic amino-acids (Arg-X-Lys-Arg) at which proteolytic cleavage of the precursor molecule occurs. So that it does not induce membrane fusion during transport out of the cell, this "fusion peptide" is probably sequestered in the center of a multimeric structure, most likely

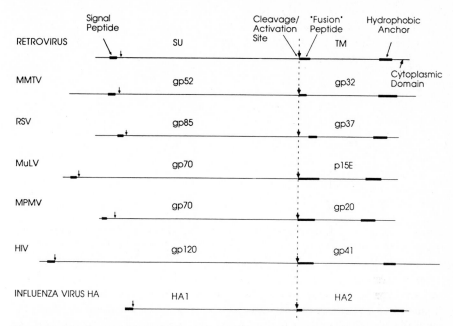

Fig. 1. Functional organization of retroviral envelope gene products. *Horizontal lines* represent the polypeptide chain translated from the *env* open reading frame, their lengths being proportional to that of the polypeptide. *Filled boxes* represent functional hydrophobic or uncharged regions, *small arrows* the site of signal peptidase cleavage. The functional organization of human influenza virus hemaglutinin protein (H2 subtype-A/Jap/307/57; GETHING et al. 1980) is shown for comparison

comprised of three or four SU-TM heterodimers that assemble prior to transport out of the rough endoplasmic reticulum (RER). This trimeric structure must thus dissociate after binding its receptor molecule in order to allow the fusion sequence to function.

The conservation of functional regions and their organization within these *env* gene products extends beyond the retrovirus family to that of other viruses, of which the HA protein in influenza virus is an example (Fig. 1). This similarly sized glycosylated protein, for which a three-dimensional structure has been determined, also possesses the three functional hydrophobic domains mentioned above. The HA precursor itself is cleaved to HA-1 and HA-2 polypeptides which function in binding receptor molecules and in fusing viral and cell membranes, respectively. Analyses of potential secondary structural features for the retroviral *env* gene products predict a similar distribution of α-helices and β-sheets within the SU and TM proteins of Rous sarcoma virus (RSV) as is seen in HA-1 and HA-2 (J. WHITE, personal communication), and a predictive analysis of the primary amino acid sequences of several retroviral TM proteins is consistent with their folding in a similar way to the influenza HA-2 protein (Fig. 2; GALLAHER et al. 1989). Nevertheless, the lack of conservation in the positions of cysteine residues throughout the two proteins and the distinctly different morphologies of the *env*

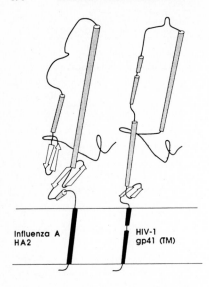

Influenza A
HA2

HIV-1
gp41 (TM)

Fig. 2. Schematic predicted structure of the TM protein of HIV-1 and influenza virus. *Solid cylinder* membrane-spanning helix; *hatched cylinder*, extracellular α-helix; *directional arrows, β*-sheet Predicted structures taken from GALLAHER et al. (1989)

and HA complexes under the electron microscope suggest that at the three-dimensional level these similarities may be superficial. Meaningful structural comparisons will ultimately require X-ray crystallographic information on the retroviral *env* gene products.

2 Biosynthesis of Retroviral *env* Gene Products

The genetic organization of replication competent retroviruses, 5'-*gag-pol-env*-3', requires that the *env* gene be translated from a spliced, subgenomic mRNA. In the majority of retroviruses, this moves an initiating methionine codon at the beginning of the *env* ORF close to the 5'-end of the mRNA. In the avian sarcoma/leukosis viruses, however, the splicing event fuses the strong initiation codon from the *gag* ORF in-frame with the *env* gene sequences. The nascent Env protein of this virus is thus a fusion protein containing the first 6 amino acids (aa) from the *gag* gene product.

2.1 Protein Translocation—Signal Peptide Function

The *env* mRNA is translated as are most membrane-spanning or secreted proteins on membrane-bound polyribosomes. The initial step that introduces the nascent polypeptides into the secretory pathway is mediated by the interaction of a sequence of amino acids (the signal sequence) within the polypeptide and a component of the cellular transport machinery—the signal recognition particle (SRP)/docking protein complex (reviewed by WALTER and LINGAPPA 1986). In the retroviral *env* gene products, the hydrophobic signal peptide is generally located in a longer (30–100 aa) leader sequence (Fig. 1). The function of these sometimes numerous additional amino acids (see, for example, MMTV) is unknown. However, normal biosynthesis and translocation were observed in experiments in which the HA signal peptide was substituted for the entire RSV *env* leader sequence (PEREZ et al. 1987a); it thus seems unlikely that they have a required function in the translocation process. Furthermore, the *env*-derived signal peptides can substitute for the signal peptides of other membrane proteins (HUNTER 1988), and during the transduction of oncogenes by certain retroviruses the recombination event has resulted in fusion of the *env* signal peptide and the oncogene product (HANNICK and DONOGHUE 1984; RAINES et al. 1985). In the case of the *sis* oncogene, this fusion has been shown to be essential for oncogene function, since mutations within the *env*-derived signal sequence prevented transformation (HANNICK and DONOGHUE 1984). The length of the hydrophobic domain of the signal sequence appears to be critical for its function since mutations in this region of the RSV *env* gene product which shortern it by one or two amino acids reduced the efficiency with which it directed molecules across the RER by 50% and 95%, respectively (WILLS et al. 1983). Mutations which remove the signal peptide entirely result in the synthesis of a cytoplasmically located product that is rapidly degraded (HUNTER 1988).

During translation of the nascent *env* gene product, a host protease-mediated cleavage event removes the entire signal/leader peptide. The site of this cleavage is specified by amino acid residues within the signal peptide itself (VON HEIJNE 1983, 1984, 1985; PERLMAN and HALVORSON 1983), and a mutational analysis of the RSV *env* gene sequences in this region confirmed that amino acid changes C-terminal to the cleavage site, including the second amino acid of the site itself, had no effect on the efficiency with which cleavage occurred (HARDWICK et al. 1986).

The exact nature of the translocation complex through which membrane and secreted proteins are moved into the lumen of the RER is not known, and questions remain as to whether transport occurs through a protein channel or through the lipid bilayer itself. The driving force for translocation also remains obscure, but it is clearly unlinked from translation since short secreted proteins that must already have been released from the ribosome undergo SRP-dependent translocation (MEYER 1985). Studies on the paramyxovirus fusion protein and the RSV *env* gene product have suggested that the forces involved in folding the molecule into its final tertiary structure might be responsible for pulling the nascent molecule through the membrane (HUNTER 1988; PATERSON and LAMB 1987).

2.2 Stop Translocation/Anchor Sequences

A stretch of hydrophobic amino acids that varies in length from 23 (HIV) to 36 (MMTV) aa and is located near the C-terminus of the TM protein sequences stops translocation through the RER bilayer and anchors the molecule in the membrane. Mutations that result in translational termination prior to this sequence yield soluble secreted forms of the retroviral *env* gene product (PEREZ et al. 1987b; STEPHENS and COMPANS 1986; KOWALSKI et al. 1987; BERMAN et al. 1988b; DUBAY et al. 1988), formally proving the anchor function for this region. In most cases, this stop transfer/anchor domain consists of an uninterrupted string of apolar residues, but in HIV and other lentiviruses it is punctuated by a single basic arginine or lysine residue (SONIGO et al. 1985; PAYNE et al. 1987b). This is consistent with experiments in which an arginine residue, inserted by site-directed mutagenesis into the middle of the RSV *env* anchor domain, had no affect on the stop transfer or membrane anchor functions of this region. The mutant protein in this case, however, was unstably expressed on the cell surface and rapidly transported to lysosomes for degradation (DAVIS and HUNTER 1987). It is possible that additional protein-protein interactions stabilize the lentiviral *env* gene products in the membrane.

In an attempt to determine the minimal functional length for the RSV anchor domain, DAVIS, SHAW and HUNTER (manuscript in preparation) constructed a series of internal deletions within the hydrophobic domain, reducing its length from 27 aa to as few as 5. Surprisingly, *env* gene products with a hydrophobic domain as short as 16 aa still arrested translocation and spanned the membrane; however, such proteins were much less stable on the cell surface and were rapidly endocytosed and degraded (HUNTER 1988; DAVIS et al. 1987). It seems likely then that this region plays additional roles to those of stopping translocation and anchoring the molecule in the membrane (see below).

2.3 Cytoplasmic Domains

One consequence of the bitopic character of retroviral *env* gene products is that a stretch of amino acids extends into the cytoplasm of the cell. This cytoplasmic domain is generally quite short (22–38 aa) although in HIV-1 it extends to 150 aa. Since the cytoplasmic residues are ultimately located in the interior of the virion, it was postulated that they might interact with capsid proteins during virion assembly (GEBHARDT et al. 1984). However, the insertion of a stop codon in place of that for the first residue of the cytoplasmic domain of the RSV TM protein (i.e., to generate a polypeptide lacking a cytoplasmic domain) had no effect on the transport of the protein to the membrane, its incorporation into virions, or the infectivity of the virus (PEREZ et al. 1987b). At least in RSV then, this region is not required for glycoprotein/capsid recognition. Experiments using the truncated anchor domain mutants described above suggest that sequences within this hydrophobic anchor region of the TM protein might need to interact with capsid proteins during assembly (MILLER, DAVIS, and HUNTER, manuscript in preparation). In MuLV, after virion assembly, the viral-encoded protease cleaves the bulk of the cytoplasmic domain from the TM polypeptide (p15E) to yield a truncated p15E (frequently called p12E) and the so-called R peptide (SUTCLIFFE et al. 1980); whether this cleavage is essential for virus maturation is not known.

Studies on the long cytoplasmic domain of the HIV-1 gp41 have yielded different results from those in the avian system and point to at least three functional subdomains in this region (DUBAY et al. 1988). The results of inserting a series of stop codons along the length of the cytoplasmic domain are consistent with theoretical analyses of the primary amino acid sequence of this region which predict that the C-terminal 90 aa of gp41 fold into two interlocking amphipathic helices (VENABLE et al. 1989). Despite the hydrophilic amino acid content of this region, the high hydrophobic moment of these helices raises the possibility that they span the lipid bilayer. This is supported by in vitro translation experiments in the presence and absence of membranes, which indicate that the C-terminus of gp41 is inaccessible to site-specific antibodies (HAFFAR et al. 1988). Mutagenic analyses also suggest that a hydrophilic region, conserved within the gp41s of different HIV-1 isolates, is also essential for virus infectivity although its exact role is not understood (DUBAY et al. 1988). Surprisingly, some isolates of HIV-2 and SIV have a naturally occurring stop codon within the TM protein cytoplasmic domain that truncates it to less than 20 aa (HIRSCH et al. 1987; GUYADER et al. 1987). However, SIV isolates with truncated forms of the TM protein appear to result from mutation and selection during propagation in an unnatural (human) host cell; growth of these SIV isolates in monkey lymphocytes maintains a full-length, 41kD, TM. Since evidence has been presented for a recent sooty mangabe origin for HIV-2 (HIRSCH et al. 1989), shorter versions of the TM protein in isolates of this virus may reflect similar selective pressures. HIV-1 proviruses containing an identical mutation are noninfectious (DUBAY et al. unpublished; J. MULLINS, personal communication). Clearly much remains to be understood of the role of this region in HIV/SIV replication.

2.4 Glycosylation

In the course of cotranslational transfer into the lumen of the RER, retroviral *env* gene products are modified by the addition of oligosaccharide side chains through N-linked glycosylation of asparagine residues in the nascent polypeptide. Since oligosaccharide residues are added as the protein is translocated (ROTHMAN et al. 1978), the first detectable translation product of the *env* gene is thus a core-glycosylated precursor from which the signal peptide has already been cleaved; the nonglycosylated polypeptide is never observed in a normal infection. Following transport to the Golgi complex, a majority of the high mannose core oligosaccharides are modified by trimming of mannose residues and addition of N-acetyl-glucosamine, galactose, and fucose residues (KORNFELD and KORNFELD 1985), to yield both complex and hybrid carbohydrate side chains (HUNT et al. 1979; GEYER et al. 1988). Residues at certain sites on the glycoprotein appear to remain unmodified during transit through the Golgi complex and retain their high-mannose, endoglycosidase-sensitive form in the mature protein (PINTER and HONNEN 1984; BRADAC and HUNTER 1986; GEYER et al. 1988).

The number and distribution of N-linked glycosylation sites varies widely between different retroviruses. HIV-1 has as many as 30 of the canonical Asn-X-Ser/Thr oligosaccharide addition sites, with the majority (25) located in gp120. Mouse mammary tumor virus (MMTV) on the other hand has only four potential N-linked glycosylation sites, and these are distributed evenly between gp52 and gp37. For the most part there is little conservation of the positions at which carbohydrate is added between different groups of retrovirus. However, within a particular retrovirus group highly conserved carbohydrate residues can be observed (PATARCA and HASELTINE 1984; WILLEY et al. 1988b). These may reflect a specific requirement for carbohydrate in the structure/function of the glycoprotein.

The role of carbohydrate side chains in glycoprotein biosynthesis, transport, and stability has been a point of much discussion. While oligosaccharide side chains themselves probably do not act as signals for transport to the cell surface, they may at least in some cases provide the hydrophilicity required to drive or stabilize correct protein folding which in turn may be a prerequisite for protein transport and protein function. Removal of a highly conserved carbohydrate addition site within the gp120 of HIV resulted in a normally transported but inactive glycoprotein and loss of virus infectivity. However, infectious revertants of the mutant virus did not regain the missing carbohydrate residue but instead contained a second site mutation that presumably compensated for structural changes induced by the primary mutation (WILLEY et al. 1988b). In addition, treatment of virus-producing cells with inhibitors of glycosylation or of enzymes involved in carbohydrate processing can reduce virus infectivity significantly even under conditions in which the modified glycoproteins are efficiently incorporated into virions (BLOUGH et al. 1986; GRUTERS et al. 1987; WALKER et al. 1987; MONTEFIORI et al. 1988). Carbohydrate may also play a structural role in the mature retroviral envelope protein since enzymatic removal of carbohydrate from the HIV gp120 reduced its ability to bind the CD4 receptor (MATTHEWS et al. 1987); however, the basis for this loss of activity is not clear. It is likely that carbohydrate, through masking of susceptible residues, also enhances the stability of the glycoprotein by providing protection from proteolytic enzymes. As will be discussed later, this masking may also reduce the immunogenicity of the protein, presumably by preventing immunoreactive cells from interacting with polypeptide epitopes (ELDER et al. 1986).

While the bulk of the discussion above has concentrated on N-linked oligosaccharides, recent experiments have indicated that a variety of mammalian retroviral *env* gene products are also modified by the addition of O-linked sugars (PINTER and HONNEN 1988). The role and requirements for this posttranslational modification are presently unknown.

2.5 Protein Folding and Intracellular Transport

Retroviral glycoproteins are exported to the cell surface by the same mechanisms as cell-encoded membrane proteins, since they utilize the cell's transport machinery—the so-called secretory pathway. However, the exact nature of the mechanisms by which cells send membrane-bound and secreted proteins to their proper subcellular locations remain unknown. While it is generally thought that "sorting signals" are composed of protein, it has been difficult to determine whether some feature of the native tertiary structure of the protein or a specific peptide sequence is involved in targeting proteins (for a review of these issues, see HUNTER 1988). The importance of a tertiary structure for protein transport is clear since disruption of a polypeptide's normal folding can completely prevent its transport from the ER (GETHING et al. 1986; KREIS and LODISH 1986), and the simplest explanation for the phenotypes of a variety of conditional and nonconditional membrane protein transport mutants would be that they alter the tertiary structure of the mature protein. Studies of the RSV *env* gene product have indicated that prior to transport from the ER, the precursor molecules oligomerize into what appear to be trimer structures (EINFELD and HUNTER 1988; EINFELD and HUNTER 1989). Since the rate of oligomer formation correlates well with the rate of transport to the Golgi complex and since a mutant *env* gene product that is not transported from the ER does not form oligomers (WILLS et al. 1984; EINFELD and HUNTER 1988), it is likely that this event is a prerequisite for intracellular transport. The formation of an oligomeric structure may also provide structural rigidity to the Env protein complex and provide a mechanism for sequestering a potentially active fusion peptide (see below). Given the similarity of retroviral *env* genes, it seems likely that other retroviral glycoproteins will form analogous oligomeric structures.

After transport of the oligomeric *env* precursor to the Golgi complex, two major modifications occur: (a) the mannose-rich carbohydrate side chains are modified (as described above), and (b) the precursor molecules are cleaved by a host-derived protease into the individual SU and TM proteins. The latter cleavage occurs immediately after a series of basic amino acid residues (PEREZ and HUNTER 1987; GALLAHER 1987) that are highly conserved in different retroviruses. This places at or close to the N-terminus of the TM protein an apolar string of amino acids that are predicted, by analogy with the fusion proteins of other enveloped viruses and from mutational analyses, to be involved in mediating membrane fusion (DICKSON et al. 1984a; KOWALSKI et al. 1987; GALLAHER 1987).

Mutagenesis of the cleavage site of the RSV *env* gene product has indicated that two host enzymes exist in the Golgi complex: one which cleaves preferentially after the Lys-Arg sequence and a second which less efficiently can cleave at dibasic residues (i.e., Arg-Arg) (PEREZ and HUNTER 1987). A double mutation in the RSV *env* gene which encodes a Ser-Arg-Glu-Arg cleavage site in place of the wild-type Arg-Arg-Lys-Arg cannot be cleaved intracellularly and when substituted into a proviral genome renders the virus noninfectious—cleavage of the precursor is thus a prerequisite for virus infectivity. Since the mutated site retains arginine residues, it can be cleaved extracellularly by the addition of trypsin with infectivity at least partially restored (DONG, PEREZ and HUNTER, manuscript in preparation). A similar study in which multiple mutations were introduced into the HIV-1 cleavage site also showed a correlation between the inhibition of cleavage and loss of virus infectivity (MCCUNE et al. 1988).

Cleavage of the precursor is probably accompanied by a conformational change in which the activated fusion peptide is sequestered inside the glycoprotein oligomer until after receptor binding. The exact location within the Golgi complex at which cleavage occurs has not been determined; studies with RSV and REV are consistent with this occurring in a late (trans) compartment of this organelle (WILLS et al. 1984; TSAI et al. 1988), but recent studies with HIV-1 have suggested that cleavage of its *env* gene product might occur prior to addition of complex carbohydrate (GEYER et al. 1988). In some retroviruses, RSV for example, the mature products of cleavage are covalently joined through disulfide linkages in an SU-TM heterodimer (LEAMNSON and HALPERN 1976). In other retroviruses, however, only a fraction of the virion glycoproteins appear to be covalently linked (e.g., MuLV; LEAMNSON et al. 1977; WITTE et al. 1977) or are held together entirely by noncovalent forces (e.g., HIV, M-PMV; ROBEY et al. 1987; BRADAC and HUNTER 1986). The latter arrangement allows the SU protein to be readily shed from the virus (ROBEY et al. 1986).

Following the complex series of modifications, the mature *env* complex is transported from the trans-Golgi reticulum to the plasma membrane where it can be incorporated into assembling virions. In fibroblastic and lymphoid cells this may be a relatively unregulated process, but in epithelial cells, which have apical and basolateral surface membranes with distinctive membrane protein compositions, all retroviral glycoproteins studied to date are transported exclusively to the basolateral membrane (ROTH et al. 1983a, b; STEPHENS et al. 1986). It is possible that since this membrane is also the site of virus assembly and release that basolateral transport might provide a mechanism by which retroviruses establish a systemic versus localized infection.

2.6 Glycoprotein Assembly

As we have pointed out above, the assembly and release of lipid-enveloped virus particles does not require the presence of viral glycoproteins (reviewed by DICKSON et al. 1984a); however, such bald particles are noninfectious for normally susceptible target cells. The mechanism that specifies incorporation of retroviral glycoproteins into assembling virions is not understood. This appears to be a specific event since host cell membrane proteins are inefficiently incorporated into virus; nevertheless, the nature of the glycoprotein/capsid protein interactions have not been defined. In the avian retroviruses cross-linking of the TM protein and the MA protein of the capsid has been reported (GEBHARDT et al. 1984), and since glycoproteins lacking a cytoplasmic domain are still efficiently incorporated into virions, it seems likely that if such TM-MA interactions are essential, they must occur within the hydrophobic anchor domain of the TM protein (PEREZ et al. 1987b). Preliminary experiments with mutants in this region support this hypothesis (MILLER, DAVIS, and HUNTER, manuscript in preparation), and it is interesting that the gp65 glycoprotein of the murine spleen focus forming virus (SFFV), which has an altered anchor domain and no cytoplasmic domain, is not incorporated into virions (PINTER and HONNEN 1985). Studies utilizing site-directed mutagenesis of both the *env* and *gag* genes together with the construction of chimeric glycoproteins should shed light in this area.

2.7 Virus Entry

Once incorporated into the virus particle the glycoproteins play a critical role in virus entry into a new target cell. The SU protein binds to a specific receptor on the target cell, thereby defining the host range of the virus. In the avian retroviruses at least two distinct regions within the central portion of the SU polypeptide contribute to host-range definition (see Sect. 3), consistent with this being a binding pocket composed of multiple polypeptide chains; however, the nature of the receptor is unknown. There are very few retroviruses for which the receptor molecule has been unequivocally defined; the best characterized receptor is that of the HIV/SIV group of lentiviruses. These viruses utilize the CD4 molecule found predominantly on lymphocytes of the T helper class (reviewed by SATTENTAU and WEISS 1988). The binding constant for the gp120/CD4 interaction is extremely high ($K_d = 4 \times 10^{-9} M/1$; LASKY et al. 1987) in contrast to that observed for influenza virus HA/sialic acid binding event ($K_d = 1 \times 10^{-3} M/1$). It is likely that a conformational change occurs shortly after receptor binding (perhaps as a result of the binding event itself) which results in the disassembly of the glycoprotein oligomer and exposure of the sequestered fusion peptide. An interaction of the latter with the cell membrane is postulated to result in viral membrane/cell membrane fusion (WHITE et al. 1983; GALLAHER 1987), and the viral nucleocapsid is introduced into the cytoplasm of the cell. For the majority of retroviruses this latter event does not require a low pH environment (STEIN et al. 1987; MADDON et al. 1988; J. WHITE, personal communication; M. SOMMERFELT, personal communication), and the mechanisms which trigger fusion peptide activation are not known. MMTV, in contrast, appears to resemble the HA of influenza virus in that cells expressing the gp52/gp36 protein can be stimulated to undergo cell fusion after a brief exposure to low pH (REDMOND et al. 1984). For MuLV, compounds which increases the pH of endosomes interfere with virus infectivity (ANDERSON and NEXO 1983). For these murine retroviruses then, it is possible that the glycoprotein complex undergoes a pH-induced conformational change analogous to that seen with the HA trimer (SKEHEL et al. 1982; DOMS et al. 1986). Much remains to be understood about the processes involved in the binding/fusion events of the retrovirus replication cycle.

3 Avian Sarcoma/Leukosis Virus *env* Gene Products

Avian retroviruses of the sarcoma/leukosis virus group (e.g., RSV and avian leukosis virus) were among the first retroviruses to be described. Over the past 80 years these viruses have been a rich source of material for genetic, biologic, and biochemical studies. This is especially true for studies of the viral *env* gene, which actually represents a group of allelic sequences that encode proteins capable of interacting with different host cell receptors. The comparative analysis of viruses with different alleles (known as virus subgroups) has provided an opportunity to examine sequences important for interaction with the host cell receptor and a means for evaluating the role of the *env* gene products in pathogenesis.

The *env* gene encodes a protein of approximately 600 aa. The initial translation product is rapidly glycosylated to give a protein with an apparent molecular mass of 92kD. This precursor is cleaved to give two proteins (gp85 and gp37) which remain linked by disulfide bridges. One, gp85, is external to the virus particle (the SU protein) while gp37 spans the viral envelope as an integral membrane protein (the TM protein) (reviewed in DICKSON et al. 1984a).

3.1 Host-Range Determinants

Careful analysis of the pattern of virus infectivity in cells derived from different chicken embryos led to the discovery of a pattern of susceptibility and resistance to infection (reviewed in VOGT 1977; WEISS 1984). Viruses showing the same pattern of infectivity are grouped together in subgroups. Chicken cells are classified by their resistance to infection by a specific subgroup virus; for example, C/A indicates chicken cells resistant to subgroup A viruses, and C/O indicates susceptibility to all virus subgroups. Genetic crosses between chickens with different susceptibilities showed that susceptibility is a dominant trait and that the patterns of virus infectivity could be explained by three different loci, termed *tv-a*, *tv-b*, and *tv-c*, encoding determinants of susceptibility to different viruses. There is also evidence that *tv-b* may have different alleles that affect the efficiency of virus infection in a susceptible cell (CRITTENDEN and MOTTA 1975; BROWN and ROBINSON 1988b).

These results have generally been interpreted to indicate that the chicken loci encode receptors for the different virus subgroups, with resistance to infection indicating the absence of a specific receptor. If each locus is present in all chickens, then resistance to a given strain may indicate homozygosity for an allele that cannot function as a receptor. The evidence that these loci encode the virus receptor is incomplete. Binding assays for the SU protein (gp85) or whole virus to susceptible and resistant cells show preferential binding to susceptible cells; however, the level of discrimination in binding is small compared with the level of discrimination seen using infectivity (PIRAINO 1967; CRITTENDEN 1968; MOLDOW et al. 1979). Identification of the host cell receptors for these and most retroviruses has been difficult but remains an area of active interest.

While three chicken loci involved in susceptibility to infection have been identified, the corresponding chicken viruses have been divided into five subgroups (A through E) (reviewed in VOGT 1977; WEISS 1984). The subgroups are distinguished by their ability to infect chicken cells derived from animals carrying different susceptibility loci (host range), by similarities in the pattern of neutralization by antibodies, and by their ability to interfere with infection by a superinfecting virus. Virus subgroups A, B, and C are dependent on the presence of the host loci *tv-a*, *tv-b*, and *tv-c*, respectively, for infection and do not interfere with superinfection by viruses from the different subgroups. Subgroup D viruses use the same receptor as subgroup B viruses, show incomplete interference by subgroup B viruses, and are also able to infect mammalian cells, albeit at a low level. Subgroup E viruses also appear to use the same receptor as subgroup B viruses but are unable to interfere with superinfection by a subgroup B virus (presumably because of a lower affinity of the subgroup E SU protein for the host cell receptor). Several other viruses with a different host range (e.g. subgroups F and G) have been isolated after passage of an avian sarcoma-leukosis virus through cells of another avian species. These viruses appear to have acquired a new host range as the result of recombination with sequences of the heterologous host.

The genetic locus in the viral genome responsible for determining subgroup specificity was identified as the *env* gene using T_1 oligonucleotide mapping of viral genomes that had recombined to acquire a new host range (JOHO et al. 1975; WANG et al. 1976; COFFIN et al. 1978). In the past few years the nucleotide sequences of the *env* gene region of several virus isolates have become available (see below), and the precise location within the nucleotide sequence of the region encoding the mature *env* gene products has been determined by sequence analysis of the SU and TM proteins (HUNTER et al. 1983). A comparison of these sequences, particularly within the domain encoding the SU protein (gp85), has provided a first look at the molecular basis of subgroup specificity.

At present, nucleotide sequence data are available for all or part of the *env* region for two subgroup A viruses (BOVA et al. 1986, 1988), three subgroup B viruses (DORNER et al. 1985; KAN et al. 1985; BOVA et al. 1986), one subgroup C virus (SCHWARTZ et al. 1983), one subgroup D virus (BOVA et al. 1988), and one subgroup E virus (DORNER et al. 1985; BOVA et al. 1986). A comparison of these sequences reveals that regions of sequence heterogeneity are clustered. Five such regions have been identified: three short regions (6–12 aa in length) named vr1, vr2, and vr3; and two larger stretches of sequence heterogeneity named hr1 and hr2 (30–50 aa in length). Sequence similarity between the conserved domains is usually greater than 90%, while the level of similarity in the variable domains is generally around 50%. However, even within the regions of sequence heterogeneity there are conserved amino acids, frequently at positions containing proline, glycine, and cysteine. Since these amino acids play a large role in determining protein structure (i.e., turns and disulfide bonds), it is likely that the SU proteins from the different subgroup viruses have similar overall structures within both the conserved domains and the heterogeneous regions, with the differences being confined to the amino acid sequence and length of similarly placed loops. It can be anticipated that these loops, either extended on the surface of the protein or forming the sides of pits, will be the regions that interact with domains on the host-cell receptor. A diagramatic representation of the sequence organization of the *env* gene is shown in Fig. 3.

Recombinant viruses have been used to probe the specific sequence requirements involved in subgroup specificity and the potential interactions between the different variable regions. A series of recombinants have been constructed showing that for all subgroups the major determinants of subgroup specificity lie within the portion of the viral genome spanning the five variable regions (BOVA et al. 1986, 1988; DORNER and COFFIN 1986). Even greater detail of this region has come from the analysis of a naturally occurring recombinant between a subgroup B and a subgroup E virus, NTRE-4, and similar recombinants constructed in vitro (DORNER et al. 1985; DORNER and COFFIN 1986). NTRE-4 contains approximately 200 bases of sequence derived from a subgroup E virus, spanning the hr2 domain in the background of a subgroup B virus. NTRE-4 has the normal host range of a subgroup B virus but is also able to infect turkey cells (which are resistant to subgroup B viruses but are susceptible to subgroup E viruses) (TSICHLIS et al. 1980). These results show a direct role for hr2 in determining the host range, presumably by interacting with the host-cell receptor.

Further analysis of recombinant viruses suggests that vr1 does not play a role in determining the host range (DORNER and COFFIN 1986). Also, since sequence variability associated with vr2 is confined to subgroup B viruses, this region is not a major determinant of host range. However, both hr1 and vr3 can affect the host range, although the role of vr3 is more subtle than that of hr1 and hr2 (DORNER and COFFIN 1986). In addition to NTRE-4 there are two other examples of viruses with apparent mixtures of hr1 and hr2 domains, although in neither case is the biologic significance of the recombinant genome structure known. A variant viral genome has been detected in the Prague C RSV stock which has a subgroup C-like sequence with subgroup E sequences in the position of hr2, analogous to the structure of NTRE-4 (SCHWARTZ et al. 1983). A viral genome cloned from the B77 RSV stock is similar to a subgroup A virus but has subgroup C sequences in the position of hr1 (BOVA, SHANK and SWANSTROM, unpublished observation). Although most of the recombinants tested that mix hr1 and hr2 domains from different subgroups were not viable (DORNER and COFFIN 1986), the appearance

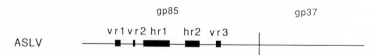

Fig. 3. Structure of the avian sarcoma/leukosis virus *env* gene product. Both gp85 and gp37 are derived from the primary translation product. A late step in the maturation of the viral glycoproteins is a cleavage separating the two proteins. The position of this cleavage is shown by the *vertical line*. *Solid blocks* indicate the positions of the regions of sequence variability seen in the gp85 domain when comparing the *env* gene sequences from viruses of different subgroups

of such viruses in nature suggests that certain combinations of hr1 and hr2 can have special properties that at least permit maintenance in a virus stock. Whether these novel *env* genes will confer an altered host range as in the case of NTRE-4 is not yet known.

Certain isolates of the ASLV group (subgroup D and the B77 strain of subgroup C) are able to infect mammalian cells although the infection does not result in the release of new virus. This ability is determined by the *env* gene product (DUFF and VOGT 1969; BOETTIGER et al. 1975). One feature of subgroup D viruses is that they utilize the subgroup B receptor but have an extended host range that includes mammalian cells. The nucleotide sequence of the subgroup D SU coding domain confirms the similarity to subgroup B viruses (BOVA et al. 1988). Analysis of molecular recombinants suggests that the ability to penetrate mammalian cells is the result of amino acid changes resulting in an unstable glycoprotein that is fusogenic in the absence of the normal receptor (C. BOVA and R. SWANSTROM, unpublished observation).

3.2 Antigenicity

The host immune response to infection by viruses of the ASLV group is variable. However, two types of virus neutralization response can be discerned that are the result of the *env* gene product. One response recognizes determinants on the viral glycoprotein that are common to all viruses within a subgroup (and common neutralization properties is one of the criteria for inclusion within a subgroup). A second type of response that is seen is highly specific to the virus used to infect with no appearance of a significant neutralization response to other viruses even within the same subgroup; this response is called type-specific.

The subgroup-specific neutralization response correlates closely with host-range specificity and thus is likely to be another manifestation of the sequence variability that determines the host range (reviewed in VOGT 1977). The type-specific neutralization response probably has two components, antigenic variability among viruses within the same subgroup and a variable response by a host to a subset of epitopes that may or may not vary between isolates. In one study of two subgroup A viruses, type-specific epitopes were shown to reside within the same domain of the SU protein that spans the host-range determinants (BOVA et al. 1988). Sequence comparison of the two viruses and comparison of three subgroup B viruses with each other revealed seven small domains of sequence variability within the gp85 domain that are candidate sites for type-specific heterogeneity (BOVA et al. 1988).

Glycosylation can affect protein stability and antigenicity. The SU and TM proteins have numerous potential asparagine-linked oligosaccharide attachment sites (14 in the Prague C strain of RSV), most of which contain carbohydrate (HUNTER et al. 1983). The positions of these potential glycosylation sites are largely conserved within the SU domain encoded within the *env* gene sequences analyzed. The exceptions are two subgroup A viruses which each lack three sites (BOVA et al. 1988).

3.3 Pathogenicity

One type of pathogenesis that is correlated with *env* host range determinants is transient cell killing in culture. Viruses of the B, D, and F subgroups kill cells as a result of massive reinfection after the initial infection (WELLER et al. 1980). Cell death is correlated with the appearance of large amounts of unintegrated viral DNA and is blocked by the addition of neutralizing antibodies after the initial infection. In examining cell killing by a subgroup B virus, analysis of recombinants between subgroup B and E viruses showed that cytopathicity correlated with utilization of the subgroup B receptor (DORNER and COFFIN 1986). This indicates that either a high level of utilization of the subgroup B receptor is cytotoxic or that reinfection utilizing the B receptor is very efficient and the subsequent high level of virus replication is cytotoxic. Presumably, subgroup D viruses are cytotoxic because they use the subgroup B receptor; similar studies have not been done with a subgroup F virus. The cytotoxicity of subgroup B and D viruses correlates with the ability of these viruses to cause anemia after infection of 8-day-old chicks (SMITH and SCHMIDT 1982). Subgroups A, C, and F were reported not to cause anemia. KOTLER and colleagues have recently isolated a virus from chickens that causes hemangiomas. In addition, this virus also causes cell killing in culture, and this cell killing is apparently the result of the viral glycoprotein interacting with the host cell at a very early stage of infection (M. KOTLER, personal communication). A more detailed discussion of pathogenic mechanisms has recently appeared (TEMIN 1988).

Infection with avian leukosis virus is associated with several other disease syndromes. One that appears to be mediated by subgroup specificity is lymphoblastoid infiltration of the thyroid and pancreas. Four different subgroup C isolates caused a similar syndrome that was not seen with viruses representing the other subgroups (CARTER and SMITH 1984).

A role for the *env* gene product in oncogenicity has been inferred after comparing the frequency and spectrum of disease caused by avian leukosis viruses of different subgroups (PURCHASE et al. 1977). Subgroup A viruses were found to cause the highest frequency of disease, which was usually lymphoid leukosis but included a broad spectrum of different neoplasias. The other viruses tested caused either a lower frequency of disease, which was primarily lymphoid leukosis, or no disease at all. Using molecular recombinants BROWN et al. (1988) have shown that infection with a virus with the subgroup A *env* gene induces lymphoid leukosis at a rate two- to fourfold that of a virus with the subgroup E *env* gene. This higher disease rate is correlated with earlier replication in the target tissue, the bursa, and the subgroup A *env* gene also encodes determinants that result in a pattern of tissue tropism that is distinct from both subgroup B and E viruses (BROWN et al. 1988; BROWN and ROBINSON 1988a).

Subgroup F viruses cause a rapid and unusual disease, and a role for the subgroup F *env* gene product in disease specificity can be inferred from experiments using recombinant viruses. Infection with subgroup F viruses frequently leads to the rapid appearance of a nonclonal proliferative disorder in the lung (CARTER et al. 1983; SIMON et al. 1984). Using molecular recombinants, the major determinant of disease specificity was localized to the *env* gene region (SIMON et al. 1987).

The presence of endogenous viruses can have a variety of biological consequences. First, the endogenous sequence can be rescued by an exogenous virus with one outcome being the acquisition of a new host range. Chicken cells frequently carry remnants of subgroup E, RAV-0-like viruses, which can recombine with an exogenous virus to give a new virus with a subgroup E host range (HANAFUSA et al. 1970; HAYWARD and HANAFUSA 1975; COFFIN et al. 1978). Second, expression of a subgroup E SU protein encoded by an endogenous virus protects the cell from superinfection by a virus from the same subgroup (ROBINSON et al. 1981). Finally, expression of viral *env* sequences from an endogenous virus can affect the host immune response to infection by exogenous viruses of a different subgroup. Animals expressing a subgroup E SU protein become tolerant to certain viral antigens. Subsequent infection with an exogenous virus results in a decreased immune response compared with animals that do not express endogenous viral sequences. In certain strains of chickens, the tolerance protects the animal from a wasting syndrome that is associated with a more vigorous immune response (CRITTENDON et al. 1982, 1984; HALPERN et al. 1983). If the tolerance to subgroup E SU antigens is brought about by infection of embryos with RAV-0, then the effect of tolerance is more dramatic, resulting in a higher incidence of neoplasia with the subsequent infection by an exogenous virus (CRITTENDEN et al. 1987). Certain aspects of this system are reminiscent of observations made in the mouse system with ecotropic and MCF viruses (see below).

When a copy of the viral *env* gene is in the germline and is expressed in the somatic tissue, the animal can be resistant to infection by a virus that uses the same receptor (ROBINSON et al. 1981). Congenital infection with a subgroup A virus (SALTER et al. 1986, 1987) has been used to isolate a chicken strain that carries a defective viral genome in the germline and expresses the subgroup A *env* gene in the somatic tissue. These animals show no evidence of lymphoid leukosis after infection with a subgroup A virus and appear to be refractory to infection (L. CRITTENDEN, personal communication). This approach provides a method for developing animals that are genetically resistant to infection.

4 Murine Leukemia Virus *env* Gene Products

The murine leukemia virus (MuLV) *env* gene encodes a protein of approximately 650 aa. This protein is rapidly glycosylated and the signal sequence removed so that the initial precursor detected has an apparent molecular mass of 80 kD. The precursor is cleaved at an internal position to give the SU protein (gp70) and the TM protein (p15E), a fraction of which remain linked by at least one disulfide bond (reviewed in DICKSON et al. 1984a). Some of the p15E molecules are further cleaved near the C-terminus, apparently by the viral protease, to give a smaller protein, p12E (DURBIN and MANNING 1984; CRAWFORD and GOFF 1985; KATOH et al. 1985). The feline leukemia virus (FeLV) *env* gene product is similar to the MuLV *env* gene product in size and organization.

4.1 Host-Range Determinants

Murine leukemia viruses (MuLV) present a wide array of biological phenomena, some of which are related to the viral *env* gene. Much work has been done to characterize and classify these viruses (reviewed in TEICH 1984). However, there are a number of "exceptions" to the current classification schemes, and it is likely that there will be future refinements. In the following paragraphs each of the five well-characterized host-range classes (subgroups), as determined by the viral *env* gene product, is considered.

4.1.1 Ecotropic Viruses

These viruses were the first class of MuLVs to be identified. They efficiently infect mouse cells but not cells originating from nonrodent species. Some of the more well-known murine retroviruses like the exogenous viruses Moloney MuLV (Mo-MuLV) and Friend MuLV (F-MuLV), and the endogenous virus AKV are members of this class. Many inbred mouse strains contain germline copies of viruses with an ecotropic *env* gene. In a screen of 54 inbred strains of mice, JENKINS et al. (1982) detected 30 strains with one endogenous copy of viral DNA with an ecotropic *env* gene and 12 strains with multiple copies (between 2 and 6). Ecotropic viruses appear to represent a heterogeneous collection of *env* gene sequences, and amino acid sequences vary by up to 25% among M-MuLV, F-MuLV, and AKV (see KOCH et al. 1984). In addition, there is a distinct ecotropic sequence family represented by the Fv-4 restriction (interference) locus (KOZAK et al. 1984; IKEDA et al. 1985). Both of these ecotropic *env* gene families appear to have their new origin in certain wild populations of *Mus musculus* found in Asia (KOZAK and O'NEILL 1987). Recently, another divergent ecotropic virus (Ho-MuLV) was isolated from a different mouse species, *Mus hortulanus* (VOYTEK and KOZAK 1988).

4.1.2 Amphotropic Viruses

Like ecotropic viruses, amphotropic viruses are able to infect murine cells, but they have an extended host range in that they are also able to infect cells from certain other species. Hybridization studies have failed to detect any amphotropic-like *env* sequences in the germline of the mouse (O'NEILL et al. 1987). Amphotropic viruses have been isolated from some feral mouse populations but not from common inbred strains.

4.1.3 Xenotropic Viruses

This class of viruses is enigmatic in that their genomes are widely distributed in the germline of inbred strains of mice (between 5 and 16 copies) (O'NEILL et al. 1986; STOYE and COFFIN 1988), but they do not efficiently infect mouse cells derived from these strains. Xenotropic viruses do inefficiently infect cells derived from a variety of wild mice (ISHIMOTO et al. 1977, KOZAK 1985). Like amphotropic viruses, xenotropic viruses can infect certain cells of nonmurine origin, although the pattern of infectivity in cells from heterologous species is distinct from that of amphotropic viruses. Germline copies of viruses with xenotropic-like *env* sequences are widely distributed in wild mice of Asian and Eastern European origin (KOZAK and O'NEILL 1987).

4.1.4 MCF Viruses

These viruses were originally called mink cell focus inducing viruses because of their ability to induce foci on mink cells. They have also been called dualtropic or polytropic to reflect their ability to infect cells of both murine and nonmurine origin. They are most frequently referred to as MCF or polytropic viruses. Their designation as a separate subgroup was originally based on their host range for infection of cells from nonmurine species, which is distinct from both amphotropic and xenotropic viruses. MuLV-like elements with *env* sequences related to the MCF *env* gene are the most abundant of the MuLV-related elements in the germline of inbred strains of mice, ranging from 20 to greater than 30 copies in different strains (STOYE and COFFIN 1988). Wild mice from western Europe, the Mediterranean, and North America frequently have sequences related to the MCF virus *env* gene present in the germline (KOZAK and O'NEILL 1987).

MCF viruses have been isolated only after infection by an ecotropic virus, suggesting that the endogenous MCF-related sequences are either poorly expressed or defective. MCF viruses appear as recombinants of ecotropic viruses after growth of these viruses in certain strains of mice. Thus, MCF viruses represent recombinants within *env* between the infecting virus and viral genomes within the mouse genome to generate a virus with an altered host range (reviewed in COFFIN 1984; FAMULARI 1983; STOYE and COFFIN 1985). DNA sequence analysis of the *env* gene region of endogenous viral genomes has shown that there are two related but distinct families of sequences within this virus subgroup (STOYE and COFFIN 1987). These two groups have been referred to as polytropic and modified polytropic. Comparisons of their biological characteristics and of *env* gene sequences have revealed that several endogenous MCF *env* gene sequences can serve as donors in recombination events to generate viruses with a polytropic host range (EVANS and CLOYD 1984; REIN and SCHULTZ 1984; EVANS and CLOYD 1985; STOYE and COFFIN 1987). It is likely that the recombination events that generate MCF viruses involve reverse transcription of heterodermic genomes (COFFIN 1979). MCF-related transcripts have been detected in various mouse tissues, and these or related transcripts could serve as the source of MCF *env* sequences (OLIFF et al. 1983; KHAN et al. 1987; LAIGRET et al. 1988).

4.1.5 10A1 Virus

There is one example of a variant amphotropic virus (10A1) that has acquired polytropic-like sequences. This virus has enhanced leukemogenicity and an expanded host range compared to its amphotropic parent (RASHEED et al. 1982; LAI et al. 1982; OTT et al., 1990).

4.1.6 Env/Receptor Interactions

The above subgroups are based on features of host range from cells of different species origin. These subgroups can also be derived from interference patterns. When interference patterns were tested using NIH3T3 cells, clear groupings of ecotropic, amphotropic, MCF viruses and the 10A1 virus could be made (REIN 1982; REIN and SCHULTZ 1984). These four subgroups of viruses are also able to infect mouse cells expressing a xenotropic *env* gene product, indicating that each uses a receptor that cannot be competitively bound by the xenotropic glycoprotein (REIN and SCHULTZ 1984). Thus, both the host range differences and interference patterns indicate that these five subgroups of viruses probably utilize distinct host-cell receptors.

Genetic loci that determine susceptibility have been mapped in the mouse genome. In inbred strains separate loci of susceptibility, presumably representing the genes for the virus receptors, have been mapped for ecotropic virus (*Rec*-1 on chromosome 5), amphotropic virus (*Ram*-1 on chromosome 8), and MCF virus (*Rmc*-1 on chromosome 1) (GAZDAR et al. 1977; KOZAK 1983). Although xenotropic viruses will not infect cells from inbred strains of mice, they will infect cells derived from wild mice or different species of mice (HARTLEY and ROWE 1975; LANDER and CHATTOPADHYAY 1984; KOZAK 1985). The genetic locus for this susceptibility maps near the gene for the polytropic MCF virus receptor, suggesting that an allele of this gene can serve as the receptor for both MCF and xenotropic viruses (KOZAK 1985). It is likely that xenotropic viruses spread in the germline in a mouse background that had this receptor but that the allele of this gene which functions as the xenotropic virus receptor has been lost in the inbred strains. The receptor for the 10A1 virus has not been mapped although it is distinct from the receptors used by the other subgroups of virus (REIN and SCHULTZ 1984).

MuLV gp70 can be isolated in a form that retains its ability to bind specifically with the receptor on susceptible cells (DeLARCO and TODARO 1976). The specificity of this interaction has led to a series of studies characterizing the receptor molecule (for example, see JOHNSON and ROSNER 1986 and references therein). However, our clearest view of the viral receptor has been obtained using a genetic approach. The gene encoding the mouse ecotropic receptor has recently been cloned (ALBRITTON et al. 1989). The predicted amino acid sequence is very hydrophobic, suggesting numerous transmembrane domains. There is no obvious sequence similarity between this protein and any known protein.

The ability to use different host cell receptors should be reflected in sequence differences in the viral *env* gene product. A large number of different *env* gene

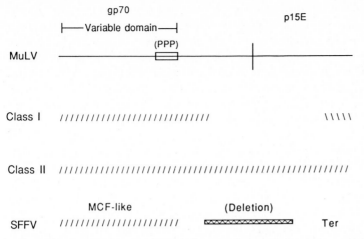

Fig. 4. Structure of MuLV *env* gene products. During their synthesis a cleavage event occurs (indicated by the *vertical line*) to separate the protein into the gp70 domain and the p15E domain. (Most of the sequence heterogeneity seen among the different gene sequences is located within the N-terminal portion of gp70 (indicated by the *bracket labeled Variable domain*). A proline-rich region (*boxed and labeled PPP*) is found near the center of the gp70 domain. The approximate positions of substitutions found in the class I and class II polytropic MCF viruses are shown. The regions shown with *forward slashes* indicate recombination with endogenous MCF-like sequences. The region with the *backward slash* indicates recombination with xenotropic-like sequences. In the SFFV genome the N-terminal domain is shown in *slashes* to indicate sequence similarity with MCF viruses. The position of the *deletion* that removes the gp70/p15E processing site is indicated as is the position of the premature termination codon (*Ter*)

sequences are now available for MuLV, although most of these are from ecotropic and MCF viruses. Sequence alignments between ecotropic, MCF, and xenotropic *env* genes have revealed some detail of the sequence organization (for examples, see KOCH et al. 1984; O'NEILL et al. 1985; STOYE and COFFIN 1987). The sequence organization of the MuLV *env* gene is shown in Fig. 4.

The N-terminal two-thirds of the gp70 domain contains most of the sequence variability and presumably the determinants for receptor interaction. The last third of gp70 and all of p15E are much more highly conserved. In the N-terminal variable domain ecotropic viruses are the most dissimilar, showing 40% or less sequence similarity with the other viruses. This dissimilarity is emphasized by the presence of several insertions of between 10 and 34aa in the ecotropic *env* sequence relative to the MCF and xenotropic *env* sequences. The xenotropic and MCF *env* sequences are much more similar in this region, with greater than 80% sequence similarity and no significant deletions or insertions. The sequence of an amphotropic virus *env* has also been determined (OTT et al. 1990). It is similar to that of the MCF/xenotropic viruses in that it does not have the additional sequences found in the ecotropic viruses; however, there is some sequence divergence in the variable N-terminal domain (approximately 75% sequence similarity with xenotropic and MCF *env* sequences), with several smaller insertions in the amphotropic sequence.

The variable N-terminal domain is separated from the more conserved C-terminal domain by a short stretch of variable amino acids which maintain a high proline content (approximately 30%). Whether this unusual sequence represents a structural determinant in the glycoprotein or an important determinant of receptor specificity is not known. That this proline-rich region may be involved in interactions with the receptor is suggested by the recombinant virus 10A1. The N-terminal variable region of this virus is similar to that of an amphotropic virus except for the proline-rich region, which is similar to an MCF virus. Virus 10A1 is able to use the amphotropic virus receptor as well as a novel receptor on mouse cells, suggesting that this combination of sequences has resulted in the acquisition of a new receptor specificity (OTT et al. 1990).

There are several observations which have yet to be accounted for with the above classification scheme. First, not all virus isolates placed within a subgroup have the same host range on heterologous cells (CLOYD et al. 1985). Second, certain recombinant viruses have the host range of one subgroup but the interference properties of another subgroup (CLOYD and CHATTOPADHYAY 1986). Third, sequence comparisons suggest that the known ecotropic viruses may themselves be recombinants, implying that the original ecotropic parent has not been identified (STOYE and COFFIN 1987). Fourth, and most perplexing, is the observation that the patterns of interference seen in NIH3T3 cells are altered in other cells, for example the SC-1 cell line derived from a wild mouse or a cell line derived from *Mus dunii* (CHESEBRO and WEHRLY 1985). An understanding of these and other phenomena related to host range will have to await detailed understanding of the effect of Env sequence heterogeneity on receptor interaction and the isolation of what is likely to be a very polymorphic set of virus receptors from the host cell.

4.2 Antigenicity

The natural antigenicity of viral glycoproteins has been examined in two important settings using MuLV. First, mapping of specific antigenic domains along the Env protein length has provided information about structural determinants. Second, analysis of the immune response, both humoral and cellular, has permitted an evaluation of the utility of immunization as a tool for controlling retroviral infection.

The general topology of the MuLV glycoprotein has been examined using a combination of localization of antigenic determinants, partial proteolytic cleavage, changes in apparent molecular weight under reducing conditions, peptide mapping, and protein sequencing. These approaches have led to the localization of sequences that correlate with the polytropic host range to the N-terminal portion of gp70 (PINTER et al. 1982; PINTER and HONNEN 1983; SCHULTZ et al. 1983; PINTER and HONNEN 1984) and to the placement of the disulfide link between gp70 and p15E to near the C-terminus of gp70 (PINTER et al. 1982; NIMAN and ELDER 1982). Another feature of the viral glycoprotein is that its antigenicity is to a significant extent influenced by the presence of its carbohydrate sidechains. Antibodies made to the glycosylated protein react less well with the deglycosylated protein (ALEXANDER and ELDER 1984), although recognition of neutralizing epitopes appears less sensitive to the presence of carbohydrates (ELDER et al. 1986).

Early work with MuLV showed that immunization can be an effective approach to limiting retrovirus infection and its associated disease. Immunization with either live or killed virus or with the purified Env glycoprotein has been shown to result in protective immunity (for example, see MAYYASI and MOLONEY 1967; HUNSMANN et al. 1981). In addition, passive immunization with antibodies against virus can also block the appearance of disease (HUEBNER et al. 1976; SCHAFER et al. 1977; NOBIS and JAENISCH 1980). The effect of this passive immunization appears to be to block the appearance of infected cells in the bone marrow early in life (BUCKHEIT et al. 1987).

More recently, alternative approaches to immunization have been tested. Using a vaccinia vector that expresses the Friend virus *env* gene, EARL et al. (1986) showed that mice could be immunized against rapid disease onset caused by the Friend virus complex. After virus challenge, the immunized mice showed the presence of both neutralizing antibodies and cytotoxic T cells.

4.3 Pathogenicity

In the family of MuLVs there are isolates that cause disease and isolates that are not pathogenic. The diseases caused range from an acute erythroproliferative disease, to lymphoproliferative disease that appears after a long latency, to peripheral neuropathy. Many factors come into play in determining whether a virus is pathogenic. The most important determinant is the viral LTR which strongly influences both the ability to cause disease and the type of disease caused (see MAJORS, this volume). The importance of the LTR is probably multifaceted but due in part to the growth rate of the virus (in addition to being a major determinant of tissue tropism). Since virtually any region of the genome can affect the growth rate, this may be the explanation for the observation that disease determinants can appear at multiple places along the viral genome (DESGROSEILLERS and JOLICOEUR 1984; OLIFF et al. 1984; HOLLAND et al. 1985a; JOLICOEUR and DESGROSEILLERS 1985). However, recombinant viruses with polytropic sequences in the *env* gene appear prominently in some MuLV-induced diseases.

4.3.1 Role of MCF Viruses in MuLV-Induced Lymphoproliferative Diseases

4.3.1.1 *Disease with Long Latency*

MCF viruses are implicated in MuLV-induced T-cell lymphomas in mice by three observations: (a) co-infection of an ecotropic and an MCF virus can accelerate the onset of disease (CLOYD et al. 1980, 1981; GREEN et al. 1980; O'DONNELL et al. 1981); (b) during infection by an ecotropic virus (either exogenous infection or through activation of an endogenous virus), recombinant polytropic viruses appear during the latent period before disease, and expression of these viruses is prominent in the disease tissue (for example, see KAWASHIMA et al. 1976; FAMULARI and CIEPLENSKY 1984; HERR and GILBERT 1984); (c) MCF viruses can be isolated which are themselves highly oncogenic in the absence of ecotropic virus (CHATTOPADHYAY et al. 1989), although this is generally not the case. However, the precise role of MCF viruses in the disease process and the significance of a virus with an altered host range remain unclear.

In high leukemic strains of mice, ecotropic virus is expressed early in life. The ecotropic virus serves as parent to two distinct types of recombinants with distinct biological properties (ROWE et al. 1980; LUNG et al. 1980; reviewed in COFFIN 1984; FAMULARI 1983; STOYE and COFFIN 1985). Recombinants are initially detected in the spleen (EVANS 1986; EVANS and MALIK 1987); these viruses have acquired most of the *env* gene (gp70 and p15E domains) apparently as a single substitution from an endogenous polytropic viral genome (Fig. 4) (LUNG et al. 1980, 1983). They are called class II recombinants and typically are not pathogenic, although class II recombinants isolated from the CWD strain of mice are able to accelerate leukemia (THOMAS et al. 1986). Class II viruses are found later in the thymus, presumably as the result of virus spread (EVANS and MALIK 1987). Here another type of recombinant appears, one that has acquired contiguous LTR and C-terminal p15E sequences from a xenotropic-like endogenous virus and has polytropic sequences within gp70 but over a smaller region than is seen in the class II viruses (ROMMELAERE et al. 1978; LUNG et al. 1980; BUCHHAGEN et al. 1980; THOMAS and COFFIN 1982; THOMAS et al. 1984; QUINT et al. 1984). This type of recombinant virus, which is composed of sequences acquired from at least two separate recombination events, is called class I virus (Fig. 4). It is usually able to accelerate leukemia (ROWE et al. 1980). An ecotropic virus with only LTR and C-terminal p15E xenotropic-like sequences has been detected (THOMAS and COFFIN 1982; HERR and GILBERT 1983), but whether this virus recombines with a class II virus or with endogenous polytropic sequences to form a class I virus is not known.

An important step in the formation of thymic lymphomas is the insertional activation of a cellular proto-oncogene. While tumor tissue may be infected with multiple viruses, the virus responsible for the insertional activation event has a central role in the disease process. In Mo-MuLV-induced lymphomas, both the ecotropic Mo-MuLV and its recombinant MCF virus are capable of functioning as the agent of insertional activation (CUYPERS et al. 1984; SELTEN et al. 1984; STEFFEN 1984). In the spontaneous tumors of AKR mice, recombinant viruses are found in the tumor tissue, suggesting that MCF viruses are mediating the insertional activation event (QUINT et al. 1981; YOSHIMURA and BREDA 1981; CHATTOPADHYAY et al. 1982; YOSHIMURA and LEVINE 1983; HERR and GILBERT 1983; CORCORAN et al. 1984). In both of these cases it is probably the enhancer (either the Mo-MuLV enhancer or the enhancer derived from the xenotropic-like parent of class I polytropic viruses) that is the important determinant of the target tissue and of insertional activation (HOLLAND et al. 1985b; and see MAJORS, this volume).

It is difficult to assess the importance of MCF viruses in the disease process since these recombinants always appear after infection of mice even after infection by highly virulent strains of ecotropic MuLV (THOMAS 1986). Two systems have provided clues to the role of MCF viruses in the disease process. One approach is to examine the pathogenicity of an ecotropic virus in the complete absence of MCF-like sequences. Such a system is available in rats, and there Mo-MuLV causes T-cell lymphomas through insertional activation in a manner that parallels the process in mice (STEFFEN 1984). A second system is to follow the disease process under circumstances in which the replication of MCF viruses is inhibited. Certain strains of mice express an MCF-like glycoprotein on the cell surface, and this expression is correlated with a 30- to 100-fold reduction in the growth of MCF viruses, presumably through viral interference (RUSCETTI et al. 1981a; BASSIN et al. 1982; HARTLEY et al. 1983; BULLER et al. 1987). The locus responsible for this phenomenon is called $Rmcf^r$. GISSELBRETCH et al. (1978) made the observation that DBA/2 mice (which carry the $Rmcf^r$ allele) are resistant to leukemia induced by Mo-MuLV, suggesting a role for MCF viruses in the generation of T-cell lymphomas in mice. However, other host factors can limit the replication of Mo-MuLV in the absence of the $Rmcf^r$ allele, making it difficult to attribute the lack of disease solely to the $Rmcf^r$ locus. In contrast, ROWE and HARTLEY (1983; J. HARTLEY, personal communication) have shown that the replication and leukemogenicity of two highly virulent ecotropic viruses (SL3 and Gross Passage A) are not affected by the $Rmcf^r$ locus. Also, in the $Rmcf^r$ background endogenous ecotropic viruses show pathogenic potential that results in a broad range of proliferative diseases, including T-cell lymphomas (MUCENSKI et al. 1986, 1987). Taken together, these results suggest that there is nothing intrinsic to the disease process that requires the presence of an MCF virus. This appears to be true for virus-induced T-cell lymphoma, as described above, and for virus-induced non-T-cell lymphomas.

Because of the use of different mouse strains with different genetic backgrounds (for both mouse and viral genes) it is difficult to generalize on the role of MCF viruses in the disease. It is likely that the growth rate of the virus in the target tissue is a contributing factor. The generation of class I viruses leads to a more rapid appearance of the same disease (T-cell lymphoma) that appears in the absence of MCF viruses (MUCENSKI et al. 1987). Thus, the recombinant MCF virus may be more virulent in some cases than its ecotropic parent. The relative contributions of the gp70 substitution and the p15E/U3 substitution need to be assessed in a mouse background in which the production of recombinant viruses is low. Several mouse strains derived from crosses between AKR and DBA have been developed which appear to be deficient for the appearance of MCF viruses (MUCENSKI et al. 1987), and another mouse strain, 129, appears to lack the ability to donate the xenotropic-like sequences that appear in the p15E/U3 region (QUINT et al. 1984). Mouse strains like these should aid in defining the role of different portions of recombinant viral genomes in the disease process.

The role of MCF viruses in disease cannot be understood solely in terms of replication rates in the target tissue. This can be seen in the observation that the presence of the parental ecotropic virus accelerates the rate of T-cell lymphoma development by the recombinant MCF virus (CLOYD et al. 1981). MCF viruses may contribute in other ways to the disease process. An altered form of the polytropic Env protein appears to be mitogenic (see below), and this activity could increase the likelihood of tumor development. The MCF virus or the ecotropic virus could shield the other genome from the immune system (or expand the host range) through pseudotyping (SITBON et al. 1985) or perhaps by inducing tolerance. Target-cell specificity may be determined in part by the substitution within gp70, although this is not apparent from virus binding studies (CLOYD 1983). One model has been suggested in which one virus type stimulates growth of cells in the immune system while the second virus type, by abrogating interference, increases the rate of a second infectious event which leads to insertional activation of a proto-oncogene (DAVIS et al. 1987). Finally, the peculiar sequence arrangement in class I viruses, representing multiple recombination events, points to unknown selective pressures at work that result in the appearance of these unusual viruses.

There is no evidence of a role for MCF viruses in the generation of non-thymic leukemias that appear after a long latency. The viral genomes present in B-cell and myeloid leukemias are almost always of ecotropic origin (BEDIGIAN et al. 1984; SILVER 1984; ZIJLSTRA et al. 1986; MUCENSKI et al. 1987). As with MuLV-induced T-cell lymphomas, the non-T-cell leukemias also appear to be mediated by the insertional activation of cellular oncogenes (SILVER and KOZAK 1986; MUCENSKI et al. 1988).

4.3.1.2 *Acute Disease*

By virtue of their LTRs certain strains of MuLV (including the Friend and Rauscher strains) replicate well in cells of the erythroid lineage (see MAJORS, this volume). As a result, these viruses cause a different spectrum of diseases. Friend MuLV appears to cause three separate diseases (two early and one late) in certain strains of mice when infection is carried out in newborns. The first early disease is a rapid onset hemolytic anemia with the appearance of increased numbers of reticulocytes (SITBON et al. 1986). It has been proposed that there is an increased turnover of reticulocytes (or their precursors) due to infection by the virus and that this is a primary cause of the anemia. Splenomegaly is observed and is thought to be the result of compensatory splenic erythropoiesis. Recombinants between different strains of F-MuLV which differ in their ability to induce early anemia showed that the *env* gene is an important determinant in the ability to cause disease (SITBON et al. 1986). The hemolytic anemia is followed by the second early disease with reduced reticulocyte counts and continued splenomegaly but now as the result of blocked erythropoiesis due to erythroleukemia. Finally, in mice surviving (or resistant to) these first two diseases, myeloid and lymphoid leukemias (and rarely erythroid leukemias) appear after a significant latency (SHIBUYA and MAK 1982; CHESEBRO et al. 1983; SILVER 1984). These tumors have F-MuLV genomes frequently integrated near a specific region of the mouse genome (SILVER 1984; SILVER and KOZAK 1986).

Virus-induced early erythroleukemia, the second disease that appears, seems to require a F-MCF recombinant virus. There is a correlation between the absence of MCF virus and the absence of erythroleukemia in some strains of mice (RUSCETTI et al. 1981, 1982; SHIBUYA and MAK 1982; CHESEBRO et al. 1983; SILVER 1984). Some F-MCF virus isolates (and the similar Rauscher MCF viruses) can induce erythroleukemia (ISHIMOTO et al. 1981; VAN GRIENSVEN and VOGT 1980; CHESEBRO et al. 1984; VOGT et al. 1985), and some apparently nonpathogenic isolates are pathogenic after co-infection with an amphotropic or ecotropic virus (RUSCETTI et al. 1981). It is possible that virus-induced early erythroleukemia may be polyclonal in nature since the disease can appear rapidly (10 weeks), and truly tumorigenic cells are only occasionally found (OLIFF et al. 1981; SHIBUYA and MAK 1982). However, this point needs to be addressed since it will distinguish between polyclonal activation, perhaps mediated by the polytropic *env* gene product, and insertional activation as the virus-dependent step in rapid erythroleukemia.

4.3.2 Spleen Focus Forming Virus

The original Friend and Rauscher virus isolates contained a mixture of viruses. In addition to the replication competent F-MuLV and R-MuLV, a defective viral genome was found. This virus has been designated spleen focus forming virus (SFFV). The SFFV genome encodes a defective glycoprotein which has undergone several alterations (see Fig. 4). First, there is a one base insertion near the end of p15E which results in a shift in the reading frame and premature termination. Termination occurs immediately after the presumed membrane spanning region and results in the loss of the cytoplasmic tail. Second, there is a deletion that removes the cleavage site between p15E and gp70; this results in the synthesis of a protein 52 K in size which contains sequences derived from the gp70 domain and the p15E domain. Finally, the *env* sequence is a recombinant with ecotropic-like sequences at its C-terminus and polytropic-like sequences at its N-terminus (reviewed in RUSCETTI and WOLFF 1984). Strains of Friend virus containing SFFV cause an acute disease very similar to that caused by the replication competent F-MuLV; however, in the presence of SFFV, disease will occur when infection is carried out in adult mice whereas F-MuLV is acutely pathogenic only in newborn mice. Analysis of both constructed and natural mutants has provided genetic evidence that the *env* domain of the SFFV genome encodes the protein responsible for the disease (LINEMEYER et al. 1982; RUTA et al. 1983; MACHIDA et al. 1984, 1985; LI et al. 1986, 1987).

The pathogenic potential of SFFV is profoundly influenced by its helper virus (JONES et al. 1988). Therefore, the clearest view of the intrinsic oncogenic potential of SFFV comes from studies in which the defective SFFV genome is rescued using a packaging cell line so that infection can take place in the absence of any helper virus. Under these circumstances, infection causes transient erythroblastosis that regresses (BERGER et al. 1985; BESTWICK et al. 1985; WOLF and RUSCETTI 1985; SPIRO et al. 1988). The erythroblastosis is accompanied by mild splenomegaly and the appearance of foci of erythroblastosis in the spleen. There is a low probability that one of these clones will further expand to form an erythroleukemia (WOLF et al. 1986; SPIRO et al. 1988). The erythroleukemia that develops is clonal, with SFFV genomes appearing in a restricted region of the mouse genome (SPIRO et al. 1988). SFFV genomes are also integrated at a specific locus in tumors induced by the Friend virus complex (MOREAU-GACHELIN et al. 1988). Surprisingly, the site of insertion by SFFV in these tumors is not disrupted in F-MuLV erythroleukemia. These results can be interpreted as the SFFV glycoprotein acting as a polyclonal stimulator of erythroblasts early in disease followed by the outgrowth of a rare cell that has undergone some genomic alteration, presumably activation of a cellular oncogene. For both F-MuLV and SFFV it is likely that the MCF sequences that are prominent in each infection, either as recombinants of F-MuLV or as part of the SFFV genome, play an important role in changing the growth properties of the erythroblast during the early stage of the disease.

A clue to the role of the SFFV glycoprotein in early disease comes from the observation that there are variants of SFFV which cause different types of disease. One variant causes polycythemia (SFFV$_P$), while the other variant causes anemia (SFFV$_A$). This difference has been attributed to the establishment of an erythropoietin-independent state in erythroblasts infected with SFFV$_P$ while erythroblasts infected with SFFV$_A$ retain some erythropoietin-dependence (HOROSZEWICZ et al. 1975; LIAO and AXELRAD 1975; STEINHEIDER et al. 1979; HANKINS and TROXLER 1980). Sequences encoded within the 3'-portion of the *env* gene are responsible for the different phenotypes (CHUNG et al. 1987).

In cells infected with SFFV$_P$, gp52 is detected, as is a more modified form of the protein, gp65, with the larger form but not the smaller form found on the surface of the cell. In SFFV$_A$-infected cells the intracellular gp52 form is found along with a small amount of a larger form (gp60); however, neither form has been detected on the cell surface (RUSCETTI et al. 1981b; reviewed in RUSCETTI and WOLF 1984). In an analysis of SFFV$_P$ mutants it was noted that retention of the pathogenic phenotype was correlated with the ability to be expressed on the cell surface suggesting gp65 may function on the surface of the cell (LI et al. 1987); however, mutants with a normal C terminus (i.e., the cytoplasmic domain) make a protein that is found on the cell surface but the protein is not transforming (SRINIVAS et al. 1987). A majority of SFFV$_P$ gp52 remains intracellular with only a small amount reaching the plasma membrane; the SFFV-encoded protein is not associated with helper virus particles (RACEVSKIS and KOCH 1978; RUSCETTI et al. 1979; DRESLER et al. 1979; RUSCETTI et al. 1981b, SRINIVAS and COMPANS 1983). In addition, secreted forms of both the SFFV$_A$ and SFFV$_P$ glycoprotein have been detected (RACEVSKIS and KOCH 1978; PINTER and HONNEN 1985). At this time it is not clear which form of the protein, intracellular, surface or secreted, is mediating transformation.

4.3.3 Hind Limb Paralysis

Certain strains of MuLV induce hind limb paralysis after infection of susceptible mice. One example is an isolate of MuLV obtained from the brain of a paralyzed wild mouse which has this feature (reviewed in GARDNER 1978, 1985). Using molecular recombinants the determinant for paralysis induction was localized to the *env* gene domain which has a sequence that within gp70 is significantly divergent from other ecotropic viruses (DESGROSEILLERS et al. 1984; RASSART et al. 1986). Molecular recombinants within *env* have shown that several domains within *env* are necessary to obtain the full phenotype (PAQUETTE et al. 1989). No role for recombinant MCF viruses has been found in this disease (OLDSTONE et al. 1983). Surprisingly, no difference has been found in the extent of virus replication in a strain of mice that is resistant to disease compared with one that is sensitive (McATEE and PORTIS 1985).

Certain temperature-sensitive strains of MuLV are also able to induce hind-limb paralysis (McCARTER et al. 1977; WONG et al. 1983; BILELLO et al. 1986). In one group of mutants the ability to cause this disease correlates with the temperature-sensitive processing of the viral glycoprotein to its mature form (WONG et al. 1983). One of these mutants (ts1) has been shown to replicate more efficiently in the CNS and in neuron-rich cultures compared with its parental strain (WONG et al. 1985). The use of molecular recombinants has shown that the disease determinant maps to the *env* gene region (YUEN et al. 1985), and sequencing studies have shown that only four amino acid differences are present between the neurovirulent strain and other related but nonneurovirulent strains (SZUREK et al. 1988)

4.3.4 Immunosuppressive Activity of p15E

Retrovirus infection is frequently associated with immune suppression. To a certain extent this may be the result of virus growing in cells involved in the immune response. However, other factors may contribute to immune suppression. The transmembrane protein of several mammalian C-type viruses has been shown to be potentially immunosuppressive (reviewed in SNYDERMAN and CIANCIOLO 1984). An active sequence has been localized to a hydrophilic domain located on the outside of the membrane, and in vitro immunosuppressive activity is associated with a peptide having a sequence from this region (CIANCIOLO et al. 1985; RUEGG et al. 1989). However, a direct role for these sequences in promoting immunosuppression during virus replication has not been demonstrated, and at least one test in vivo for immunosuppression mediated by p15E failed to show activity (SCHMIDT and SNYDERMAN 1988).

5 Feline Leukemia Virus *env* Gene Products

Based on neutralization and interference properties FeLV isolates can be classified into three subgroups (A, B, and C) (reviewed in TEICH 1984). Differences in host range parallel the subgroup classification: subgroup A viruses have the most restricted host range; subgroup B and C viruses have a more extended host range. Viruses from these different subgroups have a curious association in the wild, with subgroup A viruses frequently found alone, and subgroup B and C viruses always found in association with a subgroup A virus, and sometimes all three found together. Subgroup B viruses are fairly common, while subgroup C viruses are rare. Subgroup B viruses arise as the result of recombination between an infecting subgroup A virus and endogenous virus-like elements in the cat genome (OVERBAUGH et al. 1988a). There are between 15 and 20 endogenous subgroup B-related sequence elements (STEWART et al. 1986). The subgroup C viruses are probably also recombinants (RUSSELL and JARRETT 1978; J MULLINS, personal communication), but the nature of the endogenous sequences donating this host-range determinant is not known. Sequence comparisons of the gp70 domain of different subgroups show that subgroups A and C are more similar to each other (88% sequence similarity) than either is to the subgroup B sequence (80% sequence similarity) (see, for example, DONAHUE et al. 1988).

Less is known in this system about the temporal relationship between the appearance of recombinant viruses and the onset of disease. Subgroup A viruses appear to be pathogenic after a long latency, and disease is associated with insertional activation or transduction of the c-*myc* oncogene (LEVY et al. 1984a; MULLINS et al. 1984; NEIL et al. 1984; FORREST et al. 1987). The appearance of lymphoproliferative disease is more strongly associated with, but not restricted to, the presence of an A/B mixed infection (JARRETT et al. 1978), and experimental infection with a cloned subgroup B virus can cause a variety of diseases within a year of infection (cited in DONAHUE et al. 1988). Most strikingly, infection with a subgroup C virus is associated with rapidly appearing aplastic anemia (HOOVER et al. 1974; MACKEY et al. 1975; JARRETT et al. 1984; RIEDEL et al. 1986). The disease determinant for aplastic anemia has been localized to a small portion of the genome that includes the N-terminal domain of the SU protein encoded within the *env* gene (RIEDEL et al. 1988).

In addition to causing proliferative disorders, infection with FeLV is commonly associated with the induction of severe immunodeficiency. The appearance of disease is associated with a variant form of the viral genome and the appearance of unintegrated viral DNA in the affected tissue (MULLINS et al. 1986). Sequence changes associated with the ability to induce immunodeficiency have been localized to the *env*/LTR region (OVERBAUGH et al. 1988b). In this variant three nucleotide changes in the LTR domain were seen, while eleven amino acid codon changes and a 6 codon deletion and a similarly sized insertion were found within *env*. The glycoprotein of this variant virus has an altered pattern of posttranslational processing which results in changes in its antigenicity (POSS et al. 1989). It is possible that the altered glycoprotein is itself pathogenic, that its inefficient processing is toxic to the infected cell, or that there is inefficient establishment of interference. There are now several examples from different retroviruses that suggest important changes in the biology of a virus can be attributed to subtle changes in the glycoprotein sequence. Thus, mammal tropism associated with RSV, neurotropism associated with some strains of MuLV, and immunodeficiency associated with FeLV may have a common feature of a glycoprotein that is partially defective. Perhaps the functional heterogeneity seen in these examples represents one of the consequences of selection for sequence heterogeneity by the immune system.

FeLV has been actively studied as a system amenable to vaccination. A variety of vaccines have been tested including live virus, inactivated virus, virus-producing cells, gp70, and gp70 in a glycoside matrix (iscom) (see OSTERHAUS et al. 1985 and references therein). This work has led to the introduction of a commercial vaccine (OLSEN 1985).

6 Envelope Proteins of Other Oncoviruses

6.1 Mouse Mammary Tumor Virus

This group of endogenous and exogenous oncoviruses plays a critical role in the induction of breast adenocarcinomas in the mouse. As with other nonacute transforming oncoviruses, they do not induce tumors through expression of a virally encoded oncogene but through a rare event which activates the expression of a cellular proto-oncogene (primarily *int*-1 and *int*-2; NUSSE and VARMUS 1982; PETERS et al. 1983; DICKSON et al. 1984b). The envelope gene of MMTV encodes two polypeptides, gp52 (SU) and gp36 (TM), which form a fringe of spikes on the surface of the virion that is much denser than that seen in most of the other oncoviruses and consistent with a larger number of molecules per virion. Chemical cross-linking and electron microscopy studies suggest that these glycoprotein spikes are formed from a trimeric arrangement of gp52/gp36 molecules (RACEVSKIS and SARKAR 1980).

6.1.1 Host-Range Determinants

Host range studies on MMTV have been hampered by the fact that the virus is only marginally infectious for cells in culture. The tissue specificity of the virus for mammary epithelial cells appears to be a reflection of transcriptional control sequences in the viral LTR rather than viral glycoprotein/receptor interactions, since transgenic mice bearing the *myc* oncogene under the control of MMTV 3′ regulatory sequences developed tumors with a high frequency in the mammary gland in addition to other tissues (STEWART et al. 1984). Also, studies employing pseudotypes of VSV that contained the *env* gene product of MMTV demonstrated a similar efficiency of plaque formation on both mammary epithelial and embryo cells from a variety of mouse strains (ZAVADA et al. 1977; HILKENS et al. 1983). In the studies of ZAVADA et al. (1977), VSV pseudotypes capable of infecting mink but not human, rat, or bat cells were also found to be present after infection of MMTV-producing GR- or C3H-derived cells. The "ecotropic" MMTV envelope component was induced from 10 to 20-fold after treatment of the MMTV-producing cells with dexamethasone (ZAVADA et al. 1977) and from cell hybrid studies appeared to bind a receptor (*MTVR*-1) encoded on mouse chromosome 16 (HILKENS et al. 1983). The molecular identity of this receptor molecule remains to be determined.

6.1.2 Antigenicity

Sera from mammary tumor-bearing mice contain antibodies that are capable of neutralizing the "ecotropic" MMTV/VSV pseudotypes (ZAVADA et al. 1977; HILKENS et al. 1983) and that are cytotoxic for MMTV-producing cells (SCHOCHETMAN et al. 1979). These natural antibodies could differentiate between pseudotypes formed from the C3H, GR, and RIII strains of MMTV indicating that each has distinct type-specific neutralizing epitopes, but radioimmunoassays with the same sera also demonstrated the presence of group (all three strains) and class (C3H and GR) specific determinants on the viral glycoprotein gp52 (SCHOCHETMAN et al. 1979). Monoclonal antibodies to gp52 yielded a similar antigenic relationship (MASSEY et al. 1980). Sequence comparisons of the C3H and GR gp52 proteins indicate that these two polypeptides differ primarily in a stretch of 7 aa (nos. 80–86) that presumably are responsible for the type-specific differences between the two strains (MAJORS and VARMUS 1983).

6.2 Primate D-type Retroviruses

In 1970 a virus with many characteristics of MMTV was isolated from a mammary tumor of a rhesus monkey (CHOPRA and MASON 1970). This virus (Mason Pfizer monkey virus, M-PMV) is a horizontally transmitted exogenous virus of the rhesus monkey and represents the prototype virus of the D-type retroviruses, a group which includes endogenous viruses of the langur and squirrel monkeys and an increasing number of exogenous immunosuppression-inducing isolates from macaque species (DANIEL et al. 1984; MARX et al. 1984, 1985; STROMBERG et al. 1984). The *env* gene of this group of viruses encodes a polypeptide of approximately 570 aa that is processed to yield the gp70 (SU) and gp20 (TM) molecules found in the virion. There are 10 carbohydrate addition sites on gp70 and a single site on gp20, all of which appear to be occupied (SONIGO et al. 1986; BRADAC and HUNTER 1986).

6.2.1 Host-Range Determinants

This group of viruses has a fairly narrow host range, primarily infecting macaque and human cells (reviewed FINE and SCHOCHETMAN 1978). However, there appears to be little tissue specificity for infection, since these viruses can infect fibroblasts and lymphoid cells of both T- and B-cell lineage. Through the use of VSV pseudotypes and the capacity of members of this virus group to induce syncytium formation, SOMMERFELT and WEISS (1990) have shown that all of the D-type isolates utilize a common receptor as assessed by the establishment of viral interference. Cells infected by a D-type virus are also resistant to infection by VSV or MuSV pseudotypes of baboon endogenous virus (BaEV) and the related RD114 (SOMMERFELT and WEISS 1990; CHATTERJEE and HUNTER, unpublished). The basis of this phenomenon may lie in a common origin for the *env* gene of these divergent species. A comparison of the *env* genes of M-PMV and the avian reticuloendotheliosis-associated virus (REV-A) showed 33% identity in the SU and 61% identity in the TM domains, with a stretch of 46 identical residues that encompass the "immunosuppressive peptide" region of the latter protein (SONIGO et al. 1986). REV-A is an unusual avian virus, since it is highly related to mammalian and particularly to primate C-type viruses including BaEV (HUNTER et al. 1978; OROSZLAN et al. 1981). Indeed, a comparison of 40 N-terminal residues of the BaEV TM protein with those of REV-A and M-PMV revealed 79% and 81% identity, respectively. Since the *gag-pol* region of MPMV appears to have been derived from a progenitor to the endogenous murine A- or B-type viruses, it seems likely that the D-type family arose by recombination of such sequences with a primate C-type *env* gene (SONIGO et al. 1986).

6.2.2 Antigenicity

Macaques that recover from infection with a D-type retrovirus develop neutralizing antibodies. These have been used to classify serologically the various D-type isolates associated with immunosuppressive disease in this monkey species, and 5 distinct serotypes have been identified (P. MARX, personal communication). This classification is consistent with nucleotide sequence comparisons which show different isolates varying by as much as 15% in the SU domain (SONIGO et al. 1986; POWER et al. 1986; THAYER et al. 1987). Macaques can be protected against persistant viremia and lethal immunosuppressive disease after challenge with the immunosuppressive D-type viruses by immunization with large amounts of formalin-inactivated virus (MARX et al. 1986).

6.2.3 Pathogenicity

Although M-PMV was isolated from a mammary tumor, attempts to induce tumors by inoculation of the virus into rhesus monkeys and other primates have been unsuccessful (FINE and SCHOCHETMAN 1978). Although rhesus monkeys neonatally inoculated with M-PMV or M-PMV-infected cells did not develop tumors, many developed severe lymphadenopathy, weight loss, and thymic atrophy, and a large proportion of inoculated animals succumbed to secondary viral or bacterial pneumonia (FINE et al. 1975). These results became particularly pertinent when D-type retroviruses were associated with an immune deficiency syndrome of macaques. This disease, analogous to the human acquired immune deficiency syndrome (AIDS), has been recognized in macaque monkeys at several primate centers in the USA (DANIEL et al. 1984; MARX et al. 1984, 1985; STROMBERG et al. 1984).

The molecular basis of the immunodeficiency disease induced by the D-type retroviruses is not clearly understood. However, a role for the *env* gene in this process has been suggested from its sequence homologies with that of REV. An amino acid sequence that is shared by many retroviral TM proteins has been linked to the immunosuppressive properties of this protein (CIANCIOLO et al. 1985), and the sequences that are most highly conserved between the REV-A and M-PMV *env* gene products center around this immunosuppressive sequence. The divergence of the SU domains of the two viruses, while obviously stemming from a common origin, implies that the sequence conservation within gp20 is essential to the success of the viral infection. The immunosuppressive properties of the envelope glycoprotein of REV-A are well described (CARPENTER et al. 1977, 1978a, b; RUP et al. 1979), and it is possible that similar mechanisms are operating with the primate viruses (SONIGO et al. 1986).

6.3 Human T-cell Leukemia Viruses

Human T-cell leukemia viruses serotypes 1 and 2 (HTLV-I and HTLV-II) comprise the first two retroviruses isolated from humans. HTLV-I is the first naturally occurring retrovirus linked with human malignancy (POIESZ et al. 1980) and is etiologically associated with adult T-cell leukemia/lymphoma (ATLL). The full spectrum of diseases in which HTLV-I may play a role has not yet been fully realized. The virus has been linked to tropical spastic paraparesis (GESSAIN et al. 1985) and less convincingly with multiple sclerosis (KOPROWSKI et al. 1985; HAUSER 1986). The TM glycoprotein, gp21E, has been shown to have amino acid homology with p15E of murine leukaemia virus which in vitro demonstrates some immunosuppressive effects (CIANCIOLO et al. 1984, 1985; RUEGG et al. 1989), although the involvement of this sequence in HTLV pathogenesis in vivo is not clear. Unlike the related bovine leukemia virus (BLV), HTLV-I is not subject to antibody-independent lysis by human complement (HOSHINO et al. 1984); thus, the SU glycoprotein, gp46, is adapted to preserve the integrity of the virion envelope in human plasma. HTLV-II infection, in comparison with HTLV-I, has been thought to be rare, the virus being first isolated from a T-cell hairy leukaemia (KALYANARAMAN et al. 1982). However, recent serological data indicate that infection with this virus may be widespread (LEE et al. 1989; G. SHAW, personal communication). The mechanism by which HTLV enters cells in vivo is not clear. HTLV-I may infect cells either by direct fusion with the plasma membrane in a pH-independent manner or using receptor-mediated endocytosis in a pH-dependent mechanism. This may vary depending on the cell type used (McCLURE et al. 1990). HTLV-I has been shown to integrate randomly into the host genome at sites not located near any known oncogenes. There are more proviral copies present in cells infected in vitro compared with in vivo.

6.3.1 Host-Range Determinants

HTLV-I can bind to and infect a wide variety of different cell types in vitro (NAGY et al. 1983; CLAPHAM et al. 1983; KRITCHBAUM-STENGER et al. 1987), although only T and B cells are susceptible to virally induced transformation (CHEN et al. 1984). The T-cell tropism of the virus is not therefore at the level of receptor expression; instead post-penetration events are also involved in determining HTLV's host range. Although in vitro infection of nonlymphoid cells has been achieved in human osteosarcoma cells (HOS) and human tumor cells (HT1080), it is not clear whether nonlymphoid cells are infected in vivo. In addition to binding assays, syncytial and pseudotype assays have been employed to determine functional receptor gene expression and HTLV host range. The viral envelope glycoprotein gp46 is thought to interact with available receptors on the surface of susceptible cells. One consequence of this interaction is the formation of multinucleate syncytia following cell fusion. Cells chronically infected with a retrovirus demonstrate the phenomenon of receptor interference, in that their receptors are no longer available at the cell surface either due to blockage by surface viral envelope glycoproteins or to down modulation or regulation of receptor gene expression. Thus, the cells become resistant to superinfection or cell fusion induced by the same or any other virus that utilizes the same cell surface receptor. HTLV-I and II were postulated to share the same cell surface receptor in this way (WEISS et al. 1985). Further supportive evidence that HTLV-I and -II utilize the same cell surface receptor was obtained following the assignment of the HTLV-I and HTLV-II receptor gene to human chromosome 17 (SOMMERFELT et al. 1988). As HTLV receptors are constitutively expressed on human cells and murine cells are relatively resistant, human-mouse somatic cell hybrids segregating human chromosomes could be employed to assign the receptor gene to a specific human chromosome. The receptor shared by both HTLV-I and HTLV-II remains to be identified. There have been numerous candidates including the IL-2 receptor α-chain recognized by tac-specific antibodies (LANDO et al. 1983). At present there are no reagents available for the β-chain. Cells that lack tac expression are, however, susceptible to HTLV infection. The gene encoding the tac antigen has been assigned to human chromosome 10: no chromosome assignment has yet been made for the β-chain gene.

6.3.2 Antigenicity/Pathogenicity

HTLV-I and -II comprise two serotypes (NAGY et al. 1984), although there may be some cross-neutralizing epitopes (CLAPHAM et al. 1984). ATLL is mainly a disease of adults which usually progresses rapidly once diagnosed. There is no associated viremia as the leukemic cells produce little virus. Due to the low cell-free infectivity, the mode of horizontal transmission is probably via secretion of infected cells in seminal fluid or mother's milk as well as following transfusion of infected blood. Infection is often clustered within families, with vertical transmission of the virus from mother to child across the placenta and via lactation. Children rarely express antibodies; however, if infected by transfusion of infected blood, they will elicit an antibody response. Only 0.05%–1% of infected individuals go on to develop ATLL; the virus therefore remains latent for reasons which are not yet fully understood.

7 Envelope Proteins of Nonprimate Lentiviruses

The lentivirus subfamily of retroviruses derives its name from the slow time course of the infections they induce in primates and other mammals (SIGURDSSON 1954a, b; HAASE 1975). This group of viruses, which includes visna-maedi of sheep, caprine arthritis encephalitis virus (CAEV), equine infectious anemia virus (EIAV), and HIV, cause chronic diseases affecting the lungs, nervous system, joints, hematopoietic and immune systems of humans and animals. Since all the lentiviruses persist and spread despite host immune responses, the viral glycoproteins and the host response to them play a significant role in the disease pathogenesis.

The prototype lentiviruses, visna and maedi, derive their Icelandic names from the major symptoms of the neurological and pulmonary diseases that they cause in sheep. The same virus, in fact, is responsible for both maedi, the more common chronic interstitial pneumonia, and visna, a chronic demyelinating encephalomyelitis that leads to wasting and progressive paralysis (reviewed in HAASE 1975). Additional viruses related to visna have been isolated from sick sheep and goats. These include Zwoegerziekte (DE BOER 1975) and progressive pneumonia virus (PPV; KENNEDY et al. 1968) of sheep and the related but distinct CAEV (CORK et al. 1974). CAEV induces a syndrome characterized by leuko-encephalomyelitis in young goats (CORK et al. 1974), occasional pneumonia and mastitis, and, predominantly, a progressive arthritis in older animals; a variety of related caprine viruses have been isolated throughout the world (reviewed by CHEEVERS and McGUIRE 1988). Another extensively studied nonprimate lentivirus, EIAV, causes a chronic, relapsing disease of horses characterized by recurrent episodes of clinical illness and progressive development of immune-mediated lesions (CHEEVERS and McGUIRE 1985). More recently, two lentiviruses have been isolated from cats and cows, which because of their potential involvement in immunosuppressing the host (both induce prolonged lymphadenopathy in host animals) and their similarities to human viruses have been called feline immunodeficiency virus (FIV; PEDERSEN et al. 1987) and bovine immunosuppressive virus (BIV; GONDA et al. 1987).

Both an analysis of virion polypeptides and an examination of the *env* coding regions of the nonprimate lentiviruses have shown that the major surface glycoprotein (SU) and the membrane spanning component (TM) are larger than those of the oncoviruses. The terminally glycosylated SU polypeptide of the visna-maedi/CAEV group has an apparent molecular mass of 135 kD, while the TM protein is approximately 45 kD (SCOTT et al. 1979; SONIGO et al. 1985). Both are cleaved from a core glycosylated precursor of approximately 150 kD (CHEEVERS et al. 1988). The SU protein of EIAV, on the other hand, is only 90 kD (PAREKH et al. 1980), which primarily reflects a reduced number of carbohydrate addition sites (12 vs 24) on a somewhat shorter polypeptide chain (RUSHLOW et al. 1986).

7.1 Host-Range Determinants

The prototype visna virus replicates most efficiently in ovine cells, particularly those of the sheep choroid plexus (SCP), but can infect primary cells from many vertebrate species (THORMAR and SIGURDSARDOTTIR 1962; HARTER et al. 1968). In SCP cells the virus induces multinucleate cell formation which can be used as the basis for a quantitative assay (HARTER and CHOPPIN 1967a, b). Both CAEV and EIAV show more restricted host ranges, the former being restricted to goat synovial membrane cells or macrophages (NARAYAN et al. 1980) and the latter to equine leukocytes (KOBAYASHI and KONO 1967), although a fibroblast-adapted form of EIAV has been propagated (MALMQUIST et al. 1973). These studies indicate that distinct cell receptors exist for each of these viruses, but no information is available on their likely identity.

7.2 Antigenicity

The major viral polypeptide to which the immune response of the infected host is directed is likely to be the SU protein since it is exposed on the outer surface of the virion and of the infected cell. However, the nature of the response to this protein and subsequent effects of the immune response on virus antigenicity differ between visna, CAEV, and EIAV.

Goats naturally infected with CAEV produce binding antibodies to all viral polypeptides within a few weeks post-infection, but they do not neutralize virus infectivity (KLEVJER-ANDERSON and McGUIRE 1982). However, neutralizing antibodies of very low titer (mostly 1:2) can be detected 1–5 years post-infection (McGUIRE et al. 1988). Neutralizing antibodies can be induced more rapidly by administering virus with large amounts of *M. tuberculosis*, but the response is narrowly restricted to the immunizing strain, suggesting that a single type-specific epitope is being recognized (NARAYAN et al. 1984). More recent studies suggest that the highly sialylated nature of the CAEV gp135, which appears to result from both *N*- and *O*-linked carbohydrate structures, might mask potentially neutralizing epitopes on the viral glycoprotein, thereby reducing the immunogenicity of the molecule. Treatment of virus with neuraminidase had no affect on infectivity but enhanced the kinetics of virus neutralization by goat antibodies (HUSO et al. 1988).

Despite the low titers of neutralizing antibody found in infected goats, antigenic variation within the neutralizing epitopes has been observed concomitant with its appearance. These antigenic variants, isolated from synovial fluid, are resistant to neutralization by the circulating antibody, but in two cases antigenic variation was followed by the appearance of neutralizing antibody to the new variant (ELLIS et al. 1987; McGUIRE et al. 1988). McGUIRE and coworkers have suggested that the characteristics of the neutralizing response and the appearance of antigenic variants may contribute to the recurrence and progression of arthritis seen in CAEV-infected goats. Thus, they suggest that despite a vigorous immune response to CAEV, the failure of antibody against gp135 to limit the spread of infection could result in a large pool of infected cells which could be replenished by the emergence of antigenic variants (McGUIRE et al. 1988).

Visna virus differs from CAEV in that it induces neutralizing antibodies, but virus can still be obtained from the animal by cocultivation of peripheral blood leukocytes. Thus, cell-associated virus can coexist indefinitely with neutralizing antibody in the plasma. Since the kinetics of virus neutralization are slower than those for virus infection of macrophage monocytes, NARAYAN and colleagues have suggested that this might account for continued cell-cell spread in the presence of an active immune response (KENNEDY-STOSKOPF and NARAYAN 1986). In addition, in infected animals, antigenic variants of the virus develop that are resistant to neutralization by early sera (NARAYAN et al. 1978). Similar viruses can be isolated at low frequency ($< 1 \times 10^{-7}$) in in vitro experiments under the selection pressure of neutralizing antibody (DUBOIS-DALQ et al. 1979). Analyses of the variants from infected animals identified changes in the peptide maps of gp135 (SCOTT et al. 1979) and nucleotide sequence changes within the *env* gene that correlated with the degree of antigenic variation (CLEMENTS et al. 1980, 1982; BRAUN et al. 1987). STANLEY et al. (1987) carried out a more detailed antigenic analysis of these variants through the use of a panel of monoclonal antibodies that recognized five partially overlapping epitopes on gp135 and identified major changes in several of these epitopes. Changes could even be detected in isolates that were still neutralized by polyclonal sheep sera. While these experiments suggest a role for antigenic variation in the persistence and progression of the disease, other observations do not support this as the primary basis for visna virus persistence; antigenic variants are in the minority during chronic visna-induced disease (THORMAR et al. 1983), and they do not replace the infecting serotype (SCOTT et al. 1979; LUTLEY et al. 1983). Thus, mechanisms must exist whereby the parental virus persists. The level of gene expression in infected cells may, in fact, be the most important contributor to the persistence of disease. Most infected cells harbor the virus in a latent state in which viral antigens are produced in insufficient quantities for the detection and destruction of the infected cell by the immune surveillance mechanisms (HAASE et al. 1977). Evidence for this type of infection in monocytes has led to the proposal of a trojan horse mechanism for virus spread (PELUSO et al. 1985), in which latently infected leukocytes carry the viral genome into a variety of other tissues.

For EIAV, evidence for the role of antigenic variation in virus dissemination and persistence is much stronger. In the process of EIAV-induced disease, there are cycles of infection in which cell-free virus can be isolated from the serum or plasma, and each new virus isolate from a cycle is resistant to neutralization by antibodies that neutralized previous isolates (KONO et al. 1973; MONTELARO et al. 1984). The basis for this change in virus antigenicity was initially mapped to the viral glycoproteins gp90 and gp45 by changes in glycoprotein mobility on polyacrylamide gel electrophoresis and by peptide and glycopeptide mapping (MONTELARO et al. 1984; SALINOVICH et al. 1986). It correlates with nucleotide sequence changes within the *env* gene of the virus where there appear to be variable, hypervariable, and conserved coding regions (SALINOVICH et al. 1986; PAYNE et al. 1987a). While the overall amino acid divergence within the *env* gene of different isolates ranges from 1.3% to 3.4%, changes in the variable and hypervariable regions within the middle of gp90 range from 2.7% to 8.5% and 2.8% to 20%, respectively. As in HIV (see below), a majority (75%) of the nucleotide changes in the *env* gene result in amino acid changes. Considerable variation in the number and location of carbohydrate addition sites was seen in different isolates (PAYNE et al. 1987a), correlating well with the previous reports of glycopeptide and mobility changes associated with antigenic variation.

The recurrent fevers and anemia that characterize EIAV infection can follow one another rapidly (sometimes only 14 days apart) but nevertheless are associated with new neutralization-resistant variants of the virus (PAYNE et al. 1987b). This structural variation observed within the glycoproteins appears to be a random and noncumulative process since each isolate has a unique subset of variant peptides, nucleotide changes (PAYNE et al. 1987b), and epitope reactivity (HUSSAIN et al. 1987). However, since the starting stocks for these experiments were obtained by endpoint dilution of virus, it remains possible that some of the variants, present as minor population in the initial stock, were selected during the course of the disease.

Even with EIAV, antigenic variation does not appear to be the sole basis for virus persistence and spread. By the end of the first year, cyclic replication of EIAV is replaced by an inapparent carrier state in which continued dissemination of the virus within the animal, and to new hosts, occurs through latently infected leukocytes (CHEEVERS and McGUIRE 1988). Termination of viremia in EIAV infections requires active immune-surveillance mechanisms since foals suffering from combined immunodeficiency and that lack functional B and T cells are unable to eliminate virus from their plasma (PERRYMAN et al. 1988).

In all of the above nonprimate lentivirus systems, antigenic variation within the envelope glycoproteins is an event closely linked to the progression of disease.

While the relative importance of its role in the disease process may differ between viruses, it clearly provides a mechanism for continued virus replication in the face of an unimpeded immune response and exacerbates the problem of developing vaccines against these viruses.

8 Envelope Proteins of Primate Lentiviruses

While the nonprimate lentivirus group contains viruses that have been known for over 75 years to cause disease, their primate counterparts have only recently been recognized. Nevertheless, since the first reports of AIDS in 1981 (GOTTLIEB et al. 1981; FRIEDMAN-KIEN et al. 1982), when it was characterized by unexplained opportunistic infections and aggressive Kaposi's sarcoma in young males, the disease has reached epidemic proportions and 5–10 million persons worldwide are estimated to have been infected by HIV, the causative agent of the disease. This novel human retrovirus was first suggested to be the causative virus after its isolation from an individual suffering from lymphadenopathy (LAV; BARRÉ-SINOUSI et al. 1983). It was later identified as the causative agent of AIDS itself and was isolated from patients suffering from this syndrome (HTLV-III; POPOVIC et al. 1984; GALLO et al. 1984; ARV; LEVY et al. 1984b). Shortly after the discovery of HIV, a related retrovirus was isolated from captive macaques suffering from an AIDS-like syndrome (DANIEL et al. 1985). Initially named STLV-3, this virus is now referred to as SIV by analogy to HIV, and additional strains of the virus have been isolated from several species of African monkeys. Serological studies in West Africa identified persons whose sera reacted strongly to SIV but weakly to HIV, arguing for infection by a virus more closely related to SIV (BARIN et al. 1985). In 1986, CLAVEL et al. (1986a, b) reported the isolation of a virus termed LAV-2 from African patients dying from AIDS. Sequence comparisons showed that this was a novel virus isolate with only 40% nucleotide sequence homology to HIV-1 and 75% nucleotide sequence homology to SIV (GUYADER et al. 1987; CHAKRABARTI et al. 1987). Reports of additional West African isolates most closely related to LAV-2 (ALBERT et al. 1987; CLAVEL et al. 1987; KONG et al. 1988) demonstrate the presence in West Africa of a second group of AIDS retroviruses now termed HIV-2. As with other lentiviruses such as visna, HIV induces disease over an extended period of time (the incubation period for AIDS is between 5 and 10 years) and as we will discuss below can establish an inapparent infection during the initial years after exposure.

Perhaps more so than in any other retrovirus, the envelope glycoproteins of this group of primate lentiviruses appear to play a critical role in defining the pathobiology of the disease. As discussed further below, they define the narrow host range of the virus that is integral in specifying the nature of the disease it induces; they mediate a cytopathic effect that can result in a lytic infection or syncytium formation of target cells; and because the SU domain (gp120) is readily lost from the TM domain (gp41) in the glycoprotein complex, it can mediate an immune-mediated killing of uninfected target cells.

Electron microscopic studies of nascently assembled virions indicate that approximately 70–80 glycoprotein knobs are arranged in a symmetrical fashion on the surface of the virion (GELDERBLOM et al. 1987); thus, it is likely that a specific interaction between the underlying icosahedral capsid structure and the glycoprotein complex exists. As we discussed earlier, the TM polypeptide of these viruses has an extraordinarily long cytoplasmic domain (> 150 aa) and muta-genic analyses suggest that at least in HIV-1 it performs several functions (KOWALSKI et al. 1987; DUBAY et al. 1988).

8.1 Host-Range Determinants

The identity of the host cell-encoded receptor molecule(s) that allow attachment and entry is obscure for the majority of retroviruses. However, shortly after its identification as the causative agent of AIDS, evidence was presented to indicate that the receptor for HIV is the CD4 antigen (also known as T4). This 60 kD molecule, originally described as a cell surface marker for the helper/inducer subset of mature lymphocytes, plays an important role in immune recognition and may be involved in the process of T-cell activation itself (reviewed by SWAIN 1983; SATTENAU and WEISS 1988). It is also expressed on a variety of cell types besides T cells including monocytes and other phagocytic cells.

A major feature of AIDS is a selective depletion of the CD4-bearing helper/inducer population of lymphocytes (GOTTLIEB et al. 1981). This hallmark of the disease correlates with a selective tropism by HIV for infection of that subset of CD4 + lymphocytes in vitro (KLATZMANN et al. 1984). The dependence of HIV on CD4 antigen for infection was first demonstrated directly by using monoclonal antibodies to CD4, which could block HIV infectivity in a variety of in vitro assays. DALGLEISH et al. (1984) showed that these monoclonal antibodies could prevent both the formation of syncytia that result from mixing HIV-infected cells with CD4 + uninfected cells and the infection of cells with VSV pseudotypes carrying the HIV envelope protein. Similarly, monoclonal anti-bodies to CD4 could block infection of peripheral blood lymphocytes by HIV (KLATZMANN et al. 1984) and inhibit the binding of fluoresceinated HIV to CD4 + cells (McDOUGAL et al. 1985). The process of HIV-1 binding to CD4 + cells involves the formation of a complex between the gp120 molecule of the virus and CD4; immunoprecipitation with antisera to either molecule coprecipitates the other (McDOUGAL et al. 1986a). Measurements of the affinity constant for this reaction have shown that gp120 and CD4 form a high affinity complex with a dissociation constant of approximately $4 \times 10^{-9} M/l$ (LASKEY et al. 1987). Direct evidence for CD4 being the receptor for HIV came from the work of MADDON et al. (1986), who demonstrated that, in CD4- HeLa cells, transfection and expression of the cDNA for human CD4 rendered these normally resistant cells permissive for HIV infection.

Down-regulation of surface CD4 molecules is observed after exposure of CD4 + T cells to phorbol esters or appropriate antigen-bearing target cells (HOXIE et al. 1986; ACRES et al. 1986), and initial experiments by MADDON et al. (1986) suggested that following CD4 binding, HIV entry into the cell involved endocytosis. However, the demonstration that HIV enters cells through a pH-independent mechanism (STEIN et al. 1987; MCCLURE et al. 1988) together with the observation that mutations within the cytoplasmic domain of the CD4 molecule which severely impair endocytosis have no effect on HIV infectivity (BEDINGER et al. 1988; MADDON et al. 1988) indicate that HIV can enter cells by direct fusion of the viral envelope with the cell plasma membrane.

The CD4 molecule consists of several different structural domains: an extracellular region containing four immunoglobulin-like domains, a transmembrane region, and a highly charged cytoplasmic domain (MADDON et al. 1985). The region of CD4 which binds to gp120 was initially mapped indirectly with monoclonal antibodies to CD4 (SATTENAU et al. 1986) and through a similar analysis of nonhuman primate cells that are susceptible to infection with HIV (MCCLURE et al. 1987). An epitope essential for HIV binding has since been mapped by immunologic and molecular analyses to the first immunoglobulin loop of CD4, and genetic analyses of gp120/CD4 binding suggest that the molecular interactions center around amino acid residues 45–51 within this region (LANDAU et al. 1988; JAMESON et al. 1988; PETERSON and SEED 1988; CLAYTON et al. 1988). Molecularly engineered forms of the CD4 molecule that lack the hydrophobic anchor domain and are thus secreted from the cell bind efficiently to gp120 or intact virus even when the truncation leads to secretion of just the first two immunoglobulin-like domains (BERGER et al. 1988; RICHARDSON et al. 1988). A number of investigators have used a genetically engineered soluble form of CD4 to inhibit HIV replication and syncytium formation (SMITH et al 1987; FISHER et al. 1988; HUSSEY et al. 1988; DEEN et al. 1988; TRAUNECKER et al. 1988), and this approach is currently being investigated for its antiviral therapeutic potential in vivo. Initial studies in rhesus monkeys indicate that administration of soluble CD4 can reduce the level of replicating virus in SIV-infected animals (WATANABE et al. 1989).

A mutational analysis of the gp120 coding region of HIV by KOWALSKI et al. (1987) showed that a region at the C-terminus of gp120 is involved in CD4 binding. Three distinct regions of the SU protein were defined within which mutations reduced or abrogated binding. These regions were contained in discontinuous, conserved sequences of the gp120 molecule, confirming the importance of tertiary structure in CD4 binding (MCDOUGAL et al. 1986b). A more precise definition of at least a subset sequence involved in the CD4 binding site was obtained by LASKEY et al. (1987), who used a monoclonal antibody that could block binding, to immuno-affinity purify a cleavage fragment of gp120. Amino acid sequence analysis located the epitope to residues 397–439, and site-directed mutations within this region prevented CD4 binding, suggesting that the sequences within this region are directly involved in the receptor binding region of gp120.

While the CD4 molecule is essential for virus attachment to cells, questions remain as to whether it is sufficient for virus entry, since transfection of mouse cells with the cDNA for human CD4 allows virus binding but not infection (MADDON et al. 1986). Since HIV can replicate in murine cells if the provirus is transfected into them (ADACHI et al. 1986; LEVY et al. 1986), it seems likely that this block is at the stage of membrane fusion. It is possible that for gp41 to initiate this fusion step, the fusion peptide must interact with an additional cell membrane protein.

8.2 Antigenicity

The envelope glycoproteins of the primate lentiviruses represent a major target of the humoral immune response (BARIN et al. 1985), and, paradoxically, high titered antibodies to this surface component of the virus (as assessed by membrane fluorescence or RIA) are found even in advanced AIDS patients (WEISS et al. 1985). However, the titer of neutralizing antibody in these patients' sera is generally quite low (WEISS et al. 1985), may decline as the disease progresses (ROBERT-GUROFF et al. 1985), and does not result in the abrogation of viral persistence in the responding individual. Despite the fact that the *env* gene sequence of different HIV isolates is highly variable, these human sera are broadly cross-neutralizing even for viral strains that differ by more than 15% in their *env* gene sequences (WEISS et al. 1986). In contrast, experimental HIV infection of chimpanzees results in a highly restricted, strain-specific neutralizing response (RUSCHE et al. 1988; GOUDSMIT et al. 1988a). Similarly, moderate-titered, type-specific neutralizing antibody was induced in goats, horses, and chimpanzees immunized with purified viral gp120 (ROBEY et al. 1986; ARTHUR et al. 1987), and type-specific responses have been seen in other animals administered genetically engineered envelope peptides of HIV (CHAHN et al. 1986; LASKEY et al. 1986; PUTNEY et al. 1986).

Interestingly, a region towards the C-terminus of gp120 (residues 303–330) appears to be the major, strain-specific, immunodominant neutralizing epitope seen by these recipients (PALKER et al. 1988; RUSCHE et al. 1988; GOUDSMIT et al. 1988a; MATSUSHITA et al. 1988). This neutralization epitope is located within a hypervariable region of gp120 and putatively exists as a loop between two cysteine residues (amino acids 296 and 331) connected by a disulfide bond. The peptide can completely block the neutralizing activity of serum from goats immunized with the PB1 region of gp120 from bacteria or with recombinant gp160. It can also block the neutralizing activity of serum from chimpanzees infected with HIV-1 (RUSCHE et al. 1988). Moreover, a significant percentage of sera from HIV-infected individuals react with peptides from this region (PALKER et al. 1988); the antibodies appear within 6 months of seroconversion and persist (GOUDSMIT et al. 1988b). While antibodies to this immunodominant epitope are effective at neutralizing virus, they do not block CD4 binding to gp120 (LINSLEY et al. 1988; SKINNER et al. 1988). It is likely therefore that they prevent a conformational change within the envelope complex that is required for membrane fusion to occur following receptor binding.

The broader cross-neutralizing human sera appear to contain antibodies that recognize several conserved domains on the envelope proteins (Ho et al. 1987). Rabbit antibodies to a peptide from one of these conserved regions of gp120 (residues 254–274) were efficient at neutralizing three different isolates but did not prevent virus binding to CD4-positive cells. It thus appears to target sequences that function in a post-binding process (Ho et al. 1988). Nevertheless, neutralization by sera from from HIV-infected individuals can involve blocking of CD4 binding (SKINNER et al. 1988). One region within gp41 (residues 598–609) is recognized by greater than 99% of sera from HIV-infected individuals (GNANN et al. 1987). This series of residues is just C-terminal to the so-called immunosuppressive peptide (ISP) of gp41. Antibodies to a peptide in the ISP region itself are found almost exclusively in asymptomatic, infected individuals, suggesting that they may confer some protection against the immunosuppressive aspects of infection (KLASSE et al. 1988).

Less information is available on the cellular immune response to the HIV envelope proteins. Virus-specific cytotoxic T lymphocytes (CTL) that can kill cells expressing either *env* or *gag* polypeptides are found in HIV-infected individuals (WALKER et al. 1987; PLATA et al. 1987) and may in fact contribute to inflammatory responses in the host (PLATA et al. 1987). However, these responses appear to be somewhat defective when compared with those against other viruses in the same individuals (WAHREN et al. 1987). Studies from human volunteers vaccinated with a recombinant vaccinia virus expressing gp160 of HIV indicated that CTL capable of recognizing two regions of gp120 (residues 112–114 and 428–443), predicted to be T-cell epitopes, were present (BERZOFSKY et al. 1988); however, an extended analysis of other regions of gp120 and gp41 was not carried out. CTL can also be demonstrated after vaccination of macaques and chimpanzees with vectors expressing the HIV *env* gene (ZARLING et al. 1986, 1987). Similar studies in mice have suggested that at least in this host a portion of the humoral immunodominant epitope (residues 307–322) is also a major CTL epitope (TAKAHASHI et al. 1988). In addition to CTL, both antibody-dependent, cell-mediated and NK/K immune responses to gp120 can be observed in HIV-seropositive patients (TYLER et al. 1989; WEINHOLD et al. 1988). Such activities may represent a primary cytotoxic response to the virus in this disease.

A major concern in attempting to augment the host's immune response to HIV or in the development of vaccines against the virus has been the level of variation observed throughout the genome and particularly within the *env* gene of different isolates (WONG-STAAL et al. 1985; HAHN et al. 1985; ALIZON et al. 1986; WILLEY et al. 1986; STARCICH et al. 1986). A sequence comparison of the envelope genes of the BH10 and ARV2 isolates revealed over 17% amino acid sequence difference in Env compared with only 6% in Gag (STARCICH et al. 1986). Furthermore, in *gag* and *pol*, most nucleotide changes are due to point mutations, whereas in *env* there are clustered changes involving in-frame deletions, insertions and duplications. The majority of changes in *gag* and *pol* are in the third nucleotide position of codons, but in *env* more than half the point mutations occur in the first and second nucleotide positions, which results in a high frequency of amino acid changes (STARCICH et al. 1986). Despite the high level of variability in the HIV envelope, there are regions that are highly conserved that presumably have important functional roles. For example, all 18 cysteines within gp120 and most in gp41 are conserved in most viruses (MODROW et al. 1987), suggesting that these residues are critical in maintaining a correct tertiary structure. Similarly, the CD4 binding domain has been mapped to conserved regions toward the C-terminus of gp120 (LASKY et al. 1987; KOWALSKI et al. 1987).

Studies have recently addressed the question of genetic variation of HIV in infected individuals as the disease progresses. In one study in which virus was isolated from persistently infected individuals over a period of 2 years, nucleotide changes were detected throughout the genome, including deletion and insertions as well as substitution mutations, and mutations were more frequent in *env* (10^{-3} nucleotide substitution per site per year) than in *gag* and *pol* (10^{-4}) (HAHN et al. 1986). These rates of variation resemble those recently described for visna virus, and EIAV (PAYNE et al. 1987a); BRAUN et al. 1987), and, as with the latter virus, variants appeared to arise randomly rather than sequentially with time. HIV variation within a single infected individual can be extensive with isolates varying by as much as 25% (SAAG et al. 1988). It seems likely that this plasticity of the HIV genome contributes to its persistence and continued spread in the host by allowing escape from the humoral immune response (ROBERT-GUROFF et al. 1986) and by generating virus that preferentially propagates in phagocytic cells (GARTNER et al. 1986; KOYANAGI et al. 1987). It should be noted, however that recent studies employing PCR amplification of viral DNA sequences in peripheral blood lymphocytes indicate that essentially nonmutated parental viral genomes remain the most prevalent form in these cells despite the high level of variation observed in isolated viruses (G. SHAW, personal communication).

A variety of approaches has been taken in an attempt to develop a vaccine against HIV. Since there is no available nonhuman primate in which HIV infection induces the disease observed in AIDS patients, two main strategies have been followed: (a) vaccination of chimpanzees, the only primate source susceptible to HIV-1 infection and persistence, and (b) use of SIV and its related immunodeficiency disease for vaccine development and testing (DESROSIERS 1989; P. MARX, personal communication). Because of the limited number of chimpanzees available, it is likely that studies will concentrate on the latter approach over the next several years. Experiments with chimpanzees have to date been disappointing. Immunization of these animals by a variety of mechanisms yields, as described above, primarily type-specific neutralizing responses to the immunizing strain but more importantly no protection to challenge even with the same strain of virus (HU et al. 1987; BERMAN et al. 1988a). Studies in the SIV system employing inactivated whole virus preparations for immunization are more encouraging and have shown that some macaques vaccinated in this way can be protected from challenge with SIV, although in the majority of the animals it was still possible to isolate virus from peripheral blood lymphocytes (DESROSIERS et al. 1989; P. MARX, personal communication). Even in these virus positive animals, however, both virus load and the rate of disease progression appear to be reduced. The general ability of the lentivirus group to infect phagocytic cells or lymphocytes and enter a down-regulated state may be a critical component in SIV avoiding the immune response in these virus-positive vaccinated animals, since similar approaches have been successful in protecting macaques completely from the immunosuppressive D-type retroviruses (MARX et al. 1986).

8.3 Pathogenicity

Although the clinical hallmark of AIDS is a progressive deterioration of immune competence due to a progressive loss of CD4 + helper/inducer lymphocytes (FAUCI 1988), the precise mechanisms involved in both cell cytopathicity and immune cell depletion remain unclear. However, the viral glycoproteins clearly play critical and probably multiple roles in these processes. Studies in which HIV proviral DNA was transfected into susceptible CD4-bearing cells showed conclusively that HIV alone was capable of eliciting a cytopathic effect and death in these cells (FISHER et al. 1985). High level expression of the HIV *env* gene, in the absence of the other viral structural genes, resulted in syncytia formation and the loss of viability in such cells, indicating that the glycoproteins alone can play a major role in cell cytopathicity (SODROSKI et al. 1986; LIFSON et al. 1986). While syncytium formation may contribute to a reduction in cell viability, it does not appear to be the main basis of the cell killing since mutations within the *env* gene can abrogate cell killing without affecting cell fusion (FISHER et al. 1986), and HIV is cytopathic in some cells in the absence of cell fusion (SOMASUNDARAN and ROBINSON 1987). Chronic expression of the HIV *env* gene in cytolysis-sensitive cells reduced CD4 expression and conferred a cytolysis-resistant phenotype to the host cell such that persistent infection rather than cell lysis followed infection with HIV. Treatment of these persistently infected cells with phorbol esters resulted in stimulation of virus replication followed by cytolysis without syncytia formation (STEVENSON et al. 1988). In addition, the HIV glycoprotein has a direct effect on the sodium/potassium balance in infected cells which may be related to the viral cytopathic effect (GARRY et al. 1988).

In vivo, additional mechanisms may be active in reducing the T helper/inducer cell population. Paradoxically, while only a very small portion of the circulating CD4 + lymphocytes (less than 1 in 10 000) express HIV mRNA or proteins at any time during the course of the disease, there is a progressive and eventually total destruction of this cell type (SHAW et al. 1984; HARPER et al. 1986). It has been suggested that progressive recruitment of uninfected T cells into Env expressing syncytia might be one mechanism through which this could occur. In addition, it has been shown that free gp120 can bind to the CD4 molecule on cells expressing this marker, making them a target for antibody-dependent cellular cytotoxicity (LYERLY et al. 1987) or class II restricted T cell-mediated cytolysis (LANZAVECCHIA et al. 1988; SILICIANO et al. 1988). Since gp120 is readily lost from the surface of virus and cells expressing the HIV Env proteins, these mechanisms could contribute in a significant way to the process of CD4 cell destruction in the course of the disease.

In summary, the glycoproteins of the primate lentiviruses continue to be a focus of research in addressing the problem of AIDS. Understanding how these highly variable molecules modulate cell surface marker expression, directly induce a cell cytopathic effect, and target both beneficial and deleterious immune responses to HIV infection will clearly play a major role in the development of therapeutic and preventative approaches to this disease.

Acknowledgements. Dr. M. Sommerfelt for her contribution of the HTLV glycoprotein section; R. Buckheit, C. Dickson, J. Dubay, L. Evans, M. Cloyd, R. Desrosiers, J. Sodroski, S. Rhee for their helpful comments; C. Bova, L. Crittendon, J. Cunningham, R. Desrosiers, R. Freidrich, W. Gallaher, R. Garry, J. Hartley, M. Kotler, C. Kozak, P. Marx, J. Mullins, R. O'Neill, A. Rein, R. Smith, R. Weiss, and J. White for communication of unpublished results; and A. Gayles, J. Johnson, and S. Winn for their skillful and patient assistance in preparation of the manuscript. Our own research efforts are supported by grants from NIAID and from NCI.

References

Acres RB, Conlon PJ, Mochizuki DY, Gallis B (1986) Rapid phosphorylation and modulation of the T4 antigen on cloned helper T cells induced by phorbol myristate acetate or antigen. J Biol Chem 261: 16210–16214

Adachi A, Gendelman HE, Koenig S, Folks T, Willey R, Rabson A, Martin MA (1986) Production of acquired immunodeficiency syndrome-associated retrovirus in human and nonhuman cells transfected with an infectious molecular clone. J Virol 59: 284–291

Albert J, Bredberg U, Chiodi F, Bottiger B, Fenyo EM, Norrby E, Biberfeld G (1987) A new human retrovirus isolate of West African origin (SBL-6669) and its relationship to HTLV-IV, LAV-II, and HTLV-IIIB. Aids Res Hum Retroviruses 3: 3–10

Albritton LM, Tseng L, Scadden D, Cunningham JM (1989) A putative murine ecotropic retrovirus receptor gene encodes a multiple membrane-spanning protein and confers susceptibility to virus infection. Cell 57: 659–666

Alexander S, Elder JH (1984) Carbohydrate dramatically influences immune reactivity of antisera to viral glycoprotein antigens. Science 226: 1328–1330

Alizon M, Wain-Hobson S, Montagnier L, Sonigo P (1986) Genetic variability of the AIDS virus: nucleotide sequence analysis of two isolates from African patients. Cell 46: 63–74

Anderson KB, Nexo BA (1983) Entry of murine retrovirus into mouse fibroblasts. Virology 125: 85–98

Arthur LO, Pyle SW, Nara PL, Bess JJ, Gonda MA, Kelliher JC, Gilden RV, Robey WG, Bolognesi DP, Gallo RC, Fischinger PJ (1987) Serological responses in chimpanzees inoculated with human immunodeficiency virus glycoprotein (gp120) subunit vaccine. Proc Natl Acad Sci USA 84: 8583–8587

Barin F, McLane MF, Allan JS, Lee TH, Groopman JE, Essex M (1985) Virus envelope protein of HTLV-III represents major target antigen for antibodies in AIDS patients. Science 228: 1094–1096

Barré-Sinoussi F, Chermann JC, Rey F, Nugeyre MT, Chamaret S, Gruest J, Dauguet C, Axler-Blin C, Brun-Vezinet F, Rouzioux C, Rozenbaum W, Montagnier L (1983) Isolation of a T-lymphocyte retrovirus from a patient at risk for acquired immune deficiency syndrome (AIDS). Science 220: 868–871

Bassin RH, Ruscetti S, Ali I, Haapala DK, Rein A (1982) Normal DBA/2 mouse cells synthesize a glycoprotein which interferes with MCF virus infection. Virology 123: 139–151

Bedigian HG, Johnson DA, Jenkins NA, Copeland NG, Evans R (1984) Spontaneous and induced leukemias of myeloid origin in recombinant inbred BXH mice. J Virol 51: 586–594

Bedinger P, Moriarty A, von Borstel R, Donovan NJ, Steimer KS, Littman DR (1988) Internalization of the human immunodeficiency virus does not require the cytoplasmic domain of CD4. Nature 334: 162–165

Berger EA, Fuerst TR, Moss B (1988) A soluble recombinant polypeptide comprising the amino-terminal half of the extracellular region of the CD4 molecule contains an active binding site for human immunodeficiency virus. Proc Natl Acad Sci USA 85: 2357–2361

Berger SA, Sanderson N, Bernstein A, Hankins WD (1985) Induction of the early stages of Friend erythroleukemia with helper free Friend spleen focus-forming virus. Proc Natl Acad Sci USA 82: 6913–6917

Berman PW, Groopman JE, Gregory T, Clapham PR, Weiss RA, Ferriani R, Riddle L, Shimasaki C, Lucas C, Lasky LA, Eichberg JW (1988a) Human immunodeficiency virus type 1 challenge of chimpanzees immunized with recombinant envelope glycoprotein gp120. Proc Natl Acad Sci USA 85: 5200–5204

Berman PW, Nunes WM, Haffar OK (1988b) Expression of membrane-associated and secreted variants of gp160 of human immunodeficiency virus type 1 in vitro and in continuous cell lines. J Virol 62: 3135–3142

Berzofsky JA, Bensussan A, Cease KB, Bourge JF, Cheynier R, Lurhuma Z, Salaun JJ, Gallo RC, Shearer GM, Zagury D (1988) Antigenic peptides recognized by T lymphocytes from AIDS viral envelope-immune humans. Nature 334: 706–708

Bestwick RK, Hankins WD, Kabat D (1985) Roles of helper and defective retroviral genomes in murine erythroleukemia: studies of spleen focus-forming virus in the absence of helper. J Virol 56: 660–664

Bilello JA, Pitts OM, Hoffman PM (1986) Characterization of a progressive neurodegenerative disease induced by a temperature-sensitive Moloney murine leukemia virus infection. J Virol 59: 234–241

Blough HA, Pauwels R, De CE, Cogniaux J, Sprecher GS, Thiry L (1986) Glycosylation inhibitors block the expression of LAV/HTLV-III (HIV) glycoproteins. Biochem Biophys Res Commun 141: 33–38

Boettiger D, Love DN, Weiss RA (1975) Virus envelope markers in mammalian tropism of avian RNA tumor viruses. J Virol 15: 108–114

Bova CA, Manfredi JP, Swanstron R (1986) Env genes of avian retroviruses: nucleotide sequence and molecular recombinants define host range determinants. Virology 152: 343–354

Bova CA, Olsen JC, Swanstrom R (1988) The avian retrovirus env gene family: molecular analysis of host range and antigenic variants. J Virol 62: 75–83

Bradac J, Hunter E (1986) Polypeptides of Mason-Pfizer Monkey virus. II. Synthesis and processing of the env gene products. Virology 150: 491–502

Braun MJ, Clements JE, Gonda MA (1987) The visna virus genome: evidence for a hypervariable site in the env gene and sequence homology among lentivirus envelope proteins. J Virol 61: 4046–4054

Brown DW, Robinson HL (1988a) Influence of env and long terminal repeat sequences on the tissue tropism of avian leukosis viruses, J Virol 62: 4828–4831

Brown DW, Robinson HL (1988b) Role of RAV-0 genes in the permissive replication of subgroup E avian leukosis viruses on line 15$_B$evl CEF. Virology 162: 239–242

Brown DW, Blais BP, Robinson HL (1988) Long terminal repeat (LTR) sequences env, and a region near the 5″ LTR influence the pathogenic potential of recombinants between Rous-associated virus types 0 and 1. J Virol 62: 3431–3437

Buchhagen DL, Pederson FS, Crowther RL, Haseltine WA (1980) Most sequence difference between the genomes of the AKV virus and leukemogenic Gross A virus passaged in vitro are located near the 3′ terminus. Proc Natl Acad Sci USA 77: 4359–4363

Buckheit RW, Bolognesi DP, Weinhold KJ (1987) The effects of leukemosuppressive immunotherapy of bone marrow infectious cell centres in AKR mice. Virology 157: 387–396

Buller RS, Ahmed A, Portis JL (1987) Identification of two forms of an endogenous murine retroviral *env* gene linked to the *Rmcf* locus. J Virol 61: 29–34

Carpenter CR, Bose HR, Rubin AS (1977) Contact-mediated suppression of mitogen induced responsiveness by spleen cells in reticuloendotheliosis virus-induced tumorigenesis. Cell Immunol 33: 392–401

Carpenter CR, Kempf KE, Bose HR, Rubin AS (1987a) Characterization of the interaction of reticuloendotheliosis virus with the avian lymphoid system. Cell Immunol 39: 307–315

Carpenter CR, Rubin AS, Bose Jr. HR (1978b) Suppression of the mitogen-stimulated blastogenic response during reticuloendotheliosis virus-induced tumorigenesis: investigations into the mechanism of action of the suppressor. J Immunol 120: 1313–1320

Carter JK, Smith RE (1984) Specificity of avian leukosis virus-induced hyperlipidemia. J Virol 50: 301–308

Carter JK, Proctor SJ, Smith RE (1983) Induction of angiosarcomas by ring-necked pheasant virus. Infect Immun 40: 310–319

Chakrabarti L, Guyader M, Alizon M, Daniel MD, Desrosiers RC, Tiollais P, Sonigo P (1987) Sequence of simian immunodeficiency virus from macaque and its relationship to other human and simian retroviruses. Nature 328: 543–547

Chanh TC, Dreesman GR, Kanda P, Linette GP, Sparrow JT, Ho DD, Kennedy RC (1986) Induction of anti-HIV neutralizing antibodies by synthetic peptides. EMBO J 5: 3065–3071

Chattopadhyay SK, Cloyd MW, Linemeyer DR, Lander MR, Rands E, Lowy DR (1982) Cellular origin and role of mink cell focus-forming viruses in murine thymic lymphomas. Nature 295: 25–31

Chattopadhyay SK, Baroudy BM, Holmes KL, Fredrickson TN, Lander MR, Morse HC III, Hartley JW (1989) Biologic and molecular genetic characteristics of a unique MCF virus that is highly leukemogenic in ecotropic virus-negative mice. Virology 168: 90–100

Cheevers WP, McGuire TC (1985) Equine infectious anemia virus. Immunopathogenesis and persistence. Rev Infect Dis 7: 83–88

Cheevers WP, McGuire TC (1988) The lentiviruses: Maedi/visna, caprine arthritis-encephalitis, and equine infectious anemia. Adv Virus Res 34: 189–215

Cheevers WP, Stem TA, Knowles DP, McGuire TC (1988) Precursor polypeptides of caprine arthritis-encephalities lentivirus structural proteins. J Gen Virol 69: 675–681

Chen ISY, McLaughlin J, Golde DW (1984) Long terminal repeats of human T-cell leukemia virus II genome determine target cell specificity. Nature 309: 277–279

Chesebro B, Wehrly K (1985) Different murine cell lines manifest unique patterns of interference to superinfection by murine leukemia viruses. Virology 141: 119–129

Chesebro B, Portis JL, Wehrly K, Nishio J (1983) Effect of murine host genotype on MCF virus expression, latency, and leukemia cell type of leukemias induced by Friend murine leukemia helper virus. Virology 128: 221–233

Chesebro B, Wehrly K, Nishio J, Evans L (1984) Leukemia induction by a new strain of Friend mink cell focus-inducing virus: synergistic effect of Friend ecotropic murine leukemia virus. J Virol 51: 63–70

Chopra HC, Mason MM (1970) A new virus in a spontaneous mammary tumor of a rhesus monkey. Cancer Res 30: 2081–2086

Chung S-W, Wolff L, Ruscetti S (1987) Sequences responsible for the altered erythropoietin responsiveness in spleen focus-forming virus strain SFFV$_p$-infected cells are localized to a 678-base-pair region at the 3' end of the envelope gene. J Virol 61: 1661–1664

Cianciolo GJ, Kipnis RJ, Synderman R (1984) Similarity between p15E of a murine and feline leukemia virus and p21 of HTLV. Nature 311: 515

Cianciolo GJ, Copeland TD, Oroszlan S, Synderman R. (1985) Inhibition of lymphocyte proliferation by a synthetic peptide homologous to retroviral envelope proteins. Science 230: 453–455

Clapham P, Nagy K, Cheinsong-Popov R, Weiss RA (1983) Productive infection and cell free transmission of human T-cell leukemia virus in a non-lymphoid cell line. Science 222: 1125–1127

Clapham P, Nagy K, Weiss RA (1984) Pseudotypes of human T-cell leukemia virus types 1 and 2: Neutralization by patients' sera. Proc Natl Acad Sci USA 81: 2886–2889

Clavel F, Guetard D, Brun-Vezinet F, Chamaret S, Rey MA, Santos-Ferreira MO, Laurent AG, Dauguet C, Katlama C, Rouzioux C, Klatzmann D, Champalimaud JL, Montagnier L (1986a) Isolation of a new human retrovirus from West African patients with AIDS. Science 233: 343–346

Clavel F, Guyader M, Guetard D, Salle M, Montagnier L, Alizon M (1986b) Molecular cloning and polymorphism of the human immune deficiency virus type 2. Nature 324: 691–695

Clavel F, Mansinho K, Chamaret S, Guetard D, Favier V, Nina J, Santos FM, Champalimaud JL, Montagnier L (1987) Human immunodeficiency virus type 2 infection associated with AIDS in West Africa. N Engl J Med 316: 1180–1185

Clayton LK, Hussey RE, Steinbrich R, Ramachandran H, Husain Y, Reinherz EL (1988) Substitution of murine for human CD4 residues identifies amino acids critical for HIV-gp120 binding. Nature 335: 363–366

Clements JE, Pederson FS, Narayan O, Haseltine WS (1980) Genomic changes associated with antigenic variation of visna virus during persistent infection. Proc Natl Acad Sci USA 77: 4454–4458

Clements JE, D'Antonio N, Narayan O (1982) Genomic changes associated with antigenic variation of visna virus. II. Common nucleotide sequence changes detected in variants from independent isolations. J Mol Biol 158: 415–434

Cloyd MW (1983) Characterization of target cells for MCF viruses in AKR mice. Cell 32: 217–225

Cloyd MW, Chattopadhyay SK (1986) A new class of retrovirus present in many murine leukemia systems. Virology 151: 31–40

Cloyd MW, Hartley JW, Rowe WP (1980) Lymphomagenicity of recombinant mink cell focus-inducing murine leukemia viruses. J Exp Med 151: 542–552

Cloyd MW, Hartley JW, Rowe WP (1981) Genetic study of lymphoma induction by AKR mink cell focus-inducing virus in AKR × NFS crosses. J Exp Med 154: 450–458

Cloyd MW, Thompson MM, Hartley JW (1985) Host range of mink cell focus-inducing viruses. Virology 140: 239–248

Coffin JM (1979) Structure, replication, and recombination of retrovirus genomes: some unifying hypotheses. J Gen Virol 42: 1–26

Coffin J (1984) Endogenous viruses. In: Weiss R, Teich N, Varmus H, Coffin J (eds) Molecular biology of tumor viruses: RNA tumor viruses 2 edn. Cold Spring Harbor Laboratory, Cold Spring Harbor, p 1109

Coffin JM, Champion M, Chabot F (1978) Nucleotide sequence relationships between the genomes of an endogenous and an exogenous avian tumor virus. J Virol 28: 972–991

Corcoran LM, Adams JM, Dunn AR, Cory S (1984) Murine T lymphomas in which the cellular *myc* oncogene has been activated by retroviral insertion. Cell 37: 113–122

Cork LC, Hadlow WJ, Crawford TB, Gorham JR, Piper RC (1974) Infectious leukoencephalomyelitis of young goats. J Infect Dis 129: 134–141

Crawford S, Goff SP (1985) A deletion mutation in the 5' part of the *pol* gene of Moloney murine leukemia virus blocks proteolytic processing of the *gag* and *pol* polyproteins. J Virol 53: 899–907

Crittenden LB (1968) Observations on the nature of a genetic cellular resistance to avian tumor viruses. JNCI 41: 145–153

Crittenden LB, Motta JV (1975) The role of the *tub* locus in genetic resistance to RSV (RAV-O). Virology 67: 327–334

Crittenden LB, Fadly AM, Smith EJ (1982) Effect of endogenous leukosis virus genes on response to infection with avian leukosis and reticuloendotheliosis viruses. Avian Dis 26: 279–294

Crittenden LB, Smith EJ, Fadly AM (1984) Influence of endogenous viral (*ev*) gene expression and strain of exogenous avian leukosis virus (ALV) on mortality and ALV infection and shedding in chickens. Avian Dis 28: 1037–1056

Crittenden LB, McMahon S, Halpern MS, Fadly AM (1987) Embryonic infection with the endogenous avian leukosis virus Rous-associated virus-0 alters responses to exogenous avian leukosis virus infection. J Virol 61: 722–725

Cuypers HT, Selten G, Quint W, Zijlstra M, Maandag ER, Boelens W, van Wezenbeek P, Melief C, Berns A (1984) Murine leukemia virus-induced T-cell lymphomagenesis: integration of proviruses in a distinct chromosomal region. Cell 37: 141–150

Dalgleish AG, Beverley PC, Clapham PR, Crawford DH, Greaves MF, Weiss RA (1984) The CD4 (T4) antigen is an essential component of the receptor for the AIDS retrovirus. Nature 312: 763–767

Daniel MD, King NW, Letvin NL, Hunt RD, Sehgal PK, Desrosiers RC (1984) A new type D retrovirus isolated from the macaques with an immunodeficiency syndrome. Science 223: 602–605

Daniel MD, Letvin NL, King NW, Kannagi M, Sehgal PK, Hunt RD, Kanki PJ, Essex M, Desrosiers RC (1985) Isolation of T cell tropic HTLV-III-like retrovirus from macaques. Science 228: 1201–1204

Davis GL, Hunter E (1987) A charged amino acid substitution within the transmembrane anchor of the Rous Sarcoma virus envelope glycoprotein affects surface expression but not intracellular transport. J Cell Biol 105: 1191–1203

Davis BR, Brightman BK, Chandy KG, Fan H (1987) Characterization of a preleukemic state induced by Moloney murine leukemia virus: Evidence for two infection events during leukemogenesis. PNAS USA 84: 4875–4879

De Boer GF (1975) Zwoegerziekte virus, the causative agent for progressive interstitial pneumonia (maedi) and meningo-leucoencephalitis (visna) in sheep. Res Vet Sci 18: 15–25

Deen KC, McDougal JS, Inacker R, Folena WG, Arthos J, Rosenberg J, Maddon PJ, Axel R, Sweet RW (1988) A soluble form of CD4 (T4) protein inhibits AIDS virus infection. Nature 331: 82–84

DeLarco J, Todaro GJ (1976) Membrane receptors for murine leukemia viruses: characterization using the purified viral envelope glycoprotein. Cell 8: 365–371

DesGroseillers L, Jolicoeur P (1984) Mapping the viral sequences conferring leukemogenicity and disease specificity in Moloney and amphotropic murine leukemia viruses. J Virol 52: 448–456

DesGroseillers L, Barrette M, Jolicoeur P (1984) Physical mapping of the paralysis-inducing determinant of a wild mouse ecotropic neurotropic retrovirus. J Virol 52: 356–363

Desrosiers RC (1988) Simian immunodeficiency viruses. Annu Rev Microbiol 42: 607–625

Desrosiers RC, Wyand MS, Kodama T, Ringler DJ, Arthur LO, Sehgal PK, Letvin NL, King NW, Daniel MD (1989) Vaccine protection against simian immunodeficiency virus infection. Proc Natl Acad Sci USA 86: 6353–6357

Dickson C, Eisenman R. Fan H. Hunter E, Teich N (1984a) Protein biosynthesis and assembly. Weiss R et al. (eds) Molecular biology of tumor viruses 2 edn. Cold Spring Harbor Laboratory, Cold Spring Harbor, pp 513–648

Dickson C, Peters G, Smith R, Brookes S (1984b) Tumorigenesis by mouse mammary tumor virus may involve provirus integration in a specific region of the mouse chromosome and activation of a cellular gene. Cancer Cells 2: 195–203

Doms RW, Helenius A (1986) Quaternary structure of influenza virus hemagglutinin after acid treatment. J Virol 60: 833–839

Donahue PR, Hoover EA, Beltz GA, Riedel N, Hirsch VM, Overbaugh J, Mullins JI (1988) Strong sequence conservation among horizontally transmissible, minimally pathogenic feline leukemia viruses. J Virol 62: 722–731

Dorner AJ, Coffin JM (1986) Determinants for receptor interaction and cell killing on the avian retrovirus glycoprotein gp85. Cell 45: 365–374

Dorner AJ, Stoye JP, Coffin JM (1985) Molecular basis of host range variation in avian retroviruses. J Virol 53: 32–39

Dresler S, Ruta M, Murray MJ, Kabat D (1979) Glycoprotein encoded by the Friend spleen focus-forming virus. J Virol 30: 564–575

Dubay J, Kong L, Kappes J, Shaw G, Hahn B, Hunter E (1988) Mutational analysis of the gp41 glycoprotein Abst IV int Conf on AIDS, Stockholm, Sweden p 1517

Dubois Dalcq M, Narayan O, Griffin DE (1979) Cell surface changes associated with maturation of visna virus in antibody-treated cell cultures. Virology 92: 353–366

Duff RG, Vogt PK (1969) Characteristics of two new avian tumor virus subgroup. Virology 39: 18–30

Durbin RK, Manning JS (1984) Coordination of cleavage of gag and env gene products of murine leukemia virus: implication regarding the mechanism of processing. Virology 134: 368–374

Earl PL, Moss B, Morrison RP, Wehrly K, Nishio J, Chesebro B (1986) T-lymphocyte priming and protection against Friend leukemia by vaccinia-retrovirus env gene recombinant. Science 234: 728–731

Einfeld D, Hunter E (1988) Oligomeric structure of a prototype retrovirus glycoprotein. Proc Natl Acad Sci USA 85: 8688–8692

Einfeld D, Hunter E (1989) Oligomeric structure of retroviral envelope glycoproteins. In: Air GM, Laver G (eds) Use of X-ray crystallography in the design of antiviral agents. Academic, New York pp 00–00

Elder JH, McGee JS, Alexander S (1986) Carbohydrate side chains of Rauscher leukemia virus envelope glycoproteins are not required to elicit a neutralizing antibody response. J Virol 57: 340–342

Ellis TM, Wilcox GE, Robinson WF (1987) Antigenic variation of caprine arthritis- encephalitics virus during persistent infection of goats. J Gen Virol 63: 3145–3152

Evans LH (1986) Characterization of polytropic MuLVs from three-week-old AKR/J mice. Virology 153: 122–136

Evans LH, Cloyd MW (1984) Generation of mink cell focus-forming viruses by friend murine leukemia virus: recombination with specific endogenous proviral sequences. J Virol 49: 772–781

Evans LH, Cloyd MW (1985) Friend and Moloney murine leukemia viruses specifically recombine with different endogenous sequences to generate mink cell focus-forming viruses. Proc Natl Acad Sci USA 82: 459–463

Evans LH, Malik FG (1987) Class II polytropic murine leukemia viruses (MuLVs) of AKR/J mice: possible role in the generation of class I oncogenic polytropic MuLVs. J Virol 61: 1882–1892

Famulari NG (1983) Murine leukemia viruses with recombinant env genes: a discussion of their role in leukemogenesis. Curr Top Microbiol Immunol 103: 75–108

Famulari NG, Cieplensky D (1984) A time-crouse study of MuLV env gene expression in the AKR thymus: qualitative and quantitative analysis of ecotropic and recombinant virus gene products. Virology 132: 282–291

Fauci A (1988) The human immunodeficiency virus: infectivity and mechanisms of pathogenesis. Science 239: 617

Fine D, Schochetman G (1978) Type D primate retroviruses: a review. Cancer Res 38: 3123–3139

Fine DL, Landon JC, Pienta RJ, Kubicek MT, Valerio MJ, Loeb WF, Chopra HC (1975) Responses of infant rhesus monkeys to inoculation with Mason-Pfizer monkey virus materials. JNCI 54: 651–658

Fisher AG, Collalti E, Ratner L, Gallo RC, Wong-Staal F (1985) A molecular clone of HTLV-III with biological activity. Nature 316: 262–265

Fisher AG, Ratner L, Mitsuya H, Marselle LM, Harper ME, Broder S, Gallo RC, Wong-Staal F (1986) Infectious mutants of HTLV-III with changes in the 3′ region and markedly reduced cytopathic effects. Science 233: 655–659

Fisher RA, Bertonis JM, Meier W, Johnson VA, Vostopoulos DS, Liu T, Tizard R, Walker BD, Hirsch MS, Schooley RT, Flavell RA (1988) HIV infection is blocked in vitro by recombinant soluble CD4. Nature 331: 76–78

Forrest D, Onions D, Lees G, Neil JC (1987) Altered structure and expression of c-myc in feline T-cell tumours. Virology 158: 194–205

Friedman-Kein AE, Laubenstein LJ, Rubinstein P, Buimovici-Klein E, Marmor M, Stahl R, Spigland I, Kim KS, Zolla-Pazner S (1982) Disseminated Kaposi's sarcoma in homosexual men. Ann Intern Med 96: 693–700

Gallaher WR (1987) Detection of a fusion peptide sequence in the transmembrane protein of human immunodeficiency virus. Cell 50: 327–328

Gallaher WR, Ball JM, Garry RF, Griffin MC, Montelaro RC (1989) A general model for the transmembrane proteins of HIV and other retroviruses. AIDS Res Hum Retroviruses 5: 431–440

Gallione CJ, Rose JK (1983) Nucleotide sequence of a cDNA clone encoding the entire glycoprotein from the New Jersey serotype of vesicular stomatitis virus. J Virol 46: 162–169

Gallo RC, Salahuddin SZ, Popovic M, Shearer GM, Kaplan M, Haynes BF, Palker TJ, Redfield R, Oleske J, Safai B, White G, Foster P, Markham PD (1984) Frequent detection and isolation of cytopathic retroviruses (HTLV-III) from patients with AIDS and at risk for AIDS. Science 224: 500–503

Gardner MB (1978) Type-C viruses of wild mice: characterization and natural history of amphotropic, ecotropic and xenotropic murine leukemia viruses. Curr Top Microbiol Immunol 79: 215–239

Gardner MB (1985) Retroviral spongiform polioencephalomyelopathy. Rev Infect Dis 7: 99–110

Garry RF, Gottlieb AA, Zuckerman KP, Pace JR, Frank TW, Bostick DA (1988) Cell surface effects of human immunodeficiency virus. Biosci Rep 8: 35–48

Gartner S, Markovits P, Markovitz DM, Kaplan MH, Gallo RC, Popovic M (1986) The role of mononuclear phagocytes in HTLV-III/LAV infection. Science 233: 215–219

Gazdar AF, Oie H, Lalley P, Moss WW, Minna JD (1977) Identification of mouse chromosomes required for murine leukemia virus replication. Cell 11: 949–956

Gebhardt A, Bosch JV, Ziemiecki A, Friis RR (1984) Rous srcoma virus p19 and gp35 can be chemically crosslinked to high molecular weight complexes: an insight into viral association. J Mol Biol 174: 297–317

Gelderblom HR, Hausmann EH, Ozel M, Pauli G, Koch MA (1987) Fine structure of human immunodeficiency virus (HIV) and immunolocalization of structural proteins. Virology 156: 171–176

Gessain A, Barin F, Vernant JC, Gout O, Maurs L, Calender A, De The G (1985) Antibodies to human T-lymphotropic virus type-1 in patients with tropical spastic paraparesis. Lancet II: 407–409

Gething MJ, Bye J, Skehel J, Waterfield M (1980) Cloning and DNA sequence of double-stranded copies of haemagglutinin genes from H2 and H3 strains elucidates antigenic shift and drift in human influenza virus. Nature 287: 301–306

Gething M, McCammon K, Sambrook J (1986) Expression of wild-type and mutant forms of influenza hemagglutinin: the role of folding in intracellular transport. Cell 46: 939–950

Geyer H, Holschbach C, Hunsmann G, Schneider J (1988) Carbohydrates of human immunodeficiency virus. Structures of oligosaccharides linked to the envelope glycoprotein 120. J Biol Chem 263: 11760–11767

Gisselbrecht S, Pozo F, Debre P, Hurot MA, Lacombe MJ, Levy JP (1978) Genetic control of sensitivity to Moloney-virus-induced leukemias in mice. I. Demonstration of multigenic control. Int J Cancer 21: 626–634

Gnann Jr JW, Nelson JA, Oldstone MB (1987) Fine mapping of an immunodominant domain in the transmembrane glycoprotein of human immunodeficiency virus. J Virol 61: 2639–2641

Gonda MA, Braun MJ, Carter SG, Kost TA, Bess Jr. JW, Arthur LO, Van Der Maaten MJ (1987) Characterization and molecular cloning of a bovine lentivirus related to human immunodeficiency virus. Nature 330: 388–391

Gottlieb MS, Schroff R, Schanker HM, Weisman JD, Fan PT, Worlf RA, Saxon A (1981) Pneumocystis carinii pneumonia and mucosal candidiasis in previously healthy homosexual men. Evidence of a new acquired cellular immunodeficiency. N Engl J Med 305: 1425–1431

Goudsmit J, Debouck C, Meloen RH, Smit L, Bakker M, Asher DM, Wolff AV, Gibbs CJ, Gajdusek DC (1988a) Human immunodeficiency virus type 1 neutralization epitope with conserved architecture elicits early type-specific antibodies in experimentally infected chimpanzees. Proc Natl Acad Sci USA 85: 4478–4482

Goudsmit J, Thiriart C, Smit L, Bruck C, Gibbs CJ (1988b) Temporal development of cross-neutralization between HTLV-III B and HTLV-III RF in experimentally infected chimpanzees. Vaccine 6: 229–32

Green N, Hiai H, Elder JH, Schwartz RS, Khiroya RH, Thomas CY, Tsichlis PN, Coffin JM (1980) Expression leukemogenic recombinant viruses associated with a recessive gene in HRS/J mice. J Exp Med 152: 249–264

Gruters RA, Neefjes JJ, Tersmette M, de GR, Tulp A, Huisman HG, Miedema F, Ploegh HL (1987) Interference with HIV-induced syncytium formation and viral infectivity by inhibitors of trimming glucosidase. Nature 330: 74–77

Guyader M, Emerman M, Sonigo P, Clavel F, Montagnier L, Alizon M (1987) Genome organization and transactivation of the human immunodeficiency virus type 2. Nature 326: 662–669

Haase AT (1975) The slow infection caused by visna virus. Curr Top Microbiol Immunol 72: 101–156

Haase AT (1986) Pathogenesis of lentivirus infections. Nature 322: 130–136

Haase AT, Stowring L, Narayan O, Griffin D, Price DL (1977) The slow and persistent infection caused by visna virus. The role of lysogeny. Science 1954: 175

Haffar OK, Dowbenko DJ, Berman PW (1988) Topogenic analysis of the human immunodeficiency virus type 1 envelope glycoprotein, gp 160, in microsomal membranes. J Cell Biol 107:1677–1687

Hahn BH, Gonda MA, Shaw GM, Popovic M, Hoxie JA, Gallo RC, Wong-Staal F (1985) Genomic diversity of the acquired immune deficiency syndrome virus HTLV-III: different viruses exhibit greatest divergence in their envelope genes. Proc Natl Acad Sci USA 82: 4813–4817

Hahn BH, Shaw GM, Taylor ME, Redfield RR, Markham PD, Salahuddin SZ, Wong-Staal F, Gallo RC, Parks ES, Parks WP (1986) Genetic variation in HTLV-III/LAV over time in patients with AIDS or at risk for AIDS. Science 232: 1548–1553

Halpern MS, Ewert DL, Flores LJ, Crittenden LB (1983) The influence of the ev 3 locus on the inductibility of serum antibody reactivity for envelope glycoprotein group-specific determinants. Virology 128: 502–504

Hanafusa T, Hanafusa H, Miyamoto T (1970) Recovery of a new virus from apparently normal cells by infection with avian tumor viruses. Proc Natl Acad Sci USA 67: 1797–1803

Hankins WD, Troxler D (1980) Polycythemia and anemia inducing erythroleukemia viruses exhibit differential erythroid transforming effects in vitro. Cell 22: 693–699

Hannink M, Donoghue DJ (1984) Requirement for a signal sequence in biological expression of the v-sis oncogene. Science 312: 1197–1199

Hardwick JM, Shaw KES, Wills JW, Hunter E (1986) Amino-terminal deletion mutants of the Rous sarcoma virus glycoprotein do not block signal peptide cleavage but can block intracellular transport. J Cell Biol 103: 829–838

Harper ME, Marselle LM, Gallo RC, Wong-Staal F (1986) Detection of lymphocytes expressing human T-lymphotropci virus type III in lymph nodes and peripheral blood from infected individuals by in situ hybridization. Proc Natl Acad Sci USA 83: 772–776

Harter DH, Choppin PW (1967a) Cell-fusing activity of visna virus particles. Virology 31: 279–288

Harter DH, Choppin PW (1967b) Plaque assay of visna virus using a secondary cellular overlay as an indicator. Virology 31: 176–178

Harter DH, Hsu KC, Rose HM (1968) Multiplication of visna virus in bovine and porcine cell lines. Proc Soc Exp Biol Med 129: 295–300

Hartley JW, Rowe WP (1975) Clonal cell lines from a feral mouse embryo which lack host-range restriction for murine leukemia viruses. Virology 65: 138–134

Hartley JW, Yetter RA, Morse HC III (1983) A mouse gene on chromosome 5 that restricts infectivity of mink cell focus-forming recombinant murine leukemia viruses. J Exp Med 158: 16–24

Hauser SL, Aubert C, Burks JS, Kerr C, Lyon-Caen O, de The G, Brahic M (1986) Analysis of human T-lymphotropic virus sequences in multiple sclerosis tissue. Nature 322: 176–177

Hayward WS, Hanafusa H (1975) Recombination between endogenous and exogenous RNA tumor virus genes as analyzed by nucleic acid hybridization. J Virol 15: 1367–1377

Herr W, Gilbert W (1983) Somatically acquired recombinant murine leukemia proviruses in thymic leukemias of AKR/J mice. J Virol 46: 70–82

Herr W, Gilbert W (1984) Free and integrated recombinant murine leukemia virus DNAs appear in preleukemic thymuses of AKR/J mice. J Virol 50: 155–162

Hikins J, van der Zeijst B, Buijs F, Kroezen V, Bleumink N, Hilgers J (1983) Identification of a cellular receptor for mouse mammary tumor virus and mapping of its gene to chromosome 16. J Virol 45: 140–147

Hirsch V, Riedel N, Mullins JI (1987) The genome organization of STLV-3 is similar to that of the AIDS virus except for a truncated transmembrane protein. Cell 49: 307–319

Hirsch VM, Olmsted RA, Murphey-Corb M, Purcell RH, Johnson PR (1989) An African primate lentivirus (SIVsm) closely related to HIV-2. Nature 339: 389–392

Ho DD, Sarngadharan MG, Hirsch MS, Schooley RT, Rota TR, Kennedy RC, Chanh TC, Sato VL (1987) Human immunodeficiency virus neutralizing antibodies recognize several conserved domains on the envelope glycoproteins. J Virol 61: 2024–2028

Ho DD, Kaplan JC, Rackauskas IE, Gurney ME (1988) Second conserved domain of gp120 is important for HIV infectivity and antibody neutralization. Science 239: 1021–1023

Holland CA, Hartley JW, Rowe WP, Hopkins N (1985a) At least four viral genes contribute to the leukemogenicity of murine retrovirus MCF 247 in AKR mice. J Virol 53: 158–165

Holland CA, Wozney J, Chatis PA, Hopkins N, Hartley JW (1985b) Construction of recombinants between molecular clones of murine retrovirus MCF 247 and Akv: determinant of an in vitro host range property that maps in the long terminal repeat. J Virol 53: 152–157

Hoover EA, Kociba GJ, Hardy WD Jr, Yohn DS (1974) Erythroid hypoplasia in cats inoculated with feline leukemia virus. J Nat Cancer Inst 53: 1271–1276

Horoszewicz JS, Leong SS, Carter WA (1975) Friend leukemia: rapid development of erythropoietin-independent hematopoietic precursors. JNCI 54: 265–267

Hoshino H, Tanaker H, Miwa M, Okada H (1984) Human T-cell leukaemia virus is not lysed by human serum. Nature 310: 324–325

Hoxie JA, Alpers JD, Radkowski J, Huebner K, Haggarty BS, Cedarbaum AJ, Reed JC (1986) Alterations in T4 (CD4) protein and mRNA synthesis in cells infected with HIV. Science 234: 1123

Hu SL, Fultz PN, McClure HM, Eichberg JW, Thomas EK, Zarling J, Singhal MC, Kosowski SG, Swenson RB, Anderson DC, Todaro G (1987) Effect of immunization with a vaccinia-HIV env recombinant on HIV infection of chimpanzees. Nature 328: 721–723

Huebner RJ, Gilden RV, Toni R, Hill RW, Trimmer RW, Fish DC, Sass B (1976) Prevention of spontaneous leukemia in AKR mice by type-specific immunosuppression of endogenous ecotropic virogenes. Proc Natl Acad Sci USA 73: 4633–4635

Hunsmann G, Schneider J, Schulz A (1981) Immunoprevention of Friend virus-induced erythroleukemia by vaccination with viral envelope glycoprotein complexes. Virology 113: 602–612

Hunt LA, Wright SE, Etchinson JR, Summers DF (1979) Oligosaccharide chains of avian RNA tumor virus glycoproteins contain heterogeneous oligomannosyl cores. J Virol 29: 336–343

Hunter E (1988) Membrane insertion and transport of viral glycoproteins: a mutational analysis. In: Das RC, Robbin PW (ed) Protein transfer and organelle biogenesis. Academic, New York, pp 109–158

Hunter E, Bhown AS, Bennett JC (1978) Amino-terminal amino acid sequence of the major structural polypeptides of avian retroviruses: sequence homology between reticuloendotheliosis virus p30 and p30s of mammalian retroviruses. Proc Natl Acad Sci USA 75: 2708–2712

Hunter E, Hill E, Hardwick M, Bhown A, Schwartz D, Tizard R (1983) Complete sequence of the Rous sarcoma virus env gene: identification of structural and functional regions of its product. J Virol 46: 920–936

Huso DL, Narayan O, Hart GW (1988) Sialic acids on the surface of caprine arthritis-encephalitis virus define the biological properties of the virus. J Virol 62: 1974–1980

Hussain KA, Issel CJ, Schnorr KL, Rwambo PM, Montelaro RC (1987) Antigenic analysis of equine infectious anemia virus (EIAV) variants by using monoclonal antibodies: epitopes of glycoprotein gp90 of EIAV stimulate neutralizing antibodies. J Virol 61: 2956–2961

Hussey RE, Richardson NE, Kowalski M, Brown NR, Chang HC, Siliciano RF, Dorfman T, Walker B, Sodroski J, Reinherz EL (1988) A soluble CD4 protein selectively inhibits HIV replication and syncytium formation. Nature 331: 78–81

Ikeda H, Laigret F, Martin MA, Repaske R (1985) Characterization of a molecularly cloned retroviral sequence associaued with FV-4 resistance. J Virol 55: 768–777

Ishimoto A, Hartley JW, Rowe WP (1977) Detection and quantitation of phenotypically mixed viruses: mixing of ecotropic and xenotropic murine leukemia viruses. Virology 81: 263–269

Ishimoto A, Adachi A, Sakai K, Yorifugi T, Tsuruta S (1981) Rapid emergence of mink cell focus-forming (MCF) virus in various mice infected with NB-tropic Friend virus. Virology 113: 644–655

Jameson BA, Rao PE, Kong LI, Hahn BH, Shaw GM, Hood LE, Kent SB (1988) Location and chemical synthesis of a binding site for HIV-1 on the CD4 protein. Science 240: 1335–1339

Jarrett O, Hardy WD, Golder MC, Hay D (1978). The frequency of occurrence of feline leukemia virus subgroups in cats. Int J Cancer 21: 334–337

Jarrett O, Golder MC, Toth S, Onions DE, Stewart MF (1984) Interaction between feline leukaemia virus subgroups in the pathogenesis of erythroid hypoplasia. Int J Cancer 34: 283–288

Jenkins NA, Copeland NG, Taylor BA, Lee BK (1982) Organization, distribution, and stability of endogenous ecotropic murine leukemia virus DNA sequences in chromosomes of mus musculus. J Virol 43: 26–36

Johnson PA, Rosner MR (1986) Characterization of Murine-Specific Leukemia Virus Receptor from L Cells. J Virol 58: 900–908

Joho RH, Billeter MA, Weissman C (1975) Mapping of biological functions on RNA of avian tumor viruses: location of regions required for transformation and determining host range. Proc Natl Acad Sci USA 72: 4772–5776

Jolicoeur P, DesGroseillers L (1985) Neurotropic Cas-BR-E murine leukemia virus harbors several determinants of leukemogenicity mapping in different regions of the genome. J Virol 56: 639–643

Jones KS, Ruscetti S, Lilly F (1988) Loss of pathogenicity of spleen focus-forming virus after pseudotyping with AKV. J Virol 62: 511–518

Kalyanaraman VS, Sarngadharan MG, Robert-Guroff M, Miyoshi I, Blayney D, Golde D, Gallo RC (1982) A new subtype of human T-cell leukemia virus (HTLV-II) associated with a T-cell variant of hairy cell leukemia. Science 218: 571–573

Kan NC, Baluda MA, Papas T (1985) Sites of recombination between the transforming gene of avian myeloblastosis virus and its helper virus. Virology 145: 323–329

Katoh I, Yoshinaka Y, Rein A, Shibuya M, Odaka T, Oroszlan S (1985) Murine leukemia virus maturation: protease region required for conversion from "immature" to "mature" core form and for virus infectivity. Virology 145: 280–292

Kawashima K, Ikeda H, Hartley JW, Stockert E, Rowe WP, Old LJ (1976) Changes in expression of murine leukemia virus antigens and production of xenotropic virus in the late preleukemic period in AKR mice. Proc Natl Acad Sci USA 73: 4680–4684

Kennedy RC, Eklund CM, Lopez C, Hadlow WJ (1968) Isolation of a virus from lungs of Montana sheep affected with progressive penumonia. Virology 35: 483–484

Kennedy-Stoskopf S, Narayan O (1986) Neutralizing antibodies to visna lentivirus: Mechanism of action and possible role in virus persistence. J Virol 59: 37–44

Khan AS, Laigret F, Rodi CP (1987) Expression of mink cell focus-forming murine leukemia virus-related transcripts in AKR mice. J Virol 61: 876–882

Klasse PJ, Pipkorn R, Blomberg J (1988) Presence of antibodies to a putatively immunosuppressive part of human immunodeficiency virus (HIV) envelope glycoprotein gp41 is strongly associated with health among HIV-positive subjects. Proc Natl Acad Sci USA 85: 5225–5229

Klatzmann D, Champagne E, Chamaret S, Gruest J, Guetard D, Hercend T, Gluckman JC, Montagnier L (1984) T-lymphocyte T4 molecule behaves as the receptor for human retrovirus LAV. Nature 312: 767–768

Klevjer-Anderson P, McGuire TC (1982) Neutralizing antibody response of rabbits and goats to caprine arthritis-encephalitis virus. Infect Immun 38: 455–461

Kobayashi K, Kono Y (1967) Propagation and titration of equine infectious anemia virus in horse leukocyte culture. Natl Inst Anim Health Q 7: 8–20

Koch W, Zimmermann W, Oliff A, Friedrich R (1984) Molecular analysis of the envelope gene and long terminal repeat of Friend mink cell focus-inducing virus: implications for the functions of these sequences. J Virol 49: 828–840

Kong LI, Lee SW, Kappes JC, Parkin JS, Decker D, Hoxie JA, Hahn BH, Shaw GM (1988) West African HIV-2-related human retrovirus with attenuated cytopathicity. Science 240: 1525–1529

Kono Y, Kobayashi K, Fukunaga Y (1973) Antigenic drift of equine infectious anemia virus in chronically infected horses. Arch Gesamte Virusforsch 41: 1–40

Koprowski H, DeFreitas EC, Harper ME, Sandberg-Wollhaim M, Sheremata WA, Robert-Guroff M, Saxinger CW, Feinberg MB, Wong-Staal F, Gallo RC (1985) Multiple sclerosis and human T-cell lymphotropic retroviruses. Nature 318: 154–160

Kornfeld R, Kornfeld S (1985) Assembly of asparagine-linked oligo-saccharides. Annu Rev Biochem 54: 631–664

Kowalski M, Potz J, Basiripour L, Dorfman T, Goh WC, Terwilliger E, Dayton A, Rosen C, Haseltine W, Sodroski J (1987) Functional regions of the envelope glycoprotein of human immunodeficiency virus type 1. Science 237: 1351–1355

Koyanagi Y, Miles S, Mitsuyasu RT, Merrill JE, Vinters HV, Chen ISY (1987) Dual infection of the central nervous system by AIDS viruses with distinct cellular tropisms. Science 236: 819–822

Kozak CA (1983) Genetic mapping of a mouse chromosomal locus required for mink cell focus-forming virus replication. J Virol 48: 300–303

Kozak CA (1985) Susceptibility of wild mouse cells to exogenous infection with xenotropic leukemia viruses: control by a single dominant locus on chromosome 1. J Virol 55: 690–695

Kozak CA, O'Neill RR (1987) Diverse wild mouse origins of xenotropic, mink cell focus-forming, and two types of ecotropic proviral genes. J Virol 61: 3082–3088

Kozak CA, Gromet NJ, Ikeda H, Buckler CE (1984) A unique sequence related to the ecotropic murine leukemia virus is associated with the Fv-4 resistance gene. Proc Natl Acad Sci USA 81: 834–837

Kreis TE, Lodish HF (1986) Oligomerization is essential for transport of Vesicular stomatitis virus glycoprotein to the cell surface. Cell 46: 929–937

Kritchbaum-Stenger K, Poiesz BJ, Keller P, Ehrlich G, Gavalchin J, Davis B, Moore J (1987) Specific adsorption of HTLV-1 to various target human and animal cells. Blood 70: 1303–1311

Lai MMC, Rasheed S, Shimizu CS, Gardner MB (1982). Genomic characterization of a highly oncogenic env gene recombinant between amphotropic retrovirus of wild mouse and endogenous xenotropic virus of NIH Swiss mouse. Virology 117: 262–266

Laigret F, Repaske R, Boulukos K, Rabson AB, Khan AS (1988) Potential progenitor sequences of mink cell focus-forming (MCF) murine leukemia viruses: ecotropic, xenotropic, and MCF-related viral RNAs are detected concurrently in thymus tissues of AKR mice. J Virol 62: 376–386

Landau NR, Warton M, Littman DR (1988) The envelope glycoprotein of the human immunodeficiency virus binds to the immunoglobulin-like domian of CD4. Nature 334: 159–162

Lander MR, Chattopadhyay SK (1984) A Mus dunni cell line that lacks sequences closely related to endogenous murine leukemia viruses and can be infected by ecotropic, amphotropic, xenotropic, and mink cell focus-forming viruses. J Virol 52: 695–698

Lando Z, Sarin P, Megson M, Greene WC, Waldman TA, Gallo RC, Broder S (1983) Association of human T-cell leukemia/lymphoma virus with a Tac antigen marker for the human T-cell growth factor receptor. Nature 305: 733–766

Lanzavecchia A, Roosnek E, Gregory T, Berman P, Abrignani S (1988) T-cells can present antigens such as HIV gp120 targeted to their own surface molecules. Nature 334: 530–532

Lasky LA, Groopman JE, Fennie CW, Benz PM, Capon DJ, Dowbenko DJ, Nakamura GR, Nunes WM, Renz ME, Berman PW (1986) Neutralization of the AIDS retrovirus by antibodies to a recombinant envelope glycoprotein. Science 233: 209–212

Lasky LA, Nakamura G, Smith DH, Fennie C, Shimasaki C, Patzer E, Berman P, Gregory T, Capon DJ (1987) Delineation of a region of the human immunodeficiency virus type 1 gp120 glycoprotein critical for interaction with the CD4 receptor. Cell 50: 975–985

Leamnson RN, Halpern MS (1976) Subunit structure of the glycoprotein complex of avian tumor virus. J Virol 18: 956–968

Leamnson RN, Shander MHM, Halpern MD (1977) A structural protein complex in Moloney leukemia virus. Virology 76: 437–439

Lee H, Swanson P, Shorty VS, Zack JA, Rosenblatt JD, Chen I S-Y (1989) High rate of HTLV-II infection in seropositive IV drug abusers in New Orleans. Science 244: 471–475

Levy LS, Gardner MB, Casey JW (1984a) Isolation of a feline leukaemia provirus containing the oncogene *myc* from a feline lymphosarcoma. Nature 308: 853–856

Levy JA, Hoffman AD, Kramer SM, Landis JA, Shimabukuro JM, Oshiro LS (1984b) Isolation of lymphocytopathic retroviruses from San Francisco patients with AIDS. Science 225: 840–842

Levy JA, Cheng MC, Dina D, Luciw PA (1986) AIDS retrovirus (ARV-2) clone replicates in transfected human and animal fibroblasts. Science 232: 998–1001

Li J-P, Bestwick RK, Machida C, Kabat D (1986) Role of a membrane glycoprotein in Friend virus erythroleukemia: nucleotide sequences of nonleukemogenic mutant and spontaneous revertant viruses. J Virol 57: 534–538

Li J-P, Bestwick RK, Spiro C, Kabat D (1987) The membrane glycoprotein of Friend spleen focus-forming virus: evidence that the cell surface component is required for pathogenesis and that it binds to a receptor. J Virol 61: 2782–2792

Li Y, Naidu Y, Fultz P, Daniel MD, Desrosiers RC (1989) An African primate lentivirus (SIVsm) closely related to HIV-2. Nature 339: 389–392

Liao S, Axelrad AA (1975) Erythropoietin-independent erythroid colony formation *in vitro* by hemopoietic cells of mice infected with Friend virus. Int J Cancer 15: 467–482

Lifson J, Coutre S, Huang E, Engleman E (1986) Role of envelope glycoprotein carbohydrate in human immunodeficiency virus (HIV) infectivity and virus-induced cell fusion. J Exp Med 164: 2101–2106

Lifson JD, Feinberg MB, Reyes GR, Rabin L, Banapour B, Chakrabarti S, Moss B, Wong SF, Steimer KS, Engleman EG (1986) Induction of CD4-dependent cell fusion by the HTLV-III/LAV envelope glycoprotein. Nature 323: 725–728

Linemeyer DL, Menke JG, Ruscetti SK, Evans LH, Scolnick EM (1982) Envelope gene sequences which encode the gp52 protein of spleen focus-forming virus are required for the induction of erythroid cell proliferation. J Virol 43: 223–233

Linsley PS, Ledbetter JA, Kinney TE, Hu SL (1988) Effects of anti-gp120 monoclonal antibodies on CD4 receptor binding by the env protein of human immunodeficiency virus type 1. J Virol 62: 3695–3702

Lung ML, Hering C, Hartley JW, Rowe WP, Hopkins N (1980) Analysis of the genomes of mink cell focus-inducing murine type-C viruses: a progress report. Cold Spring Harbor Symp Quant Biol 44: 1269–1274

Lung ML, Hartley JW, Rowe WP, Hopkins NH (1983) Large RNase T-resistant oligonucleotides encoding p15E and the U3 region of the long terminal repeat distinguish two biological classes of mink cell focus-forming type C viruses of inbred mice. N Virol 45: 275–290

Lutley R, Petursson G, Palsson PA, Georgsson G, Klein J, Nathanson N (1983) Antigenic drift in visna. Virus variation during long term infection of Islandic sheep. J Gen Virol 64: 1433–1440

Lyerly HK, Matthews TJ, Langlois AJ, Bolognesi DP, Weinhold KJ (1987) Human T-cell lymphotropic virus IIIB glycoprotein (gp120) bound to CD4 determinants on normal lymphocytes and expressed by infected cells serves as target for immune attack. Proc Natl Acad Sci USA 84: 4601–4605

Machida CA, Bestwick RK, Kabat D (1984) Reduced leukemogenicity caused by mutations in the membrane glycoprotein gene of Rauscher spleen focus-forming virus. J Virol 49: 394–402

Machida CA, Bestwick RK, Kabat D (1985) A weakly pathogenic Rauscher spleen focus-forming virus mutant that lacks the carboxyl-terminal membrane anchor of its envelope glycoprotein. J Virol 53: 990–993

Mackey L, Jarrett W, Jarrett O, Laird H (1975) Anemia associated with feline leukemia infection in cats. JNCI 54: 209–217

Maddon PJ, Littman DR, Godfrey M, Maddon DE, Chess L, Axel R (1985) The isolation and nucleotide sequence of a cDNA encoding the T-cell surface protein T4: a new member of the immunoglobulin gene family. Cell 42: 93–104

Maddon PJ, Dalgleish AG, McDougal JS, Clapham PR, Weiss RA, Axel R (1986) The T4 gene encodes the AIDS virus receptor and is expressed in the immune system and the brain. Cell 47: 333–348

Maddon PJ, McDougal JS, Clapham PR, Dalgleish AG, Jamal S, Weiss RA, Axel R (1988) HIV infection does not require endocytosis of its receptor, CD4. Cell 54: 865–874

Majors JE, Varmus HE (1983) Nucleotide sequencing of an apparent proviral copy of env mRNA defines determinants of expression of the mouse mammary tumor virus env gene. J Virol 47: 495–504

Malmquist WA, Barnett D, Becvar CS (1973) Production of equine infectious anemia antigen in a persistently infected cell line. Arch Gesamte Virusforsch 42: 361–370

Marx PA, Maul DH, Osborn KG, Lerche NW, Moody P, Lowenstine LJ, Henrickson RV, Arthur LO, Gilden RV, Gravell M, London WT, Sever JL, Levy JA, Munn RJ, Gardner MB (1984) Simian AIDS: isolation of a type D retrovirus and transmission of the disease. :Science 223: 1083–1086

Marx PA, Bryant ML, Osborn KG et al. (1985) Isolation of a new serotype of simian acquired immune deficiency syndrome type D retrovirus from Celebes black macaques (Macaca nigra) with immune deficiency and retroperitoneal fibromatosis. J Virol 56: 571–578

Marx PA, Pedersen NC, Lerche NW, Osborn KG, Lowenstine LJ, Lackner AA, Maul DH, Kwang HS, Kluge JD, Zaiss CP, Sharpe V, Spinner A, Gardner M (1986) Prevention of simian acquired immune deficiency syndrome with a formalin-inactivated type D retrovirus vaccine. J Virol 60: 431–435

Massey RJ, Arthur LO, Nowinski RC, Schochetman G (1980) Monoclonal antibodies identify individual determinants on mouse mammary tumor virus glycoprotein gp52 with group, class, or type specificity. J Virol 34: 635–643

Matsushita S, Robert GM, Rusche J, Koito A, Hattori T, Hoshino H, Javaherian K, Takatsuki K, Putney S (1988) Characterization of a human immunodeficiency virus neutralizing monoclonal antibody and mapping of the neutralizing epitope. J Virol 62: 2107–2114

Matthews TJ, Weinhold KJ, Lyerly HK, Langlois AJ, Wigzell H, Bolognesi DP (1987) Interaction between the human T-cell lymphotropic virus type IIIb envelope glycoprotein gp120 and the surface antigen CD4: role of carbohydrate in binding and cell fusion. Proc Natl Acad Sci USA 84: 5424–5428

Mayyasi SA, Moloney JB (1967) Induced resistance of mice to a lymphoid strain of leukemia virus. Cancer 20: 1124–1130

McAtee FJ, Portis JL (1985) Monoclonal antibodies specific for wild mouse neurotropic retrovirus: detection of comparable levels of virus replication in mouse strains susceptible and resistant to paralytic disease. J Virol 56: 1018–1022

McCarter JA, Ball JK, Frei JV (1977) Lower limb paralysis induced in mice by a temperature-sensitive mutant of Moloney leukemia virus. JNCI 59: 179–183

McClure MO, Sattentau QJ, Beverly PCL, Hearn JP, Fitzgerald AK, Zuckerman AJ, Weiss RA (1987) HIV infection of primate lymphocytes and conservation of the CD4 receptor. Nature 330: 487–489

McClure MO, Marsh M, Weiss RA (1988) Human immunodeficiency virus infection of CD4-bearing cells occurs by a pH-independent mechanism. EMBO J 7: 513–518

McClure MO, Sommerfelt M, Marsh M, Weiss RA (1990) On the pH-dependence of mammalian retroviral infection. Virology, in press

McCune JM, Rabin LB, Feinberg MB, Lieberman M, Kosek JC, Reyes GR, Weissman IL (1988) Endoproteolytic cleavage of gp160 is required for the activation of human immunodeficiency virus. Cell 53: 55–67

McDougal JS, Mawie A, Cort SP, Nicholson JKA, Cross GD, Sheppler-Campbell JA, Hicks D, Sligh J (1985) Cellular tropism of the human retrovirus HTLV-III/LAV. I. Role of T-cell activation and expression of the T4 antigen. J Immunol 135: 3151–3162

McDougal JS, Kennedy MS, Sligh JM, Cort SP, Mawle A, Nicholson JK (1986a) Binding of HTLV-III/LAV to T4 + T-cells by a complex of the 110K viral protein and the T4 molecule. Science 231: 382–385

McDougal JS, Nicholson JK, Cross GD, Cort SP, Kennedy MS, Mawle AC (1986b) Binding of the human retrovirus HTLV-III/LAV/ARV/HIV to the CD4 (T4) molecule: conformation dependence, epitope mapping, antibody inhibition, and potential for idiotypic mimicry. J Immunol 137: 2937–2944

McGuire TC, Norton LK, O'Rourke KI, Cheevers WP (1988) Antigenic variation of neutralization-sensitive epitopes of caprine arthritis-encephalitis lentivirus during persistent arthritis. J Virol 62: 3488–3492

Meyer DI (1985) Signal recognition particle SRP does not mediate a translational arrest of nascent secretory proteins in mammalian cell-free system. EMBO J 4: 2031–2033

Modrow S, Hahn BH, Shaw GM, Gallo RC, Wong SF, Wolf H (1987) Computer-assisted analysis of envelope protein sequences of seven human immunodeficiency virus isolates: prediction of antigenic epitopes in conserved and variable regions. J Virol 61: 570–578

Moldow CF, Reynolds FH Jr, Lake J, Lundberg K, Stephenson JR (1979) Avian sarcoma virus envelope glycoprotein (gp85) specifically binds chick embryo fibroblasts. Virology 97: 448–453

Montefiori DC, Robinson WJ, Mitchell WM (1988) Role of protein N-glycosylation in pathogenesis of human immunodeficiency virus type 1. Proc Natl Acad Sci USA 85: 9248–9252

Montelaro RC, Parekh B, Orrego A, Issel CJ (1984) Antigenic variation during persistent infection by equine infectious anemia virus, a retrovirus. J Biol Chem 259: 10539–10544

Moreau-Gachelin F, Tavitian A, Tambourin P (1988) Spi-1 is a putative oncogene in virally induced murine erythroleukemias. Nature 331: 277–280

Mucenski ML, Taylor BA, Jenkins NA, Copeland NG (1986) AKXD recombinant inbred strains: models for studying the molecular genetic basis of murine lymphomas. Mol Cell Biol 6: 4236–4243

Mucenski ML, Taylor BA, Copeland NG, Jenkins NA (1987) Characterization of somatically acquired ecotropic and mink cell focus-forming viruses in lymphomas of AKXD recombinant inbred mice. J Virol 61: 2929–2933

Mucenski ML, Taylor BA, Ihle JN, Hartley JW, Morse HC III, Jenkins NA, Copeland NG (1988) Identification of a common ecotropic viral integration site, Evi-1, in the DNA of AKXD murine myeloid tumors. Mol Cell Biol 8: 301–308

Mullins JI, Brody DS, Binari RC Jr, Cotter SM (1984) Viral transduction of c-myc gene in naturally occurring feline leukaemias. Nature 308: 856–858

Mullins J, Chen C, Hoover EA (1986) Disease-specific and tissue-specific production of unintegrated feline leukaemia virus variant DNA in feline AIDS. Nature 319: 333–336

Nagy K, Clapham P, Cheinsong-Popov R, Weiss RA (1983) Human T-cell leukemia virus type 1: Induction of syncytia and inhibition of patients' sera. Int J Cancer 32: 321–328

Nagy K, Weiss RA, Clapham P, Cheingsong-Popov R (1984) Biological properties of human T-cell leukemia virus envelope antigens. In: Gallo RC (ed) Human T-cell leukemia/lymphoma virus. Cold Spring Harbor Laboratory, Cold Spring Harbor, pp 121–131

Narayan O, Griffin DE, Clements JE (1978) Virus mutation during 'slow infection'. Temporal development and characterization of mutants of visna virus recovered from sheep. J Gen Virol 41: 343–352

Narayan O, Clements JE, Strandberg JD, Cork LC, Griffin DE (1980) Biological characterization of the virus causing leukoencephalitis and arthritis in goats. J Gen Virol 59: 69–79

Narayan O, Sheffer D, Griffin DE, Clements JE, Hess J (1984) Lack of neutralizing antibodies to caprine arthritis-encephalitis lentivirus in persistently infected goats can be overcome by immunization with inactivated mycobacterium tuberculosis. J Virol 49: 349–355

Neil JC, Hughes D, McFarlane R, Wilkie NM, Onions DE, Lees G, Jarrett O (1984) Transduction and rearrangement of the myc gene by feline leukaemia virus in naturally occurring T-cell leukaemias. Nature 308: 814–820

Niman HL, Elder JH (1982) Structural analysis of Rauscher virus Gp70 using monoclonal antibodies: sites of antigenicity and P15(E) linkage. Virology 123: 187–205

Nobis P, Jaenisch R (1980) Passive immunotherapy prevents expression of endogenous Moloney virus and amplification of proviral DNA in BALB/Mo mice. Proc Natl Acad Sci USA 77: 3677–3681

Nusse R, Varmus HE (1982) Many tumors induced by the mouse mammary tumor virus contain a provirus integrated in the same region of the host genome. Cell 31: 99–109

O'Donnell PV, Stockert E, Obata Y, Old LJ (1981) Leukemogenic properties of AKR dualtropic (MCF) viruses: amplification of murine leukemia virus-related antigens on thymocytes and acceleration of leukemia development in AKR mice. Virology 112: 548–563

O'Neill RR, Buckler CE, Theodore TS, Martin MA, Repaske R (1985) Envelope and long terminal repeat sequences of a cloned infectious NZB xenotropic murine leukemia virus. J Virol 53: 100–106

O'Neill RR, Khan AS, Hoggan MD, Hartley JW, Martin MA, Repaske R (1986) Specific hybridization probes demonstrate fewer xenotropic than mink cell focus-forming murine leukemia virus env-related sequences in DNAs from inbred laboratory mice. J Virol 58: 359–366

O'Neill RR, Hartley JW, Repaske R, Kozak CA (1987) Amphotropic proviral envelope sequences are absent from the Mus germ line. J Virol 61: 2225–2231

Oldstone MBA, Jensen F, Elder J, Dixon FJ, Lampert PW (1983) Pathogenesis of the slow disease of the central nervous system associated with wild mouse virus III. Role of input virus and MCF recombinants in disease. Virology 128: 154–165

Oliff A, Ruscetti S, Douglass EC, Scolnick E (1981) Isolation of transplantable erythroleukemia cells from mice infected with helper-independent Friend murine leukemia virus. Blood 58: 244, 252–254

Oliff A, Collins L, Mirenda C (1983) Molecular cloning of Friend mink cell focus-inducing virus: identification of mink cell focus-inducing virus-like messages in normal and transformed cells. J Virol 48: 542–546

Oliff A, Signorelli K, Collins L (1984) The envelope gene and long terminal repeat sequences contribute to the pathogenic phenotype of helper-independent Friend viruses. J Virol 51: 788–794

Olsen R (1985) An innovative technique produces a feline leukemia virus vaccine. Vet Med Jan 61–64

Oroszlan S, Barbacid M, Copeland T, Aaronson SA, Gilden RV (1981) Chemical and immunological characterization of the major structural protein (p28) of MMC-1, a rhesus monkey endogenous type C virus: homology with the major structural protein of avian reticuloendotheliosis virus. J Virol 39: 845–854

Osterhaus A, Weijer K, Uytdehaag F, Jarrett O, Sundquist B, Morein B (1985) Induction of protective immune response in cats by vaccination with feline leukemia virus iscom. J Immunol 135: 591–596

Ott D, Friedrich R, Rein A (1990) Sequence analysis of amphotropic and 10A1 murine leukemia viruses: close relationship to mink cell focus-inducing viruses. J Virol 64: 757–766

Overbaugh J, Donahue P, Quackenbush S, Hoover EA, Mullins JI (1988b) Molecular cloning of a feline leukemia virus that induces fatal immunodeficiency disease in cats. Science 239: 906–910

Overbaugh J, Riedel N, Hoover EA, Mullins JI (1988a) Transduction of endogenous envelope genes by feline leukaemia virus in vitro. Nature 332: 731–734

Palker TJ, Clark ME, Langlois AJ, Matthews TJ, Weinhold KJ, Randall RR, Bolognesi DP, Haynes BF (1988) Type-specific neutralization of the human immunodeficiency virus with antibodies to env-encoded synthetic peptides. Proc Natl Acad Sci USA 85: 1932–1936

Paquette Y, Hanna Z, Savard P, Brousseau R, Robitaille Y, Jolicoeur P (1989) Retrovirus-induced murine motor neuron disease: mapping the determinant of spongiform degeneration within the envelope gene. PNAS USA 86: 3896–3900

Pareky B, Issel CJ, Montelaro RC (1980) Equine infectious anemia virus, a putative lentivirus, contains polypeptides analogous to prototype-C oncornaviruses. Virology 107: 520–525

Patarca R, Haseltine WA (1984) Similarities among retrovirus proteins. Nature 312: 496

Paterson RG, Lamb RA (1987) Ability of the hydrophobic fusion-related external domain of a paramyxovirus F protein to act as a membrane anchor. Cell 48: 441–452

Payne SL, Fang F, Liu C, Dhruva BR, Rwambo P, Issel CJ, Montelaro RC (1987a) Antigenic variation and lentivirus persistence: variations in envelope gene sequences during EIAV infection resemble changes reported for sequential isolates of HIV. Virology 161: 321–331

Payne SL, Salinovich O, Nauman SM, Issel CJ, Montelaro RC (1987b) Course and extent of variation of equine infectious anemia virus during parallel persistent infections. J Virol 61: 1266–1270

Pedersen NC, Ho EW, Brown ML, Yamamoto JK (1987) Isolation of a T-lymphotropic virus from domestic cats with an immunodeficiency-like syndrome. Science 235: 790–793

Peluso R, Haase A, Stowring L, Edwards M, Ventura P (1985) A trojan horse mechanism for the spread of visna virus in monocytes. Virology 147: 231–236

Perez LG, Hunter E (1987) Mutations within the proteolytic cleavage site of the Rous Sarcoma virus glycoprotein that block processing to gp85 and gp37. J Virol 61: 1609–1614

Perez L, Wills JW, Hunter E (1987a) Expression of the Rous sarcoma virus env gene from a simian virus 40 late-region replacement vector: effects of upstream initiation codons. J Virol 61: 1276–1281

Perez LG, Davis GL, Hunter E (1987b) Mutants of the Rous sarcoma virus envelope glycoprotein that lack the transmembrane anchor and/or cytoplasmic domains: analysis of intracellular transport and assembly into virions. J Virol 61: 2981–2988

Perlman D, Halvorson HO (1983) A putative signal peptidase recognition site and sequence in eukaryotic and prokaryotic signal peptides. J Mol Biol 167: 391–409

Perryman LE, O'Rourke KI, McGuire TC (1988) Immune responses are required to terminate viremia in equine infectious anemia lentivirus infection. J Virol 62: 3073–3076

Peters G, Brookes S, Smith R, Dickson C (1983) Tumorigenesis by mouse mammary tumor virus: evidence for a common region for provirus integration in mammary tumors. Cell 33: 369–377

Peterson A, Seed B (1988) Genetic analysis of monoclonal antibody and HIV binding sites on the human lymphocyte antigen CD4. Cell 54: 65–72

Pinter A, Honnen WJ (1983) Comparison of structural domains of gp70s of ecotropic AKV and dualtropic MCF-247 MuLVs. Virology 129: 40–50

Pinter A, Honnen WJ (1984) Characterization of structural and immunological properties of specific domains of Friend ecotropic and dual-tropic murine leukemia virus gp70s. J Virol 49: 452–458

Pinter A, Honnen WJ (1985) The mature form of the Friend spleen focus-forming virus envelope protein, gp65, is efficiently secreted from cells. Virology 143: 646–650

Pinter A, Honnen WJ (1988) O-linked glycosylation of retroviral envelope gene products. J Virol 62: 1016–1021

Pinter A, Honnen WJ, Tung J-S, O'Donnell PV, Hammerling U (1982) Structural domains of endogenous murine leukemia virus gp70s containing specific antigenic determinants defined by monoclonal antibodies. Virology 116: 499–516

Piraino F (1967) The mechanism of genetic resistance of chick embryo cells to infection by Rous sarcoma virus-Bryan strain (BS-RSV). Virology 32: 700–707

Plata F, Autran B, Martins LP, Wain-Hobson S, Raphael M, Mayaud C, Denis M, Guillon JM, Debre P (1987) AIDS virus-specific cytotoxic T-lymphocytes in lung disorders. Nature 328: 348–351

Poiesz BJ, Ruscetti FW, GAzdar AF, Bunn PA, Minna JD, Gallo RC (1980) Detection and isolation of type C retrovirus particles from fresh and cultured lymphocytes of a patient with cutaneous T-cell lymphoma. Proc Natl Acad Sci USA 77: 7415–7419

Popovic M, Sarngadharan MG, Read E, Gallo RC (1984) Detection, isolation, and continuous production of cytopathic retroviruses (HTLV-III) from patients with AIDS and pre-AIDS. Science 224: 497–500

Porter AG, Barber C, Carey NH, Hallewell RA, Threlfall G, Emtage JS (1979) Complete nucleotide sequence of an influenza virus haemagglutinin gene from cloned DNA. Nature 282: 471–477

Poss ML, Mullins JI, Hoover EA (1989) Posttranslational modifications distinguish the envelope glycoprotein of the immunodeficiency disease-inducing feline leukemia virus retrovirus. J Virol 63: 189–195

Power MD, Marx PA, Bryant ML, Gardner MB, Barr PJ, Luciw P (1986) Nucleotide sequence of SRV-1, a type D acquired immune deficiency syndrome retrovirus. Science 231: 1567–1572

Purchase HG, Okazaki W, Vogt PK, Hanafusa H, Burmester BR, Crittenden LB (1977) Oncogenicity of avian leukosis viruses of different subgroups and of mutants of sarcoma viruses. Infect Immun 15: 423–428

Putney SD, Matthews TJ, Robey WG, Lynn DL, Robert-Guroff M, Mueller WT, Langlois AJ, Ghrayeb J, Petteway S, Weinhold KJ, Fischinger PJ, Wong-Staal F, Gallo RD, Bolognesi DP (1986) HTLV-III/LAV-neutralizing antibodies to an E. coli-produced fragment of the virus envelope. Science 234: 1392–1395

Quint W, Quax W, van der Putten H, Berns A (1981) Characterization of AKR murine leukemia virus sequences in AKR mouse substrains and structure of integrated recombinant genomes in tumor tissues. J Virol 39: 1–10

Quint W, Boelens W, van Wezenbeek P, Cuypers T, Maandag ER, Selten G, Berns A (1984) Generation of AKR mink cell focus-forming viruses: a conserved single-copy xenotrope-like provirus provides recombinant long terminal repeat sequences. J Virol 50: 432–438

Racevskis J, Koch G (1978) Synthesis and processing of viral proteins in Friend erythroleukemia cell lines. Virology 87: 354–365

Racevskis J, Sarkar NH (1980) Murine mammary tumor virus structural protein interactions: formation of oligomeric complexes with cleavable cross-linking agents. J Virol 35: 937–948

Raines MA, Lewis WG, Crittenden LB, Kung HJ (1985) c-erbB activation in avian leukosis virus-induced erythroblastosis: clustered integration sites and the arrangement of provirus in the c-erbB alleles. Proc Natl Acad Sci USA 82: 2287–2291

Rasheed S, Pal BK, Gardner M (1982) Characterization of a highly oncogenic murine leukemia virus from wild mice. Int J Cancer 29: 345–350

Rassart E, Nelbach L, Jolicoeur P (1986) Cas-Br-E murine leukemia virus: sequencing of the paralytogenic region of its genome and derivation of specific probes to study its origin and the structure of its recombinant genomes in leukemic tissues. J Virol 60: 910–919

Redmond S, Peters G, Dickson C (1984) Mouse mammary tumor virus can mediate cell fusion at reduced pH. Virology 133: 393–402

Rein A (1982) Interference grouping of murine leukemia viruses: a distinct receptor for the MCF-recombinant viruses in mouse cells. Virology 120: 251–257

Rein A, Schultz A (1984) Different recombinant murine leukemia viruses use different cell surface receptors. Virology 136: 144–152

Richardson NE, Brown NR, Hussey RE, Vaid A, Matthews TJ, Bolognesi DP, Reinherz EL (1988) Binding site for human immunodeficiency virus coat protein gp120 is located in the NH2-terminal region of T4 (CD4) and requires the intact variable-region-like domain. Proc Natl Acad Sci USA 85: 6102–6106

Riedel N, Hoover EA, Gasper PW, Nicolson MO, Mullins JI (1986) Molecular analysis and pathogenesis of the feline aplastic anemia retrovirus, feline leukemia virus C-SARMA. J Virol 60: 242–250

Riedel N, Hoover EA, Dornsife RE, Mullins JI (1988) Pathogenic and host range determinants of the feline aplastic anemia retrovirus. Proc Natl Acad Sci USA 85: 2758–2762

Robert-Guroff M, Brown M, Gallo RC (1985) HTLV-III-neutralizing antibodies in patients with AIDS-related complex. Nature 316: 72–74

Robert-Guroff M, Reitz MJ, Robey WG, Gallo RC (1986) In vitro generation of an HTLV-III variant by neutralizing antibody. J Immunol 137: 3306–3309

Robey WG, Arthur LO, Matthews TJ, Langlois A, Copeland TD, Lerche NW, Oroszlan S, Bolognesi DP, Gilden RV, Fischinger PJ (1986) Prospect for prevention of human immunodeficiency virus infection: purified 120-kDa envelope glycoprotein induces neutralizing antibody. Proc Natl Acad Sci USA 83: 7023–7027

Robey WG, Nara PL, Poore CM, Popovic M, McLane MF, Barin F, Essex M, Fischinger PJ (1987) Rapid assessment of relationships among HIV isolates by oligopeptide analyses of external envelope glycoproteins. Aids Res Hum Retroviruses 3: 401–408

Robinson HL, Astrin SM, Senior AM, Salazar FH (1981) Host susceptibility to endogenous viruses: defective, glycoprotein-expressing proviruses interfere with infections. J Virol 40: 745–751

Rommelaere J, Faller DV, Hopkins N (1978) Characterization and mapping of RNase T1-resistant oligonucleotides derived from the genomes of Akv and MCF murine leukemia viruses. Proc Natl Acad USA 75: 495–499

Roth MG, Compans RW, Giusti L, Damis AR, Nayak DP, Gething M-, Sambrook J (1983a) Influenza virus hemagglutinin expression is polarized in cells infected with recombinant SV40 viruses carrying cloned hemagglutinin DNA. Cell 33: 435–443

Roth MG, Srinivas RV, Compans RW (1983b) Basolateral maturation of retroviruses in polarized epithelial cells. J Virol 45: 1065–1073

Rothman JE, Katz FN, Lodish HF (1978) Glycosylation of a membrane protein is restricted to the growing polypeptide chain but is not necessary for insertion as a transmembrane protein. Cell 15: 1447–1454

Rowe WP, Hartley JW (1983) Genes affecting mink cell focus-inducing (MCF) murine leukemia virus infection and spontaneous lymphoma in AKR F1 hybrids. J Exp Med 158: 353–364

Rowe WP, Cloyd MW, Hartley JW (1980) Status of the association of mink cell focus-forming viruses with leukemogenesis. Cold Spring Harbor Symp Quant Biol 44: 1265–1268

Ruegg CL, Monell CR, Strand M (1989) Identification, using synthetic peptides, of the minimum amino acid sequence from the retroviral transmembrane protein p15E required for inhibition of lymphoproliferation and its similarity to gp21 of human T-lymphotropic virus types I and II. J Virol 63: 3250–3256

Rup BJ, Spence JL, Haelzer JD, Lewis RB, Carpenter CR, Rubin AS, Bose HR (1979) Immunosuppression induced by avian reticuloendotheliosis virus: mechanism of induction of the suppressor cell. J Immunol 123: 1362–1370

Ruscetti S, Wolff L (1984) Spleen focus-forming virus: relationship of an altered envelope gene to the development of a rapid erythroleukemia. Curr Top Microbiol Immunol 112: 21–44

Ruscetti S, Linemeyer D, Field J, Troxler D, Scolnick EM (1979) Characterization of a protein found in cells infected with the spleen focus-forming virus that shares immunological cross-reactivity with the gp70 found in mink cell focus-inducing virus particles. J Virology 30: 787–798

Ruscetti S, Davis L, Field J, Oliff A (1981a) Friend murine leukemia virus-induced leukemia is associated with the formation of mink cell focus-inducing viruses and is blocked in mice expressing endogenous mink cell focus-inducing xenotropic viral envelope genes. J Exp Med 154: 907–920

Ruscetti SK, Field JA, Scolnick EM (1981b) Polycythaemia and anaemia-inducing strains of spleen focus-forming virus differ in post-translational processing of envelope-related glycoproteins. Nature 294: 663–665

Ruscetti S, Field J, Davis L, Oliff A (1982) Factors determining the susceptibility of NIH swiss mice to erythroleukemia induced by Friend murine leukemia virus. Virology 117: 357–365

Rusche JR, Javaherian K, McDanal C, Petro J, Lynn DL, Grimaila R, Langlois A, Gallo RC, Arthur LO, Fischinger PJ, Bolognesi DP, Putney SD, Matthews TJ (1988) Antibodies that inhibit fusion of human immunodeficiency virus-infected cells bind a 24-amino acid sequence of the viral envelope, gp120. Proc Natl Acad Sci USA 85: 3198–3202

Rushlow K, Olsen K, Stiegler G, Payne SL, Montelaro RC, Issel CJ (1986) Lentivirus genomic organization: the complete nucleotide sequence of the env gene region of equine infectious anemia virus. Virology 155: 309–321

Russell PH, Jarrett O (1978) The specificity of neutralizing antibodies to feline leukaemia viruses. Int J Cancer 21: 768–778

Ruta M, Bestwick R, Machida C, Kabat D (1983) Loss of leukemogenicity caused by mutations in the membrane glycoprotein structural gene of Friend spleen focus-forming virus. Proc Natl Acad Sci USA 80: 4704–4708

Saag M, Hahn BH, Gibbons J, Li Y, Parks ES, Parks WP, Shaw GM (1988) Extensive variation of Human Immunodeficiency Virus Type-1 in vivo. Nature 334: 440–444

Salinovich O, Payne SL, Montelaro RC, Hussain KA, Issel CJ, Schnorr KL (1986) Rapid emergence of novel antigenic and genetic variants of equine infectious anemia virus during persistent infection. J Virol 57: 71–80

Salter DW, Smith EJ, Hughes SH, Wright SE, Crittenden LB (1987) Transgenic chickens: insertion of retroviral genes into the chicken germ line. Virology 157: 236–240

Salter DW, Smith EJ, Hughes SH, Wright SE, Fadly AM, Witter RL, Crittenden LB (1986) Gene Insertion into the chicken germ line by retroviruses. Poult Sci 65: 1445–1458

Sattentau QJ, Dalgeish AG, Weiss RA, Beverley PCL (1986) Epitopes of the CD4 antigen and HIV infection. Science 234: 1120–1123

Sattentan QJ, Weiss RA (1988) The CD4 antigen: physiological ligand and HIV receptor. Cell 52: 631–633

Sattentau QJ, Clapham PR, Weiss RA, Beverley PC, Montagnier L, Alhalabi MF, Gluckmann JC, Klatzmann D (1988) The human and simian immunodeficiency viruses HIV-1, HIV-2 and SIV interact with similar epitopes on their cellular receptor, the CD4 molecule. AIDS 2: 101–105

Schafer W, Schwarz H, Thiel H-J, Fischinger PJ, Bolognesi DP (1977) Properties of mouse leukemia viruses. XIV. Prevention of spontaneous AKR leukemia by treatment with group specific antibody against the major virus gp71 glycoprotein. Virology 83: 207–210

Schmidt DM, Synderman R (1988) Retroviral protein p15E and tumorigenesis. Expression is neither required nor sufficient for tumor development. J Immunol 140: 4035–4041

Schochetman G, Arthur LO, Long CW, Massey RJ (1979) Mice with spontaneous mammary tumors develop type-specific neutralizing and cytotoxic antibodies against the mouse mammary tumor virus envelope protein gp52. J Virol 32: 131–139

Schultz A, Rein A, Henderson L, Oroszlan S (1983) Biological, chemical, and immunological studies of Rauscher ecotropic and mink cell focus-forming viruses from JLS-V9 cells. J Virol 45: 995–1003

Schwartz DE, Tizard R, Gilbert W (1983) Nucleotide sequence of Rous sarcoma virus. Cell 32: 853–869

Scott JV, Stowring L, Brahic M, Haase AT, Narayan O, Vigne R (1979) Antigenic variation in visna virus. Cell 18: 321–327

Selten G, Cuypers HT, Zijlstra M, Melief C, Berns A (1984) Involvement of c-myc in MuLV-induced T cell lymphomas in mice: frequency and mechanisms of activation. EMBO J 3: 3215–3222

Shaw GM, Hahn BH, Arya SK, Groopman JE, Gallo RC, Wong-Staal F (1984) Molecular characterization of human T-cell leukemia (lymphotropic) virus Type III in the Acquired Immune Deficiency Syndrome. Science 226: 1165–1171

Shibuya T, Mak TW (1982) Host control of susceptibility to erythroleukemia and to the types of leukemia induced by Friend murine leukemia virus: initial and late stages. Cell 31: 483–493

Sidgurdsson B (1954a) Maedi, a slow progressive pneumonia of sheep: an epizoological and pathological study. Br Vet J 110: 255–270

Sidgurdsson B (1954b) Rida, a chronic encephalitis of sheep: with general remarks on infections which develop slowly and some of their special characteristics. Br Vet J 110: 341–354

Siliciano RF, Lawton T, Knall C, Karr RW, Berman P, Gregory T, Reinherz EL (1988) Analysis of host-virus interactions in AIDS with anti-gp120 T cell clones: effect of HIV sequence variation and a mechanism for CD4 + cell depletion. Cell 54: 561–575

Silver J (1984) Role of mink cell focus-inducing virus in leukemias induced by Friend ecotropic virus. J Virol 50: 872–877

Silver J, Kozak C (1986) Common proviral integration region on mouse chromosome 7 in lymphomas and myelogenous leukemias induced by Friend murine leukemia virus. J Virol 57: 526–533

Simon MC, Smith RE, Hayward WS (1984) Mechanisms of oncogenesis by subgroup F avian leukosis viruses. J Virol 52: 1–8

Simon MC, Neckameyer WS, Hayward WS, Smith RE (1987) Genetic determinants of neoplastic diseases induced by a subgroup F avian leukosis virus. J Virol 61: 1203–1212

Sitbon M, Nishio J, Wehrly K, Chesebro B (1985) Pseudotyping of dual-tropic recombinant viruses generated by infection of mice with different ecotropic murine leukemia viruses. Virology 140: 144–151

Sitbon M, Sola B, Evans L, Nishio J, Hayes SF, Nathanson K, Garon CF, Chesebro B (1986) Hemolytic anemia and erythroleukemia, two distinct pathogenic effects of Friend MuLV: mapping of the effects to different regions of the viral genome. Cell 47: 851–859

Skehel JJ, Bayley PM, Brown EB, Martin SR, Waterfield MS, White JM, Wilson IA, Wiley DC (1982) Changes in the conformation of influenza virus hemagglutinin at the pH optimum of virus-mediated membrane fusion. Proc Natl Acad Sci USA 79: 968–972

Skinner MA, Ting R, Langlois AJ, Weinhold KJ, Lyerly HK, Javaherian K, Matthews TJ (1988) Characteristics of a neutralizing monoclonal antibody to the HIV envelope glycoprotein. AIDS Res Hum Retroviruses 4: 187–197

Smith RE, Schmidt EV (1982) Induction of anemia by avian leukosis viruses of five subgroups. Virology 117: 516–518

Smith DH, Byrn RA, Marsters SA, Gregory T, Groopman JE, Capon DJ (1987) Blocking of HIV-1 infectivity by a soluble, secreted form of the CD4 antigen. Science 238: 1704–1707

Snyderman R, Cianciolo GJ (1984) Immunosuppressive activity of the retroviral envelope protein p15E and its possible relationship to neoplasia. Immunol Today 5: 240

Sodroski J, Goh WC, Rosen C, Campbell K, Haseltine WA (1986) Role of the HTLV-III/LAV envelope in syncytium formation and cytopathicity. Nature 322: 470–474

Somasundaran M, Robinson HL (1987) A major mechanism of human immunodeficiency virus-induced cell killing does not involve cell fusion. J Virol 61: 3114–3119

Sommerfelt MA, Williams BP, Clapham PR, Solomon E, Goodfellow PN, Weiss RA (1988) Hutman T cell leukemia viruses use a receptor determined by human chromosome 17. Science 242: 1557–1559

Sommerfelt MA, Weiss RA (1990) Receptor interference groups among 20 retroviruses plating on human cells. J Gen Virol (in press)

Sonigo P, Alizon M, Staskus K, Klatzmann D, Cole S, Danos O, Retzel E, Tiollais P, Haase A, Wain-Hobson S (1985) Nucleotide sequence of the visna lentivirus: relationship to the AIDS virus. Cell 42: 369–382

Sonigo P, Barker C, Hunter E, Wain-Hobson S (1986) Nucleotide sequence of Mason-Pfizer monkey virus: an immunosuppressive D-type retrovirus. Cell 45: 375–385

Spiro C, Gliniak B, Kabat D (1988) A tagged helper-free Friend virus causes clonal erythroblast immortality by specific proviral integration in the cellular genome. J Virol 62: 4129–4135

Srinivas RV, Compans RW (1983) Membrane association and defective transport of spleen focus-forming virus glycoproteins. J Biol Chem 258: 14718–14724

Srinivas RV, Kilpatrick DR, Compans RW (1987) Intracellular transport and leukemogenicity of spleen focus-forming virus envelope glycoproteins with altered transmembrane domains. J Virol 61: 4007–4011

Stanley J, Bhaduri LM, Narayan O, Clements JE (1987) Topographical rearrangements of visna virus envelope glycoprotein during antigenic drift. J Virol 61: 1019–1028

Starcich BR, Hahn BH, Shaw GM, McNeely PD, Modrow S, Wolf, H, Parks ES, Parks WP, Josephs SF, Gallo RC, Wong-Staal F (1986) Identification and characterization of conserved and variable regions in the envelope gene of HTLV-III/LAV, the retrovirus of AIDS. Cell 45: 637–648

Steffen D (1984) Proviruses are adjacent to c-myc in some murine leukemia virus-induced lymphomas. Proc Natl Acad Sci USA 81: 2097–2101

Stein BS, Gowda SD, Lifson JD, Penhallow RC, Bensch KG, Engleman EG (1987) pH-independent HIV entry into CD4-positive T cells via virus envelope fusion to the plasma membrane. Cell 49: 659–668

Steinheider G, Seidel HJ, Kreja L (1979) Comparison of the effects of anemia and polycythemia inducing Friend virus complex. Experientia 35: 1173–1175

Stephens EB, Compans RW (1986) Nonpolarized expression of a secreted murine leukemia virus glycoprotein in polarized epithelial cells. Cell 47: 1053–1059

Stephens EB, Compans RW, Earl P, Moss B (1986) Surface expression of viral glycoproteins is polarized in epithelial cells infected with recombinant vaccinia viral vectors. EMBO J 5: 237

Stevenson M, Meier C, Mann AM, Chapman N, Wasiak A (1988) Envelope glycoprotein of HIV induces interferences and cytolysis in CD4 + cells: mechanism for persistence in AIDS. Cell 53: 483–496

Stewart MA, Warnock M, Wheeler A, Wilkie N, Mullins JI, Onions DE, Neil JC (1986) Nucleotide sequences of a feline leukemia virus subgroup A envelope gene and long terminal repeat and evidence for the recombinational origin of subgroup B viruses. J Virol 58: 825–834

Stewart TA, Pattengale PK, Leder P (1984) Spontaneous mammary adenocarcinomas in transgenic mice that carry and express MTV/myc fusion genes. Cell 38: 627–637

Stoye J, Coffin J (1985) Endogenous Viruses. In: Weiss R et al. (eds) Molecular biology of tumor viruses: RNA tumor viruses (supplement) Cold Spring Harbor Laboratory, Cold Spring Harbor, pp 357–404

Stoye JP, Coffin JM (1987) The four classes of endogenous murine leukemia virus: structural relationships and potential for recombination. J Virol 61: 2659–2669

Stoye JP, Coffin JM (1988) Polymorphism of murine endogenous proviruses revealed by using virus class-specific oligonucleotide probes. J Virol 62: 168–175

Stromberg K, Benveniste RE, Arthur LO, Rabin H, Giddens WE, Ochs HE, Morton WR, Tsai CC (1984) Characterization of exogenous type D retrovirus from a fibroma of a macaque with simian AIDS and fibromatosis. Science 224: 289–292

Sutcliffe JG, Shinnick TM, Verma IM, Lerner RA (1980) Nucleotide sequence of Moloney leukemia virus: 3′ end reveals details of replication, analogy to bacterial transposons, and an unexpected gene. Proc Natl Acad Sci USA 77: 3302–3306

Swain SL (1983) T cell subsets and the recognition of MHC class. Immunol Rev 74: 129–142

Szurek PF, Yuen PH, Jerzy R, Wong PKY (1988) Identification of point mutations in the envelope gene of Moloney murine leukemia virus TB temperature-sensitive paralytogenic mutant *ts1*: molecular determinants for neurovirulence. J Virol 62: 357–360

Takahashi H, Cohen J, Hosmalin A, Cease KB, Houghten R, Cornette JL, DeLisi C, Moss B, Germain RN, Berzofsky JA (1988) An immunodominant epitope of the human immunodeficiency virus envelope glycoprotein gp160 recognized by class I major histocompatibility complex molecule-restricted murine cytotoxic T lymphocytes. Proc Natl Acad Sci USA 85: 3105–3109

Teich N (1984) Taxonomy of Retroviruses. In: Weiss R et al. (eds) Molecular biology of tumor viruses, RNA Tumor Viruses, 2 edn. Cold Spring Harbor Laboratory, Cold Spring Harbor, pp 25–208

Temin HM (1988) Mechanisms of cell killing/cytopathic effects by nonhuman retroviruses. Rev Infect Dis 10: 399–405

Thayer RM, Power MD, Bryant ML, Gardner MB, Barr PJ, Luciw PA (1987) Sequence relationships of type D retroviruses which cause simian acquired immunodeficiency syndrome. Virology 157: 317–329

Thomas CY (1986) AKR ecotropic murine leukemia virus SL3-3 forms envelope gene recombinants in vivo. J Virol 59: 23–30

Thomas CY, Coffin JM (1982) Genetic alterations of RNA leukemia viruses associated with the development of spontaneous thymic leukemia in AKR/J mice. J Virol 43: 416–426

Thomas CY, Khiroya R, Schwartz RS, Coffin JM (1984) Role of recombinant ecotropic and polytropic viruses in the development of spontaneous thymic lymphomas in HRS/J mice. J Virol 50: 397–407

Thomas CY, Boykin BJ, Famulari NG, Coppola MA (1986) Association of recombinant murine leukemia viruses of the class II genotype with spontaneous lymphomas in CWD mice. J Virol 58: 314–323

Thormar H, Sigurdsardottier B (1962) Growth of visna virus in primary tissue cultures from various animal species. Acta Pathol Microbiol Scand 55: 180–186

Thormar H, Barshatzky MR, Arnesen K, Kozlowski PB (1983) The emergence of antigenic variants is a rare event in long-term visna virus infection in vivo. J Gen Virol 64: 1427–1432

Traunecker A, Luke W, Karjalainen K (1988) Soluble CD4 molecules neutralize human immunodeficiency virus type 1. Nature 331: 84–86

Tsai WP, Oroszlan S (1988) Novel glycosylation pathways of retroviral envelope proteins identified with avian reticuloendotheliosis virus. J Virol 62: 3167–3174

Tsichlis PN, Conklin KF, Coffin JM (1980) Mutant and recombinant avian retroviruses with extended host range. Proc Natl Acad Sci USA 77: 536–540

Tyler DS, Nastala CL, Stanley SD, Matthews TJ, Lyerly HK, Bolognesi DP, Weinhold KJ (1989) GP120 specific cellular cytotoxicity in HIV-1 seropositive individuals. Evidence for circulating CD16+ effector cells armed in vivo with cytophilic antibody. J Immunol 142: 1177–1182

Van Beveren C, Coffin J, Hughes S (1985) Nomenclature. In: Weiss R et al. (eds) Molecular biology of tumor viruses. Cold Spring Harbor Laboratory, Cold Spring Harbor, pp 559 –1222

Van Greinsven LJLD, Vogt M (1980) Rauscher "mink cell focus-inducing" (MCF) virus causes erythroleukemia in mice: its isolation and properties. Virology 101: 376–388

Venable RM, Pastor RW, Brooks BR, Carson FW (1989) Theoretically determined three-dimensional structures for amphipathic segments of the HIV-1 gp41 envelope protein. AIDS Res Hum Retro 5: 7–22

Vogt M, Haggblom C, Swift S, Haas M (1985) Envelope gene and long terminal repeat determine the different biological properties of Rauscher, Friend, and Moloney mink cell focus-inducing viruses. J Virol 55: 184–192

Vogt PK (1977) Genetics of RNA tumor viruses. In: Fraenkel-Conrat H, Wagner R (eds) Comprehensive Virology, vol. 9, Plenum, New York, pp 341–455

Von Heijne G (1983) Patterns of amino acids near signal-sequence cleavage sites. Eur J Biochem 133: 17–21

Von Heijne G (1984) Analysis of the distribution of charged residues in the N-terminal region of signal sequences: implications for protein export in prokaryotic and eukaryotic cells. EMBO J 3: 2315–2318

Von Heijne G (1985) Signal sequences. The limits of variation. J Mol Biol 184: 99–105

Voytek P, Kozak C (1988) HoMuLV: a novel pathogenic ecotropic virus isolated from the european mouse, *Mus hortulanus*. Virology 165: 469–475

Wahren B, Morfeldt-Mansson L, Biberfeld G, Moberg L, Sonnerborg A, Ljungman P, Werner A, Kurth R, Gallo R, Bolognesi D (1987) Characteristics of the specific cell-mediated immune response in human immunodeficiency virus infection. J Virol 61: 2017–2023

Walker BD, Kowalski M, Goh WC, Kozarsky K, Krieger M, Rosen C, Rohrschneider L, Haseltine WA, Sodroski J (1987) Inhibition of human immunodeficiency virus syncytium formation and virus replication by castanospermine. Proc Natl Acad Sci USA 84: 8120–8124

Walter P, Lingappa VR (1986) Mechanism of protein translocation across the endoplasmic reticulum membrane. Annu Rev Cell Biol 2: 499–516

Wang LH, Duesberg P, Kawai S, Hanafusa H (1976) The location of envelope-specific and sarcoma-specific oligonucleotides on the RNA of Schmidt-Ruppin Rous sarcoma virus. Proc Natl Acad Sci USA 73: 447–451

Watanabe M, Reimann KA, DeLong PA, Liu T, Fisher RA, Letvin NL (1989) Effect of recombinant soluble CD4 in rhesus monkeys infected with simian immunodeficiency virus of macaques. Nature 337: 267–270

Weinhold KJ, Lyerly HK, Matthews TJ, Tyler DS, Ahearne PM, Stine KC, Langlois AJ, Durack DT, Bolognesi DP (1988) Cellular anti-GP120 cytolytic reactivities in HIV-1 seropositive individuals. Lancet 1: 902–905

Weiss R (1984) Experimental biology and assay of RNA tumor viruses. In: Weiss R et al. (eds) Molecular biology of tumor viruses, RNA Tumor Viruses, 2 edn. Cold Spring Harbor Laboratory, Cold Spring Harbor, pp 209–260

Weiss RA, Clapham P, Nagy K, Hoshino H (1985) Envelope properties of human T-cell leukemia viruses. Curr Top Microbiol Immunol 115: 235–245

Weiss RA, Clapham PR, Weber JN, Dalgleish AG, Lasky LA, Berman PW (1986) Variable and conserved neutralization antigens of human immunodeficiency virus. Nature 324: 572–575

Weller SK, Joy AE, Temin HM (1980) Correlation between cell killing and massive second-round superinfection by members of some subgroups of avian leukosis virus. J Virol 33: 494–506

White J, Kielian M, Helenius A (1983) Membrane fusion proteins of enveloped animal viruses. Q Rev Biophys 16: 151–195

Willey RL, Rutledge RA, Dias S, Folks T, Theodore T, Buckler CE, Martin MA (1986) Identification of conserved and divergent domains within the envelope gene of the acquired immunodeficiency syndrome retrovirus. Proc Natl Acad Sci USA 83: 5038–5042

Willey RL, Bonifacino JS, Potts BJ, Martin MA, Klausner RD (1988a) Biosynthesis, cleavage, and degradation of the human immunodeficiency virus 1 envelope glycoprotein gp160. Proc Natl Acad Sci USA 85: 9580–9584

Willey RL, Smith DH, Lasky LA, Theodore TS, Earl PL, Moss B, Capon DJ, Martin MA (1988b) In vitro mutagenesis identifies a region within the envelope gene of the human immunodeficiency virus that is critical for infectivity. J Virol 62: 139–147

Wills JW, Hardwick JM, Shaw K, Hunter E (1983) Alteration in the transport and processing of Rous sarcoma virus envelope glycoproteins mutated in the signal and anchor regions. J Cell Biochem 23: 81–94

Wills JW, Srinivas RV, Hunter E (1984) Mutations of the Rous sarcoma virus env gene that affect the transport and subcellular location of the glycoprotein products. J Cell Biol 99: 2011–2023

Witte ON, Tsukamoto-Adey A, Weissman IL (1977) Cellular maturation of oncornavirus glycoproteins: topological arrangement of precursor and product forms in cellular membranes. Virology 76: 539–553

Wolff L, Ruscetti S (1985) Malignant transformation of erythroid cells in vivo by introduction of a nonreplicating retrovirus vector. Science 228: 1549–1552

Wolff L, Tambourin P, Ruscetti S (1986) Induction of the autonomous stage of transformation in eryhroid cells infected with SFFV; helper virus is not required. Virology 152: 272–276

Wong PKY, Soong M, MacLeod R, Gallick G, Yuen PH (1983) A group of temperature-sensitive mutants of Moloney leukemia virus which is defective in cleavage of env precursor polypeptide in infected cells also induces hind limb paralysis in newborn CFW/D mice. Virology 125: 513–518

Wong PKY, Knupp C, Yuen PH, Soong MM, Zachary JF, Tompkins WAF (1985) ts1, a paralytogenic mutant of Moloney murine leukemia virus, has an enhanced ability to replicate in the central nervous system and primary nerve cell culture. J Virol 55: 760–767

Wong-Staal F, Shaw GM, Hahn BH, Salahuddin SZ, Popovic M, Markham P, Redfield R, Gallo RC (1985) Genomic diversity of human T-lymphotropic virus type III (HTLV-III). Science 229: 759–762

Yoshimura FK, Breda M (1981) Lack of AKR ecotropic provirus amplification in AKR leukemic thymuses. J Virol 39: 808–815

Yoshimura FK, Levine KL (1983) AKR thymic lymphomas involving mink cell focus-inducing murine leukemia viruses have a common region of provirus integration. J Virol 45: 576–784

Yuen PH, Malehorn D, Knupp C, Wong PKY (1985) A 1.6-kilobase-pair fragment in the genome of the ts1 mutant of Moloney murine leukemia virus TB that is associated with temperature sensitivity, nonprocessing of $Pr80^{env}$, and paralytogenesis. J Virol 54: 364–373

Zarling JM, Morton W, Moran PA, McClure J, Kosowski SG, Hu SL (1986) T-cell responses to human AIDS virus in macaques immunized with recombinant vaccinia viruses. Nature 323: 344–346

Zarling JM, Eichberg JW, Moran PA, McClure J, Sridhar P, Hu SL (1987) Proliferative and cytotoxic T cells to AIDS virus glycoproteins in chimpanzees immunized with a recombinant vaccinia virus expressing AIDS virus envelope glycoproteins. J Immunol 139: 988–990

Zavada J, Dickson C, Weiss R (1977) Pseudotypes of vesicular stomatitis virus with envelope antigens provided by murine mammary tumor virus. Virology 82: 221–231

Zijlstra M, Quint W, Cuypers T, Radaszkiewicz T, Schoenmakers H, DeGoeda R, Melief C (1986) Ecotropic and mink cell focus-forming murine leukemia viruses integrate in mouse T, B, and non-T/non-B cell lymphoma DNA. J Virol 57: 1037–1047

Subject Index

Current Topics in Microbiology and Immunology

Volumes published since 1980 (and still available)

Vol. 134: **Oldstone, Michael B. (Ed.):** Arenaviruses. Biology and Immunotherapy. 1987. 33 figs. VII, 242 pp. ISBN 3-540-17322-6

Vol. 135: **Paige, Christopher J.; Gisler, Roland H. (Ed.):** Differentiation of B Lymphocytes. 1987. 25 figs. IX, 150 pp. ISBN 3-540-17470-2

Vol. 136: **Hobom, Gerd; Rott, Rudolf (Ed.):** The Molecular Biology of Bacterial Virus Systems. 1988. 20 figs. VII, 90 pp. ISBN 3-540-18513-5

Vol. 137: **Mock, Beverly; Potter, Michael (Ed.):** Genetics of Immunological Diseases. 1988. 88 figs. XI, 335 pp. ISBN 3-540-19253-0

Vol. 138: **Goebel, Werner (Ed.):** Intracellular Bacteria. 1988. 18 figs. IX, 179 pp. ISBN 3-540-50001-4

Vol. 139: **Clarke, Adrienne E.; Wilson, Ian A. (Ed.):** Carbohydrate-Protein Interaction. 1988. 35 figs. IX, 152 pp. ISBN 3-540-19378-2

Vol. 140: **Podack, Eckhard R. (Ed.):** Cytotoxic Effector Mechanisms. 1989. 24 figs. VIII, 126 pp. ISBN 3-540-50057-X

Vol. 141: **Potter, Michael; Melchers, Fritz (Ed.):** Mechanisms in B-Cell Neoplasia 1988. Workshop at the National Cancer Institute, National Institutes of Health, Bethesda, MD, USA, March 23–25, 1988. 1988. 122 figs. XIV, 340 pp. ISBN 3-540-50212-2

Vol. 142: **Schüpbach, Jörg:** Human Retrovirology. Facts and Concepts. 1989. 24 figs. 115 pp. ISBN 3-540-50455-9

Vol. 143: **Haase, Ashley, T.; Oldstone, Michael B. A. (Ed.):** In Situ Hybridization. 1989. 33 figs. XII, 90 pp. ISBN 3-540-50761-2

Vol. 144: **Knippers, Rolf; Levine, A. J. (Ed.):** Transforming Proteins of DNA Tumor Viruses. 1989. 85 figs. XIV, 300 pp. ISBN 3-540-50909-7

Vol. 145: **Oldstone, Michael B. A. (Ed.):** Molecular Mimicry. Cross-Reactivity between Microbes and Host Proteins as a Cause of Autoimmunity. 1989. 28 figs. VII, 141 pp. ISBN 3-540-50929-1

Vol. 146: **Mestecky, Jiri; McGhee, Jerry (Ed.):** New Strategies for Oral Immunization. International Symposium at the University of Alabama at Birmingham and Molecular Engineering Associates, Inc. Birmingham, AL, USA, March 21–22, 1988. 1989. 22 figs. IX, 237 pp. ISBN 3-540-50841-4

Vol. 147: **Vogt, Peter K. (Ed.):** Oncogenes. Selected Reviews. 1989. 8 figs. VII, 172 pp. ISBN 3-540-51050-8

Vol. 148: **Vogt, Peter K. (Ed.):** Oncogenes and Retroviruses. Selected Reviews. 1989. XII, 134 pp. ISBN 3-540-51051-6

Vol. 149: **Shen-Ong, Grace L. C.; Potter, Michael; Copeland, Neal G. (Ed.):** Mechanisms in Myeloid Tumorigenesis. Workshop at the National Cancer Institute, National Institutes of Health, Bethesda, MD, USA, March 22, 1988. 1989. 42 figs. X, 172 pp. ISBN 3-540-50968-2

Vol. 150: **Jann, Klaus; Jann, Barbara (Ed.):** Bacterial Capsules. 1989. 33 figs. XII, 176 pp. ISBN 3-540-51049-4

Vol. 151: **Jann, Klaus; Jann, Barbara (Ed.):** Bacterial Adhesins. 1990. 23 figs. XII, 192 pp. ISBN 3-540-51052-4

Vol. 152: **Bosma, Melvin J.; Phillips, Robert A.; Schuler, Walter (Ed.):** The Scid Mouse. Characterization and Potential Uses. EMBO Workshop held at the Basel Institute for Immunology, Basel, Switzerland, February 20–22, 1989. 1989. 72 figs. XII, 263 pp. ISBN 3-540-51512-7

Vol. 153: **Lambris, John D. (Ed.):** The Third Component of Complement. Chemistry and Biology. 1989. 38 figs. X, 251 pp. ISBN 3-540-51513-5

Vol. 154: **McDougall, James K. (Ed.):** Cytomegaloviruses. 1990. 58 figs. IX, 286 pp. ISBN 3-540-51514-3

Vol. 155: **Kaufmann, Stefan H. E. (Ed.):** T-Cell Paradigms in Parasitic and Bacterial Infections. 1990. 24 figs. IX, 162 pp. ISBN 3-540-51515-1

Vol. 156: **Dyrberg, T. (Ed.):** The Role of Viruses and the Immune System in Diabetes Mellitus. 1990. 15 figs. XI, 142 pp. ISBN 3-540-51918-1